THE REIGN OF KING JOHN

SIDNEY PAINTER

ARNO PRESS
A New York Times Company
New York • 1979

Editorial Supervision: Mary Kay Hamalainen

Reprint Edition 1979 by Arno Press Inc.

Copyright © 1949 by the Johns Hopkins Press

Reprinted by permission of the Johns Hopkins Press

JOHNS HOPKINS UNIVERSITY PRESS REPRINTS
ISBN for complete set: 0-405-10575-4
See last pages of this volume for titles.

Manufactured in the United States of America

THE REIGN OF KING JOHN

This is a volume in the Arno Press collection

JOHNS HOPKINS UNIVERSITY PRESS REPRINTS

*See last pages of this volume
for a complete list of titles.*

THE REIGN OF KING JOHN

THE REIGN OF KING JOHN

By
SIDNEY PAINTER

BALTIMORE
THE JOHNS HOPKINS PRESS

Copyright © 1949 by The Johns Hopkins Press, Baltimore, Md. 21218
Manufactured in the United States of America
Library of Congress Catalog Card No. 49-49221

Originally published, 1949
Second printing, 1952
Third printing, 1959
Fourth printing, 1964

Johns Hopkins Paperbacks edition, 1966, 1968

TABLE OF CONTENTS

Chapter		Page
I.	The Succession	1
II.	The King and the Magnates	17
III.	The King's Servants	57
IV.	The Royal Administration	93
V.	King John and the Church	151
VI.	King or Tyrant	203
VII.	The Seeds of Revolt	226
VIII.	Magna Carta	285
IX.	The Civil War	349
Index		379

PREFACE

This volume is the first step in an effort to write a comprehensive history of England in the time of King John. It is essentially a political and administrative history of his reign. Some day I hope to produce a companion volume under some such title as " England in the reign of King John." This would cover the numerous and fascinating phases of the history of the time that have been neglected here.

I have made no attempt in this book to deal with King John's over-seas domains, the lordship of Ireland and his continental fiefs, because I believe that they have been treated adequately by other historians. Then I have left for the later volume such subjects as military and naval institutions and the development of the common law. Excellent arguments can be advanced for putting these subjects in either volume, and this one grew large enough without them.

When someone writes a book because he wants to and deals with the subjects that interest him most, he finds it hard to explain why the result should interest others. When I started to write this volume, there was no adequate account of the reign of a mediæval English king. Now Sir Maurice Powicke's *King Henry III and the Lord Edward* has filled that gap in historical literature, and I can only hope that the *Reign of King John* can hold its place beside it. Actually this book can make only one claim for the interest of the general reader with a fondness for the Middle Ages—it attempts to delineate fully the background and immediate consequences of the issuance of Magna Carta.

No historian can ever adequately recognize his obligations to other scholars, but I should like to mention a few to whom I am particularly indebted. I have benefited far more than meagre footnote references can indicate from the works of Sir Maurice Powicke, Sir Frederick and Lady Stenton, Mr. H. G. Richardson, and Professor C. R. Cheney. I have pillaged both references and ideas from my friend and former student Mr. Fred A. Cazel, Jr. I have also made use of some material from a manuscript written by the late Professor Sydney Knox Mitchell that I am preparing for publication. In the actual writing of this volume I have been assisted by the members of the Johns Hopkins Historical Seminar who read and criticized two chapters, by my colleague Mrs. John Van Eerde who read the entire manuscript, and by Sir Maurice Powicke who gave me valuable advice on a number of difficult points. Finally I should like to express my gratitude to Miss Lilly Lavarello who, I am convinced, is without a peer as either editor or typist.

SIDNEY PAINTER

The Johns Hopkins University
October, 1949

Chapter I

THE SUCCESSION

ON APRIL 6, 1199, Richard Plantagenet, king of England, duke of Normandy and Aquitaine, and count of Anjou, died in his camp in the hills of the Limousin from a wound received ten days earlier. As the news spread over his wide lands, the criminally inclined took up their arms and went forth in search of booty. Even men of position, earls, barons, and knights, gathered their followers to settle their private grudges before a new king's peace should descend on the realm.[1] It was a glorious opportunity —the king was dead and no one knew for certain who would succeed him.

As King Richard had had no children by his wife, Berengeria of Navarre, the crown passed to his younger brothers or their representatives. Four legitimate sons of King Henry II had reached maturity—Henry, Richard, Geoffrey, and John. Henry and Geoffrey had died before their father, but Geoffrey had left a son, Arthur. Hence Richard's heir was either his brother John or his nephew Arthur. Three sets of considerations would play a part in the decision between them—the law of inheritance, the wishes of the barons and great officers of the realm, and the desires of the late king.

The question as to who was Richard's legal heir was extremely complex. The Angevin empire was not a unified state but a collection of feudal principalities. Each of these principalities—England, Normandy, Aquitaine, and Anjou—had its own law of succession. In the continental domains of the Plantagenet family this law was simply the feudal custom of the fief in question. The idea of representation by which the son is considered to take the place

---

[1] *Magna vita sancti Hugonis episcopi Lincolniensis* (ed. James F. Dimock, Rolls series), pp. 284-285; Ralph de Coggeshall, *Chronicon Anglicanum* (ed. Joseph Stevenson, Rolls series), p. 98; *Curia regis rolls* (Rolls series), I, 255, 384, 440; *Pipe roll 2 John* (Pipe roll society), p. 20; *Memoranda roll 1 John* (Pipe roll society), p. 12.

of his dead father is a comparatively sophisticated conception and was apparently just beginning to find a place in feudal custom. The author of the *Très ancien coutumier* of Normandy is aware of it but rejects it. To him " the younger son is the nearer heir to the inheritance of his father than the child of the elder brother who died before the father." [2] We have no contemporary expression of the custom of Anjou or Aquitaine. The barons of Anjou maintained that according to their custom Arthur was the rightful heir to Richard, and one can only accept their statement.[3] As to Aquitaine the ducal seat was probably not considered to be vacant. Eleanor, duchess of Aquitaine, who had brought that vast fief to her husband, Henry II, was still alive. In short it appears that John was the legal heir to the duchy of Normandy and Arthur to the county of Anjou while Aquitaine remained in the hands of its aged duchess.

The law of succession to the English crown was in a state of complete confusion. The Anglo-Saxon monarchy had been elective. Although it had been customary to select the king from among the members of the royal family, the election of a Canute and a Harold had been possible. One would expect the Norman kings to apply in their new realm the feudal customs of inheritance that prevailed in their ancestral duchy, and there is reason to believe that such was their intention. Henry I had obliged his barons to swear fidelity first to his son William and then to his daughter Matilda. Stephen had clearly considered his son Eustace his heir. But circumstances had conspired to prevent the establishment of a clear hereditary principle. Henry II had felt it necessary to crown his eldest son to assure his succession. Richard had been the first English king after the conquest who was the undisputed heir of his predecessor according to feudal custom. Hence the tradition of elective monarchy was still strong at Richard's death. The author of the *Histoire de Guillaume le Maréchal* shows clearly

---

[2] *Le très ancien coutumier de Normandie* (ed. Ernest-Joseph Tardif in *Coutumiers de Normandie*, Société de l'histoire de Normandie), pp. 12-13.

[3] Roger of Hovedon, *Chronica* (ed. William Stubbs, Rolls series), IV, 86-87; Roger of Wendover, *Flores historiarum* (ed. H. G. Hewlett, Rolls series), I, 286.

through the words he puts into the mouths of the archbishop of Canterbury and William Marshal that he believed that the great men of England had the right to select Richard's successor.[4] But even if the feudal custom of inheritance had been firmly established as governing the succession to the English crown, no clear decision between John and Arthur would have been possible. The author of the treatise on English law ascribed to Ranulf de Glanvill states that it is doubtful which of the two, uncle or nephew, the law prefers and gives the arguments on both sides. He himself favors the nephew's claim.[5]

It is obviously impossible to make any comprehensive statement as to the preferences of the prelates and barons of the Angevin empire. In all probability the majority did not care very much which of the rivals succeeded and was led by the small groups that had decided views. All that is certain is that the barons of Anjou supported Arthur while the interlocking Anglo-Norman baronage favored John. We have, however, some indications of the reasoning of the latter group. The author of the *Histoire de Guillaume le Maréchal* gives a conversation between William Marshal and Hubert Walter, archbishop of Canterbury, just after they learned of Richard's death. The archbishop supports Arthur's right, but advances no arguments. The reader is clearly intended to presume that he simply distrusted John. William Marshal presented two arguments for John. In accordance with Norman feudal custom he maintained that John was the legal heir. Then he stated that Arthur was irascible, haughty, and had bad counselors. He was besides no friend of the English.[6] As this last point was probably the vital one, it deserves analysis.

In the hope of drawing Brittany permanently into the orbit of Plantagenet power King Henry II had arranged a marriage between his third son Geoffrey and Constance, daughter and heiress of Conan IV, duke of Brittany. The barons of Brittany did not relish the prospect of being ruled by a Plantagenet, but they could

[4] *L'histoire de Guillaume le Maréchal* (ed. Paul Meyer, Société de l'histoire de France), lines 11877-11908.
[5] Glanvill, *De legibus et consuetudinibus regni Anglie* (ed. G. E. Woodbine), pp. 101-104.
[6] *Histoire de Guillaume le Maréchal*, lines 11877-11908.

offer little resistance to the power of Henry II. The dukes of Brittany had always been weak feudal suzerains, and the barons feared with reason that a duke supported by the forces of the Angevin empire would be able to expand his authority at their expense. Moreover there existed in Brittany a strong feeling of national independence, and the idea of being ruled by a foreigner was distasteful. When Duke Geoffrey died leaving his wife pregnant, the Bretons saw their opportunity. They rallied around Constance who apparently shared their feelings. The very name given to Constance's son symbolized their hopes. But if the Bretons were to maintain their duchy's independence and keep control of their future duke, they needed someone to support them against the Plantagenet power until the young prince came of age. The natural place to seek this aid was from the Capetian kings. Hence whenever there was danger that young Arthur's Plantagenet relatives would take him into their care, the Bretons entrusted him to King Philip Augustus. In short, at Richard's death Arthur was a young boy not quite twelve years old who had been brought up among the nobles of Brittany and France.

At the time of Richard's death John was in his early thirties. He could not by any stretch of the imagination be called an Englishman. He was the son of Eleanor, duchess of Aquitaine, and Henry, count of Anjou, whose Anglo-Norman mother, Matilda, had given him his claim to Normandy and England. If all John's sojourns in England were added together, it seems improbable that they would reach a total of five years. When Richard was captured on his way home from the crusade, John had formed an alliance with King Philip Augustus, and he had been suspected of contemplating a similar maneuver just before his brother's death. But John had been brought up at his father's court among the Anglo-Norman barons. His intimates, the members of his household, were Anglo-Normans. While it is clear that most of the barons and prelates of England and Normandy had no very high opinion of John, they thought of him as one of them while Arthur was a stranger.

King Richard had never shown any interest in the welfare of the Angevin empire except when it involved his favorite occupation—fighting. Nowhere is this negligence more clearly shown than in his casual treatment of the question of who was to be his successor. Before starting on his crusade in June 1190 he made no statement as to whom he considered his heir, but left his brother John in so strong a position that he could almost certainly secure the succession by force if the king were to die on the expedition. Then in October of the same year he made a treaty with Tancred, king of Sicily, in which he spoke of Arthur as his heir. This was the closest Richard ever came to a formal pronouncement on the subject. In March 1194 when the king had returned to England to find John in alliance with Philip Augustus, he had called on the barons of his court to render a judgment against his brother for treason. According to Hovedon's account John was summoned to appear within forty days to answer the charge and when he failed to do so, he was condemned to banishment from England.[7] The *Annals of Margam* say that he received three summonses to appear within forty days and then was judged to be disinherited " not only from all the lands which he had in the realm but also from all honors that he might hope or expect to have from the English crown." [8] Of these two accounts the one of Hovedon seems most likely. Richard made his request for a judgment against John on March 31. On May 12 he crossed to Normandy and soon after was reconciled with his brother at Lisieux. There was thus time for one forty-day period to expire, but not for three such periods. Moreover the statement that John was exiled from England sounds reasonable. As a matter of fact, whether from choice or from necessity, he did not revisit the island until after his brother's death. But if John had been disinherited as completely as the Margam annalist maintains, it seems impossible that even so casual a monarch as Richard could have restored to him a part of his lands and treated him as his heir without some formal announcement.

In April 1196 King Richard directed the barons of Brittany to deliver Arthur into his custody. As Brittany was a fief held of

[7] Hovedon, III, 241-242.
[8] *Annals of Margam* (ed. H. R. Luard in *Annales Monastici*, I, Rolls series), p. 24.

the duchy of Normandy, this was a perfectly proper procedure, but the Bretons refused and sent their young duke to Philip's court.[9] This incident seems to have changed Richard's views about the succession. John had been loyal to him since 1194, and Arthur was in the custody of his enemy. In the summer of 1197 Richard made an alliance with Baldwin, count of Flanders. On September 8 John issued letters patent stating that at his brother's request he had promised Baldwin that he would observe this treaty of alliance if Richard were to die. On October 16, John, once more at Richard's request, confirmed an exchange of lands between the king and the archbishop of Rouen.[10] These two incidents seem to indicate that in 1197 Richard considered John his heir.

Early in 1199 Richard and John were at odds once more, but the source of the trouble is not clear. According to Hovedon, Philip Augustus was anxious to separate the brothers. He told Richard that John had formed an alliance with him and showed him a document to prove it. Richard believed the story and seized all of John's lands, but later accepted his brother's denials and was reconciled to him.[11] This account is supported by the author of the *Magna vita sancti Hugonis*.[12] The pipe rolls do not indicate that John was disseised of any lands at that time, but that could be accounted for by a rapid recall of the royal order before it was carried out. Coggeshall states that John left Richard's court because he was short of money and had quarreled with his brother.[13] John's choice of a place of refuge would seem to indicate that he had been carrying on some sort of negotiations with Richard's foes—he proceeded to Brittany to visit his nephew Arthur and was there when he learned of his brother's death.

The last scene in this strange tale of two brothers took place in Richard's camp in the Limousin. Hovedon states that when Rich-

---

[9] Hovedon, IV, 7; William of Newburgh, *Historia rerum Anglicarum* (ed. Richard Howlett in *Chronicles of the reigns of Stephen, Henry II, and Richard I*, Rolls series), II, 463.
[10] Lionel Landon, *The itinerary of King Richard I* (Pipe roll society), pp. 121, 124, 207-208.
[11] Hovedon, IV, 81.
[12] *Magna vita sancti Hugonis*, p. 287.
[13] Coggeshall, p. 99.

ard realized that he was going to die, he called his men about him, declared John his heir, and ordered them to swear fidelity to him.[14] The king had gone into the Limousin with a slender following. In addition to his favorite mercenary captain, Mercadier, he was accompanied by William de Briouse, Thomas Basset, Peter de Stoke, Gerard de Furnival, and Geoffrey de la Celle.[15] Geoffrey de la Celle was an Angevin baron who had been Richard's seneschal of Gascony, but who was to have little connection with John. The other four were to stand high in John's favor and to profit from it largely. William de Briouse was to extend enormously his already vast lands. Thomas Basset was to have the custody of the earldom of Warwick and to be allowed to marry his daughter to the young earl. Peter de Stoke became seneschal of John's household. Gerard de Furnival received a valuable heiress for his son. These facts in themselves are interesting. But even more curious is the account of John's succession to the crown in the *Annals of Margam*. The annalist states that John was made king largely through the efforts of William de Briouse and his accomplices.[16] Professor Powicke has shown the strong probability that William de Briouse furnished the author of the *Annals of Margam* with much of his information.[17] If William said that he had been largely responsible for John's succession to the throne, was he simply boasting? Or did he and his fellows persuade Richard to make the declaration in favor of John? There is obviously one other possibility. Richard may have been casual to the last and made no declaration whatever. William and his associates may have invented the whole incident. Outside of this little group only one person of rank saw Richard before he died—his mother Queen Eleanor. And Eleanor was a lady whose conscience rarely gave her much trouble and who clearly preferred John to Arthur.[18]

[14] Hovedon, IV, 83.
[15] These men witnessed the only known charter issued by Richard at Chalus. Landon, *Itinerary*, p. 145.
[16] *Annals of Margam*, p. 24.
[17] F. M. Powicke, *The loss of Normandy* (Manchester, 1913), Appendix I.
[18] For a perhaps slightly exaggerated estimate of Eleanor's role in se-

This rather long survey of the arguments that could have been advanced in support of the claims of each of the two rivals for control of the Angevin empire seems to lead to but one reasonable conclusion—the honors lay about even between them. Any prelate or baron of the Plantagenet lands could convince himself without much difficulty that either John or Arthur was Richard's rightful heir. If either rival could eliminate the other, or, failing to do that, could obtain a secure hold on the bases of power, the royal fortresses and treasuries, he was almost certain to win the succession. The chance that one contestant might eliminate the other depended largely on conditions in Anjou and southern Touraine and on pure luck. The question as to who would get control of the royal fortresses and treasuries would be decided by the men who had possession of them—Richard's administrators.

John's situation at the time of his brother's death was extremely precarious. He was the guest of his rival Arthur and was surrounded by the latter's Bretons.[19] While Arthur was too young to make any vigorous decisions for himself, it is hard to believe that the Duchess Constance and her barons would have hesitated to seize the young duke's rival. Presumably John learned of his brother's death before the news reached his hosts. Perhaps Queen Eleanor had already informed him of Richard's wound. At any rate John quickly made his way into Anjou. The two chief royal strongholds of the region, the great fortress of Chinon that held the treasure of Anjou and the castle of Loches, were in the control of Robert de Turnham, seneschal of Anjou. Robert was an English knight who had been seneschal of Anjou under Henry II and had played a prominent part in Richard's crusade. Richard had rewarded his services with an heiress, the daughter of William Fossard, a Yorkshire baron. When John appeared at the gates of Chinon on April 14, Robert surrendered the fortress to him. There the members of Richard's household joined him and swore fidelity to him as his brother's successor.[20] Richard in his *Histoire des*

curing John's succession see Alfred Richard, *Histoire des comtes de Poitou, 778-1204* (Paris, 1903), II, 333-335.
[19] *Magna vita sancti Hugonis*, p. 287.
[20] *Ibid.* Coggeshall, p. 99; Hovedon, IV, 86; Wendover, I, 285-286.

comtes de Poitou suggests that Eleanor had persuaded Robert de Turnham to support John.[21] It seems just as likely that Robert believed John would become king of England and his interests centered in that realm.

At Chinon John was joined by the most revered prelate of England, Hugh of Avalon, bishop of Lincoln, who had been on his way to see Richard when he learned of his death and had officiated at the king's funeral in the abbey of Fontrevault. Together they journeyed to Fontrevault and on to Beaufort-en-Vallée where Richard's widow, Berengeria, was staying. There they passed Easter Sunday and there John learned how weak was his grip on Anjou.[22] Arthur had moved out of Brittany with his Breton troops and had been joined by at least part of the Angevin baronage. On that same Easter day he solemnly declared himself count of Anjou, and the castle of Angers was surrendered to him by a nephew of Robert de Turnham.[23] About the same time John heard that Philip Augustus was advancing on Maine and Anjou from the east. The next morning John returned to Fontrevault.[24] It was farther away from Arthur than Beaufort, it was near Chinon, and in all probability Richard's mercenaries under Mercadier were there. Certainly Queen Eleanor who was still at Fontrevault had a strong escort of barons from her duchy. The author of the *Magna vita sancti Hugonis* states that John was nearly captured when the Bretons seized Le Mans two days after Easter, but as John was at Beaufort on April 18 and in Fontrevault on the twenty-first it seems practically impossible that he should have been in Le Mans on the twentieth. But as his recent travelling companion, Hugh of Lincoln, was in Le Mans that day, it seems highly likely that the Bretons hoped to find John there.[25] On the twenty-second John left Fontrevault and made his way north to Normandy. Except for the fortresses held by Robert de Turnham, Anjou belonged to Arthur.

[21] Richard, *Histoire des comtes de Poitou*, II, 334.
[22] *Magna vita sancti Hugonis*, pp. 287-293.
[23] Hovedon, IV, 86; *Layettes du trésor des chartes* (ed. Alexandre Teulet, Paris, 1863-1866), I, 199.
[24] *Ibid.*, p. 200.
[25] *Magna vita sancti Hugonis*, p. 296.

Had Arthur's supporters captured John in Anjou, it seems quite likely that the young duke of Brittany might have become the master of the Angevin empire. Once John escaped from that danger, the decision lay with the officials of Normandy and England. These two feudal states were in the hands of a small group of men who were closely knit together by long association in the royal administration. The seneschal of Normandy, William fitz Ralph, was an English knight who had started his career in the household of Henry II's younger brother. He was essentially a royal servant without extensive landed power. The other dominant figure in Normandy was its metropolitan, Walter of Coutance, archbishop of Rouen, who had also attained his eminent position through faithful service to the English crown. The head of the English administration was the justiciar, Geoffrey fitz Peter. As a young man in the royal administration Geoffrey had obtained a minor heiress, Beatrice de Say. Some years later the extinction of the Mandeville earls of Essex made Beatrice one of the possible heirs to their vast estates. The fact that the last Mandeville earl had died after Richard had left England on the crusade and that Geoffrey was one of the justices left to rule the realm made certain that he would gain the inheritance. He was thus in 1199 a powerful territorial magnate as well as the justiciar. The primate of all England, Hubert Walter, archbishop of Canterbury, had been Geoffrey's predecessor as justiciar and was also a royal servant of long standing. While these four men were the dominant figures, there stood behind them a powerful group closely associated with them.

When Richard departed on his crusade he had left a group of four justices to aid his justiciar in ruling England—Geoffrey fitz Peter, William Marshal, Hugh Bardolf, and William Brewer. These men still dominated the English administration. Geoffrey fitz Peter was justiciar and sheriff of Staffordshire and Yorkshire. William Marshal, who was also a great baron through marriage to an heiress, was sheriff of Gloucestershire and Sussex. Hugh Bardolf was sheriff of Northumberland and Westmoreland. William Brewer was sheriff of Nottinghamshire and Derbyshire and custodian of the honors of Wallingford and Peverel of Nottingham.

All these men owed everything they had to the generosity of their royal masters, Henry II and Richard. They had long worked together in the royal service. Geoffrey fitz Peter, Hubert Walter, and Walter de Coutance had started their careers as clerks of the great justiciar, Ranulf de Glanvill. They were extremely likely to work together for one of the rivals for the succession. What evidence we have indicates that no one of them had any great enthusiasm for John. But they knew him and he knew them. During Richard's absence on the crusade they had cooperated with John until he went over to King Philip. He was their obvious choice for Richard's successor.

When King Richard had first realized that his wound was serious, he had despatched a messenger to inform the archbishop of Canterbury and William Marshal who were at Vaudreuil in Normandy. They were directed to take possession of the Tower of Rouen where the Norman treasure was kept.[26] There on April 10 they received the news of Richard's death and, according to the *Histoire*, decided to support John.[27] William Marshal immediately sent his favorite knight, John d'Erley, to England to carry the word to the justiciar, Geoffrey fitz Peter.[28] As soon as John heard of his brother's death, he ordered the archbishop and William Marshal to go to England to reinforce the justiciar.[29]

While it is extremely unlikely that there was much real sentiment in England in favor of Arthur, every magnate of the island whether he was English, Welsh, or Scots saw in the doubtful succession a magnificent opportunity. Outside of the group that had made their fortunes as servants of Henry II and Richard, there were few who did not nurse some grudge against the house of Plantagenet. When young Henry, duke of Normandy, had been fighting with King Stephen for the English crown, he had bought the support of many English barons by lavish promises. Most of these promises he had neglected to keep. Henry's heavy-handed rule had led to the great revolt of 1173-1174. When it was sup-

---

[26] *Histoire de Guillaume le Maréchal,* lines 11775-11814.
[27] *Ibid.,* lines 11836-11908.
[28] *Ibid.,* lines 11909-11916.
[29] Hovedon, IV, 86; Wendover, I, 285.

pressed, the defeated rebels had been punished. Hence at the death of Henry II a fair part of the English baronage was disaffected. Richard had conciliated a few of them, and his fame as a warrior made rebellion against him an unattractive idea. Very few great lords had been so indiscreet as to become involved in John's treason while Richard was a prisoner in Germany. But the barons had not forgotten their grievances and were ready to make the most of them when an opportunity appeared. Much the same thing can be said of the Welsh and the Scots. Under the strong rule of the first two Plantagenets the Welsh had been slowly but surely pushed back. The marcher lordships with their castles spread farther and farther up the river valleys into the hills. The elder brother of William, king of Scotland, had done much to assist Henry II to win the English throne. William himself had supported the baronial revolt against Henry, had been captured, and had been forced to give up most of the lands his brother had received from the English king. The disputed succession might well enable him to recover these fiefs.

It is certain that there was some disorder in England at the news of Richard's death, but it is difficult to discover how much it amounted to. The rolls contain a few references to plundering by baronial bands and one chronicler speaks of it.[30] But it seems clear that in general the disaffected barons did not actually take up arms. Probably most of the disorder was due to ordinary malefactors who took advantage of what they hoped would be a hiatus in law enforcement. The justiciar acted vigorously to restore order and maintain the authority of the government. The royal castles and the private castles that were in the king's hands were put in repair, supplied, and garrisoned. In a number of shires bands of knights and serjeants were hired as mobile police forces.[31]

When the archbishop and William Marshal reached England, they and the justiciar proceeded to conciliate the dissident barons.

[30] *Curia regis rolls*, I, 255, 384, 440; *Pipe roll 2 John*, p. 20; *Memoranda roll 1 John*, p. 12; Coggeshall, p. 98.

[31] Entries showing the cost of preparing castles for defense and hiring troops run all through the *Pipe roll* of 1199. For samples see *Pipe roll 1 John*, pp. 1, 2, 4, 22, 27, 38, 56, 58, 59, 71, 73, 78, 85, 87, 154, 163, 169, 182, 188, 200, 210, 212, 214, 242, 243, 247.

They summoned the ones whom they considered most dangerous to meet them at Northampton to discuss their grievances. This group included David, earl of Huntingdon; Ranulf, earl of Chester; Richard de Clare, earl of Hertford; William de Ferrers, earl of Derby, Waleran, earl of Warwick; Roger de Lacy, constable of Chester, and William de Mowbray.[32] The feudal importance of these men can best be grasped by considering the knight service owed to them by their vassals—over 850 fees. One can only guess as to their specific grievances. David, earl of Huntingdon, was the younger brother of King William of Scotland and may simply have represented his brother's discontent, but he was also one who had his castles razed in the revolt of 1173. Earl Ranulf's grandfather had received particularly lavish grants from Henry II as duke of Normandy. His father, Earl Hugh, had never held the possessions promised his father and had been temporarily deprived of his earldom after the great revolt. Ranulf himself was the legal husband of Constance of Brittany. Although the lady had declined to live with him, Ranulf may well have considered himself entitled to enjoy her large English estates, the honor of Richmond. Finally Ranulf's distant cousin, William de Roumar, had died in 1198 without heirs of his body, and there is reason for believing that King Richard had withheld some Roumar lands from the earl of Chester.[33] Richard de Clare had married a daughter of William, earl of Gloucester, sister of John's first wife, and he may have felt that he had not received a fair share of the Gloucester earldom. William de Ferrers' grandmother had been a sister of the last William Peverel of Nottingham who had been deprived of his barony and exiled by Henry II. William claimed a share of the honor of Peverel. Earl Waleran of Warwick's elder brother had possessed the marcher lordship of Gower, and the earl may have hoped to obtain it. Perhaps he was annoyed because the royal favorite, Hugh Bardolf, who had married the sister of John de Limesi, had failed to give the countess of Warwick who was John's

[32] Hovedon, IV, 88; Wendover, I, 285.
[33] John gave the Roumar lands in southern England to Hubert de Burgh. *Pipe roll 3 John*, p. 200; *Red book of the exchequer* (ed. Hubert Hall, Rolls series), II, 482; *Book of fees* (Rolls series), I, 79, 90.

widow her rightful dower in the Limesi estates.[34] It is difficult to account for Roger de Lacy's presence in this group. He may just have followed his lord, Ranulf of Chester, though it is possible that he resented the fact that the chief castle of his Yorkshire lands, the great fortress of Pontefract, had been kept in the king's possession.[35] William de Mowbray's father had had all his castles razed in the revolt of 1173.

William Marshal and Geoffrey fitz Peter must have had some sympathy for the plaints of the barons. While they had received a great deal from King Richard, he had withheld some things to which they felt entitled. Geoffrey had the lands of the Mandeville earls of Essex, but he had not been made an earl. William had been given the daughter and heiress of Richard fitz Gilbert de Clare, earl of Pembroke and lord of Leinster in Ireland. He had received with her the marcher lordship of Striguil with the English lands that were attached to it, but he got neither the county of Pembroke nor the title of earl.[36] At any rate John's three representatives promised the assembled barons that the new king would give each one his full rights. The barons then swore fidelity to John.[37]

Shortly after the appeasement of the English barons, messengers arrived from King William of Scotland. He demanded the counties of Northumberland and Cumberland that had been held by his brother. Apparently John's representatives had little confidence in their master's judgment. They refused to allow the king of Scotland's messengers to cross to Normandy. Instead they sent Earl David of Huntingdon to tell his brother to wait until John came to England. But John himself had already realized the desirability of coming to terms with the Scots king and had sent Eustace de Vesci whose wife was an illegitimate daughter of King William to

[34] *Curia regis rolls*, I, 130. Years later Earl Waleran's descendant sued for Gower. Powicke, *Loss of Normandy*, p. 470.

[35] *Pipe roll 1 John*, pp. 210, 212.

[36] The evidence for the retention of Pembroke by the crown when Richard gave William Marshal the lands of Isabel de Clare is slight but to me convincing. Pembroke castle was in the king's hand in 1199. *Pipe roll 1 John*, p. 182. Giraldi Cambrensis, *Opera* (ed. J. S. Brewer, J. F. Dimock, G. F. Warner, Rolls series), I, 76.

[37] Hovedon, IV, 88; Wendover, I, 285.

promise his father-in-law his rights in England.[38] It seems unlikely that John had any real intention of surrendering two counties to King William. He simply wanted to keep him quiet until he had firmly secured the English crown.

Once England seemed safely secured for John, William Marshal returned to Normandy. John had been consecrated as duke of Normandy on April 25 at Rouen by Archbishop Walter de Coutance.[39] By May 21 he was at Dieppe ready to sail for England.[40] On May 25 he landed at Shoreham and immediately proceeded to London. On May 27 he was solemnly crowned in Westminster by Hubert Walter, archbishop of Canterbury.[41] He was king of England and the succession was no longer in dispute.

The new king's first step was to reward the three men who had secured England for him. On the very day of his coronation he belted Geoffrey fitz Peter and William Marshal earls of Essex and Pembroke and presumably gave the latter the shire from which his title was derived. The same day saw Hubert Walter granted the office of chancellor.[42] A few days later one of the recently disaffected barons had his claims satisfied. On June 7 at Northampton William de Ferrers, earl of Derby, was belted by the king's own hand and granted the third penny of the pleas of his shire. The proceeding is rather curious. It was not a creation—William de Ferrers was already earl of Derby as his father had been. But he was girded with the sword of his earldom and given the third penny " as his ancestors had held it." [43] He was also granted the manor and hundred of Higham Ferrers with two subsidiary manors. This large estate that had been farmed for £140 a year was part of the honor of Peverel of Nottingham and was given to the earl to satisfy his claim on the Peverel lands. He offered and paid a sum

[38] Hovedon, IV, 88-89; Wendover, I, 285.
[39] Hovedon, IV, 87; Coggeshall, p. 99; Wendover, I, 286.
[40] *Calendar of documents preserved in France illustrative of the history of Great Britain and Ireland* (ed. J. Horace Round, Rolls series), pp. 35-36.
[41] Hovedon, IV, 89-90; Coggeshall, pp. 99-100; Wendover, I, 287-288.
[42] Hovedon, IV, 90.
[43] *Cartae antiquae rolls* 1-10 (ed. Lionel Landon, Pipe roll society), nos. 56, 60.

of 2,000 marks for the grant.[44] One other dissident baron was cared for at this time. Roger de Lacy, constable of Chester, received his castle of Pontefract, but was obliged to give his eldest son as a hostage for his good behavior.[45]

This first visit of John to his English realm was extremely brief. Once England was safely in his hands his mind turned quickly to his continental estates that were threatened by the alliance between Arthur and Philip Augustus. As his chief needs there were men and money, he summoned his feudal host and ordered the levying of a scutage of two marks per knight's fee on the tenants-in-chief who did not follow him to Normandy. He also directed his officials to collect a tallage from the royal demesnes and lands in the king's hand and demanded an aid from the prelates and ecclesiastical houses.[46] On June 20 he crossed from Shoreham to Dieppe. With him went most of the earls and barons of England.

[44] *Pipe roll 1 John*, p. 16; *Rotuli de oblatis et finibus* (ed. T. D. Hardy, Record commission), p. 3.
[45] Hovedon, IV, 91-92.
[46] See discussion by Doris Stenton in the Introduction to the Pipe roll of 1199. *Pipe roll 1 John*, xvi-xix.

CHAPTER II

THE KING AND THE MAGNATES

JOHN found the royal throne of England beset with serious problems. On every side the new king faced external foes. While the Scots king and the Welsh chieftains could not be called menaces to England as a whole, the fulfillment of their ambitions would decrease the resources of the English crown and gravely reduce its prestige. On the continent the alliance of Philip Augustus and Arthur threatened John with the loss of his fiefs held of the French crown. The internal situation was almost as cheerless. When the barons of England accepted John as Richard's heir, they did not abandon their desire to recover the lands, castles, and privileges which they believed they had been deprived of by Henry II and Richard I. They had simply accepted the assurances of John's representatives that he would conciliate them. To attempt to satisfy them completely would involve a very serious reduction in the power and resources of the royal government. This royal government itself was far from entirely satisfactory from John's point of view. Its leaders were men trained under Henry II and Richard. They were in general devoted to the crown to which they owed their high positions, but few of them had any enthusiasm for John personally. But the most serious problem that faced the new king was financial. John came to the throne in a time of rapidly rising prices. Henry II had been able to hire mercenary knights for eight pence a day—the cost to John was two shillings or two and one-half times as much. The cost of other types of troops had risen proportionately. If John was to defend his domains from his enemies, he needed to increase his revenue.

There were two types of concession by which John could hope to placate his external and internal foes—financial and political or military. But giving money or sources of revenue to the Welsh, the Scots, or the French would aggravate his financial difficulties while the surrender of castles would make it harder to resist them in war. The problem of internal conciliation was even more complicated. If the king conceded to his barons sources of revenue, his income was decreased, and if he gave them offices and castles, he lessened his ability to resist them if they resorted to rebellion. Moreover one of the chief if not the chief cause of baronial discontent was the financial exactions of the royal government.

These same problems had faced King Richard. His solution had been to wage war on his external enemies and to pay the costs by wringing every cent possible out of the people of his domain. His financial exactions were by the standards of his day utterly outrageous. Although he was generous to his brother John and a few personal friends, Richard made no concessions whatever to his barons in general. To keep them loyal or at least quiet he relied on his renown as a soldier. Richard was without doubt the ablest captain of his day. Backed by his chosen household knights and his mercenary serjeants he was invincible on the field of battle. Moreover it is important to remember that Richard's military capacity engendered admiration as well as fear. Prowess was the most highly valued virtue among the feudal aristocracy. Then too Richard was frank and open in manner and when well disposed, hearty, friendly, and jovial. He was a poet of sorts and an enthusiastic devotee of tournaments. All this appealed to the feudal taste. In short Richard was the most chivalric of kings and this tended to make men overlook his sexual licentiousness, his incredible rapacity, his ungovernable temper, and his complete indifference to the government of his realm in matters other than military. Finally men felt they could trust Richard because he was essentially too straightforward to be an effective dissembler. If Richard received you agreeably, you were in his favor. He was not one for dark and devious designs. But during the reign of this heavy-sworded and chivalrous monarch the springs of discontent welled steadily up toward the flood that was to engulf his brother.

The only characteristics that John shared with his father and brother were licentiousness and intelligence. Although Richard had scorned to use his brain for other than military purposes, in that field he had shown imagination and sound judgment. John was both imaginative and ingenious. He had a fondness for dissembling and for complicated and tortuous maneuvers. Worse yet he was afflicted with a coarse and vulgar sense of humor—an almost fatal defect in an English king. But most serious of all was his complete lack of military renown. Nowhere do we find John praised for deeds of prowess on the battlefield. In his entire reign troops under his command fought only one engagement, the relief of Mirabeau castle in 1202, and it seems clear that others were the leaders in that battle. John possessed none of the chivalric virtues. He seduced his ladies without the aid of poetry and considered tournaments a waste of man-power and a possible source of disorder. But while he lacked the attributes most admired in a feudal monarch, John was proud and avid for prestige and power. Throughout his reign he was to devote his energy and intelligence to developing the royal authority in England. Such was the man who had to face the problems left by the gay-hearted Richard.

Next to the defense of his continental fiefs from Philip Augustus the most acute of John's problems was the conciliation and control of the English baronage. Let us glance for a moment at this baronage in terms of feudal and military power, knights' fees and castles. In 1199 there were approximately 197 lay and 39 ecclesiastical baronies in England. To these 236 baronies were owed the services of some 7,200 knights' fees. But many of these baronies were very small. If one takes 30 fees as the minimum for a fair-sized barony, one finds 60 lay baronies with a total of 4,632 fees and 15 ecclesiastical with a total of 820 fees as large as this. Thus 75 per cent of the knights' fees belonged to baronies having 30 or more fees. In the 236 baronies there stood 140 castles. Of these 127 belonged to 89 lay baronies and 13 to 6 ecclesiastical ones. Not all of the 197 lay baronies were actually in the hands of barons in 1199. There were 15 baronies that had escheated to the crown. They had 1,400 knights' fees and 12 castles. Then John himself still held the earldom of Gloucester—some 300 fees and 3 castles.

While the figures cited above are vital as background for an understanding of the English baronage and hence of John's problem, they do not show that problem in the terms in which he was forced to consider it—men, their power, and their desires. At the time of Richard's death the most powerful baron in England had been John himself. In addition to the great earldom of Gloucester he held extensive lands in the royal demesne assigned to him by his brother. Next to him stood Earl Ranulf of Chester whose county palatine and the English lands attached to it contained some 200 knights' fees and who held about 50 more fees as heir of the Roumars.[1] Earl Ranulf's rapacious eye wandered hungrily over all northern England. Nor did he lack extensive and fairly plausible claims. Henry II had made his grandfather extremely lavish promises. He had granted him all the royal demesne in Staffordshire including the county borough with the overlordship of all the knights' fees except those held by the bishop of Chester and three great barons. He had also given him the castle and borough of Nottingham and the borough of Derby with several important royal manors and the overlordship over half a dozen minor barons. Finally he had granted him the escheated baronies of Lancaster, Tickhill, Eye, and Peverel of Nottingham.[2] These escheats alone were worth about £800 a year and had 292 knights' fees—almost as many fees and about twice the revenue of the earldom of Gloucester. None of the grants made by this charter were enjoyed by Earl Ranulf in 1199. Then in King Stephen's reign William I de Roumar had been earl of Lincoln. Ranulf himself had an ancient claim, partially recognized by Stephen, to Lincoln castle.[3] He also had a claim through his estranged wife Constance to the great honor of Richmond. Earl Ranulf's general policy was the same as his grandfather's. He wanted anything he could get anywhere, but he was especially anxious to build up his power in the shires adjacent to his palatinate of Chester. Here he was aided by his brother-in-law and close ally William de Ferrers, earl of Derby. Earl William had had his castles destroyed by Henry II after the great revolt, but he had some 80 knights' fees in Derbyshire and Staffordshire which was the region Earl Ranulf was most anxious to control.

Just below Ranulf of Chester in feudal power came, in the order of the number of knights' fees they possessed, six great earls—William de Albini, earl of Arundel; Richard de Clare, earl of Hert-

[1] William Farrer, *Honours and knights' fees* (London, 1924), II, 9.
[2] Thomas Rymer, *Foedera* (Record commission, London, 1816), I, 16.
[3] F. M. Stenton, *The first century of English feudalism* (Oxford, 1932), pp. 240-242.

ford; Constance, countess of Richmond; Roger Bigod, earl of Norfolk; Robert de Beaumont, earl of Leicester, and Hamelin Plantagenet, earl of Surrey. Their knights' fees ranged from the 186 of the earl of Arundel to the 140 of the earl of Surrey. But this arrangement by knights' fees must not be taken too seriously. By 1199 money income from demesne lands was certainly as important, perhaps more important, than knightly vassals. Unfortunately we have little information on baronial incomes and hence must use knights' fees for purposes of comparison. Nevertheless it is clear that the two most powerful men of this group were the earls of Arundel and Surrey. William de Albini had 110 fees attached to his castle of Arundel in Sussex and 76 more with the castles of Castle Rising and Buckenham in Norfolk. Hamelin, earl of Surrey, an illegitimate brother of Henry II, held the castle of Reigate in Surrey, extensive lands attached to the castle and rape of Lewes in Sussex, and a group of manors centering in the castles of Castle Acre in Norfolk and Conisborough in Yorkshire.[4] Earl Hamelin was well along in years and was soon, in 1202, to be succeeded by his son William de Warren. The earls of Arundel and Surrey lacked the fierce ambition of Ranulf of Chester. If the crown let them alone, they were willing to enjoy quietly their vast estates. Constance's earldom of Richmond was purely titular—it was firmly in the king's hands. Robert de Beaumont, earl of Leicester, had been a crusading companion of Richard and was apparently on good terms with John. His father had suffered imprisonment for his part in the revolt against Henry II, and the earl's chief castle, Mountsorrel, was still in the hands of the crown.[5] Roger Bigod, earl of Norfolk, was engaged in a fierce dispute with his brother over the possession of the earldom.[6] As he relied on the crown's support, he was unlikely to be troublesome. In short the only lord of this group that could be called discontented was Richard de Clare. He felt that he or his eldest son should have a larger share of the earldom of Gloucester.

The next ten barons to be glanced at in our survey are a very

[4] Farrer, *Honours and knights' fees,* III, 304-307.
[5] *Pipe roll 1 John,* p. 247.
[6] *Pipe roll 2 Richard I,* p. 101; *Curia regis rolls,* I, 93.

mixed group. Five of them were earls—William de Redvers, earl of Devon; William Marshal, earl of Pembroke; Geoffrey fitz Peter, earl of Essex; Waleran de Beaumont, earl of Warwick, and David, earl of Huntingdon. Five were great barons who had not achieved comtal rank—William de Briouse, Warin fitz Gerold, Robert fitz Walter, William de Mowbray, and Roger de Lacy. William de Redvers held the castle of Plympton in Devon with some 90 fees, the castle of Christchurch with 22 fees in Hampshire, and the Isle of Wight with Carisbrooke castle and 20 fees. This extremely powerful baron was out of favor with John for reasons that are obscure. But he was inclined to buy the royal favor with concessions. William Marshal had little feudal power in England. His strength lay in Netherwent, Pembroke, and Ireland. If his 45 fees in Wales and 100 in Ireland are added to his English lands, his knightly vassals were as numerous as those of Ranulf of Chester. Geoffrey fitz Peter and Waleran of Warwick were about equal in feudal power—about 100 knights' fees. But Geoffrey was the chief of the royal administration while Earl Waleran was inclined to stay in his estates and ignore the government. David, earl of Huntingdon, owed much of his importance to his close relationship to the king of Scotland, but he was also the brother-in-law of three English earls—Chester, Arundel and Derby—and the uncle of the earl of Hereford. Although his barony was not very large, some 95 fees, he had a strong castle and extremely extensive privileges.

Perhaps the most interesting as well as the most powerful baron in this group was William de Briouse. He had inherited from his father the rape of Bramber in Sussex with its two castles, half of the barony of Barnstaple in Devon, and the Marcher lordships of Abergavenny, and Brecon. William was extremely rapacious and high in John's favor. During the early years of John's reign he was to use the king's benevolence, ancient claims, and pure conquest to increase his lands greatly. The next baron in feudal power, Warin fitz Gerold, was hereditary chamberlain of the exchequer and a mild figure who gave no one any trouble. Robert fitz Walter had acquired two baronies during Richard's reign. One he had inherited from his father, Walter fitz Robert, and the other was the heritage of his wife, Gunora de Valognes. Robert fitz Walter was to become one of John's most bitter foes. But in 1199 he was simply a baron who wanted anything he could get on the basis of ancient claims. William de Mowbray had been one of the disaffected barons who met John's representatives in Northampton. In the twelfth century the Mowbrays had been extremely powerful lords with about 100 fees scattered in four groups. Two of these groups centered in the castles of Thirsk and Kirby Malzeard in Yorkshire, another around the castle of Brinklow in Warwickshire, while the fourth comprised most of the isle of Axholme in Lincolnshire. The rebellion against Henry II had cost them all their castles. Moreover Henry had listened favorably to the claim of a royal favorite, Robert de Stutville, to the Mowbray barony, and Robert had been bought off by giving him an important demesne manor and 10 knights' fees.[7] As a result of all this the Mowbrays had no great love for the Plantagenet kings. The last of these five barons was a most interesting figure, Roger de Lacy, constable of Chester. He had started his career as hereditary constable of the earldom of Chester. He held 8 knights' fees and the castles of Halton in Cheshire and Donington in Leicestershire of the earl of Chester. In addition he had a small fief in Lancashire. Then in 1184 his distant cousin Robert de Lacy, lord of the castle and barony of Pontefract in Yorkshire and the castle and lands of Clitheroe in Lancashire died without children. King Richard allowed Roger to have the succession for a fine of 3,000 marks.[8] Roger had a high reputation as a soldier and was valued as a captain by both Richard and John. But for some reason or other, perhaps because he was among the dissidents of 1199, John seems to have been suspicious of him until after Roger's long defense of Chateau-Gaillard in 1203.

We have now surveyed the most powerful lords of England. Each of them held over 95 knights' fees. All of them except William de Mowbray had a castle and most of them had more than one. They were the men whose support John needed most. But a few lesser lords deserve mention here because of their personal or family prestige or because they possessed the comtal dignity. William de Ferrers, earl of Derby, has been discussed in connection

[7] Hovedon, IV, 117.   [8] *Pipe roll 7 Richard I*, p. 98.

with Ranulf of Chester. He owed his importance largely to that alliance. Walter de Lacy, lord of Weobly in Herefordshire, held only some 50 fees in England, but he was lord of the great barony of Meath in Ireland. William Plantagenet, earl of Salisbury, was an illegitimate son of King Henry II and his position as John's half-brother made him a person of greater importance than his fief of 56 knights would justify. Henry de Bohun was the heir of two baronial houses—the Bohuns and the earls of Hereford. Starting as petty barons his ancestors had married their way into a position of considerable importance, and Henry was to continue this good work. As his grandfather, Miles of Gloucester, earl of Hereford, had been the recipient of extensive promises by Henry II, Henry de Bohun had claims against the crown. Baldwin de Bethune, a younger son of the advocate of Bethune who was an important vassal of the count of Flanders and held a small English barony, had been a crusading companion and prime favorite of King Richard. Through the king's favor he became the third husband of Hawise, countess of Aumale in Normandy, and lady of several English baronies. Finally there was Aubrey de Vere, earl of Oxford. The Vere barony was small, only 30 fees, but it had two strong fortresses, Castle Hedingham and Canfield in Essex. Earl Aubrey owed his comtal rank to the fact that his father had been the brother-in-law and close ally during Stephen's reign of the grasping Earl Geoffrey de Mandeville. Aubrey himself was engaged in modestly expanding his lands through marriage with the heiress of a minor Buckinghamshire baron, Walter de Bolebec.

The general policy adopted by John toward his barons was simple, obvious, and much the same as that of his predecessors. The lords he considered truly dangerous were to be weakened by every possible means. The more moderate dissidents were to be appeased as cheaply as possible. Then the power of barons considered reliable was to be built up and their fidelity reinforced by gratitude. When possible the lords whose power was to be increased to act as a counter-balance against those who were believed to be dangerous were to be barons of secondary importance. But John's deeply suspicious nature and his greed made the effective execution of this policy almost impossible. He was subject to sudden suspicions against those whose loyalty he had been most anxious to secure, and he apparently always secretly regretted the power he had felt obliged to give them. He was to turn his best friends into his most bitter foes. Conversely he was often obliged to turn to those whom he had most distrusted and to ply them with favors to gain their support.

John saw very clearly that the one man most dangerous to the royal authority in England was Earl Ranulf of Chester. His palatinate shire which he controlled completely gave him a center of power such as no other lord except perhaps William Marshal possessed. The vast estates scattered over England supplied revenue and knights. Moreover he had the military advantages of a Marcher baron. His own vassals were kept in training by the continuous contests with the Welsh. Then the Welsh were always ready to fight for pay, and the Marcher lords could easily hire bands of mercenary infantry. When one considers the ambition, greed, energy, and military reputation of the master of all this power, it is easy to understand John's position.

In the first years of the reign when the king was appeasing several of the great barons Earl Ranulf received nothing. He was in fact slapped in the face. The Roumar lands in southern England, usually called the honor of Cammel, were given to one of the few men John really trusted, his chamberlain Hubert de Burgh.[9] It was a foolish proceeding. Depriving the earl of a few scattered demesnes and fees so far from the center of his power was not going to weaken him materially, but it was bound to annoy him exceedingly. They were not lands to which he had a vague claim. In his mind they were unquestionably his as heir of the Roumars. It might be argued that John's grants to William de Ferrers were intended to please Earl Ranulf, but it seems more likely that John was attempting to wean the earl of Derby away from his dangerous brother-in-law. We have seen that one of John's first acts as king was to belt William with the sword of his earldom and allow him to offer a large fine for Higham Ferrers. In July 1202 he was

[9] *Pipe roll 3 John*, p. 200; *Red book of the exchequer*, II, 482; *Book of fees*, I, 79, 80, 90; *Rotuli litterarum clausarum* (ed. T. D. Hardy, Record commission), I, 60; *Pipe roll 8 John*, p. 135.

granted the manor and wapentake of Wirksworth and the manor of Ashborne in Derbyshire for a fee farm of £120 per year.[10] But while with one hand John was appeasing Earl William, with the other he was offending both him and the earl of Chester. William de Ferrers was one of the few great barons who did not possess a castle. There seems no doubt that to have one was one of his chief ambitions. At the very beginning of his reign John started the building of a great royal castle on the chief manor of a small escheated barony. In the years 1200, 1201, and 1202 £684 was spent on this castle of Horsley.[11] It stood about five miles north of Derby, the shire borough of William de Ferrers' county, and two from the ruins of Earl William's castle of Duffield that had been razed by Henry II. In short while John's policy may have appeased the earl of Derby to some extent, it was hardly likely to make him a firm ally of the crown against Ranulf of Chester.

While the king of England might have sound reasons for trying to curb the earl of Chester, it was a foolish policy for a duke of Normandy who was trying to defend his possessions against Philip Augustus and Arthur. Except for Robert of Leicester, William Marshal, and Hamelin de Warren, Ranulf of Chester was the only great baron of England whose Norman possessions were really important. He was hereditary viscount of the Avranchin and had fifty knightly vassals in his Norman fiefs. Moreover Earl Ranulf's wife, Constance of Brittany, had married, apparently without the formalities of divorce, Guy de Thouars, a younger brother of the viscount of Thouars. The earl had promptly found consolation with Clemence, sister of Geoffrey, lord of Fougères, a powerful Breton baron whose lands adjoined the Avranchin. The stepfather of the young lord of Fougères was another important lord of the Avranchin, Fulk Painel. In short Ranulf and his new relatives could seriously compromise the safety of a large section of John's continental possessions.

Early in 1203 the house of Fougères led by young Geoffrey's great-uncle and guardian, William, went over to King Philip.[12]

---

[10] Cartae antiquae rolls, Public Record Office; *Pipe roll 5 John*, p. 171.
[11] *Pipe roll 2 John*, pp. 7-8; *Pipe roll 3 John*, p. 89; *Pipe roll 4 John*, p. 186.
[12] Powicke, *Loss of Normandy*, p. 245.

Shortly before Easter, probably on April 3, John had procured the murder of young Arthur of Brittany whom he had captured at Mirabeau in the previous August.[13] He was in a savagely suspicious mood. He knew that he had treated Earl Ranulf badly and thought he might be plotting with his wife's relatives. On April 13 the king arrived at the great fortress of Vire in the Avranchin. There he was met by Earl Ranulf and Fulk Painel who assured him of their loyalty. Ranulf surrendered to John the royal castle of St. Pierre de Semilly that he had in his custody. Roger de Lacy, constable of Chester, agreed that if Ranulf betrayed the king, he would carry to John the fiefs he held of the earldom of Chester.[14] John's suspicions soon left him. They had, of course, been essentially ridiculous. Earl Ranulf could not hope to gain anything from King Philip that could balance the loss of his vast English fiefs. On May 8 the castle of St. Pierre de Semilly was returned to Ranulf's custody and on May 31 he was given custody of the castle of Avranches.[15] About the same time John confirmed to him the English lands that Geoffrey de Fougères had given him with his sister.[16]

Although John had apparently abandoned his suspicions about Ranulf's fidelity, he was soon to strike his cruelest blow at the earl's ambitions. Constance of Brittany had died in 1201. According to English custom a widower who had a child by an heiress was entitled to her lands for life. John very properly gave possession of the honor of Richmond to Guy de Thouars.[17] Even if Constance had never legally divorced Earl Ranulf, he had had no child by her and hence had no sound claim to her lands. Richmond belonged to Guy or to Arthur. But early in September 1203, Guy de Thouars went over to Philip Augustus. By that time Arthur had disappeared into the dungeons of John's castles—was in fact dead. The only Englishman with any claim to Richmond, feeble as his was, was Ranulf of Chester. Then on September 19 John gave

---

[13] *Ibid.*, pp. 456-457.
[14] *Rotuli litterarum patentium* (ed. T. D. Hardy, Record commission), pp. 28-29.
[15] *Ibid.*, pp. 29-30.
[16] *Rotuli chartarum* (ed. T. D. Hardy, Record commission), p. 104.
[17] *Pipe roll 4 John*, p. 64; *Rot. pat.*, pp. 4, 17, 27.

the shire of Richmond, that is the Yorkshire lands lying about Richmond castle, to Earl Robert of Leicester.[18] Once more we can only guess at what the king had in mind. In the reign of Stephen the earls of Chester and Leicester had waged savage war for control of the lands that lay between their respective seats. John may well have believed that by causing bitter enmity between Earl Ranulf and Robert of Leicester and building up the latter's power he could hold the earl of Chester in check.

Earl Ranulf's anger at the grant of Richmondshire to Robert of Leicester may well have lain behind his next brush with King John. On June 3, 1200, the king had granted his favorite baron, William de Briouse, any lands he could conquer from Welshmen who were enemies of the crown.[19] Some months before, John had solemnly confirmed to Gwenwynwyn, lord of Powis, all the lands of his inheritance.[20] In August 1200, he granted that Welsh chieftain the Marcher fortress of Whittington.[21] Gwenwynwyn was most certainly not the king's enemy. But unfortunately most of the land William de Briouse wanted was under his control, and William was not one to worry over fine points. William de Briouse himself joined John in Normandy in July 1202, and it is possible that the war with the lord of Powis was started by his sons. At any rate by the winter of 1202-1203 it was in full swing. On January 18, 1203, John informed Geoffrey fitz Peter that William de Briouse complained that Gwenwynwyn was plundering his lands and ordered the justiciar to protect William's men.[22] In August 1204 John gave Gwenwynwyn a safe conduct to go to Woodstock to meet him on September 5. Pending the conference he and the Briouse family were to observe a truce.[23] Apparently Gwenwynwyn did not go and the war continued. On December 14 John directed the sheriffs of Nottinghamshire, Yorkshire, Leicestershire, Warwickshire, and Lincolnshire to seize all the lands of Ranulf of Chester and to arrest any vassal of the earl who tried to perform service to him. The reason given was that Earl Ranulf

[18] *Ibid.*, p. 30. *Rotulis de liberate ac de misis et praestitis* (ed. T. D. Hardy, Record commission), pp. 63-64.
[19] *Rot. chart.*, p. 66.
[20] *Ibid.*, p. 63.
[21] *Ibid.*, p. 74.
[22] *Rot. pat.*, p. 23.
[23] *Ibid.*, pp. 44-45.

was in alliance with Gwenwynwyn.[24] It is, of course, impossible to say whether Earl Ranulf was aiding the Welsh prince because of his annoyance with John or whether he had simply been too slow in following the rapid turns of the king's policy in Wales.

Thus from his accession to the end of 1204 John had refused all favors to Ranulf of Chester and had even deprived him of part of his rightful inheritance. He had given Robert of Leicester the lands at which Ranulf looked most hopefully. He had openly suspected him of plotting with Philip Augustus and had seized his English lands for allying with the Welsh. One would have said that John regarded Ranulf as his worst enemy among the English barons. Then in March 1205 Earl Robert of Leicester died. Within the month John granted Earl Ranulf all Richmondshire except for the fees of Ruald fitz Alan, hereditary constable of Richmond castle, and those of one other vassal.[25] Perhaps John felt that Earl Robert's death removed the last baron who could counterbalance Ranulf and that the only course was to try to buy the earl of Chester's loyalty. Other favors soon followed. Earl Ranulf was forgiven the debts that his father had owed to Aaron of Lincoln. He was also pardoned a penalty of £100 that had been assessed against him for a novel disseisin.[26] While the relations between John and the earl never became intimate, from March 1205 to the king's death they were completely amicable.

In addition to Ranulf of Chester there was one other great baron whom John showed no desire to placate—William de Mowbray. William's grandfather, Roger, had bought off the claims of Robert de Stutville to his barony in the reign of Henry II.[27] In April 1200 John issued a charter to Robert's son, William de Stutville, promising him justice toward William de Mowbray in a suit for the entire Mowbray barony. For this and other favors granted in the same charter William promised to pay 3,000 marks.[28] William de Mowbray promptly offered John 2,000 marks that he might be treated justly in the suit.[29] The affair was settled before John and his court on January 21, 1201, at Louth in Lincolnshire.

[24] *Rot. claus.*, I, 16.
[25] *Rot. pat.*, p. 51.
[26] *Rot. claus.*, I, 30, 60.
[27] Hovedon, IV, 117.
[28] *Cartae antiquae rolls*, no. 102.
[29] *Rot. oblatis*, p. 102.

William de Mowbray gave William de Stutville nine knights' fees in addition to the ten given his father and the manor of Brinklow in Warwickshire that was valued at £12 a year.[30] According to Hovedon it was deemed proper to reopen the dispute that had been settled in Henry II's reign because the agreement between Roger de Mowbray and Robert de Stutville had never been confirmed by the crown.[31] But one can easily understand how this argument had little appeal to William de Mowbray. Whether from poverty or disinclination he made little progress in paying the 2,000 marks he had promised. In 1207 he still owed 1,940 marks.[32] In 1209 the king was attempting to collect it directly from the vassals of the Mowbray barony as an aid to pay their lord's debts.[33] William de Mowbray's hatred of John seems to have been well founded early in the reign.

An interesting intermediary case between those of the great barons who received no favors from John and the lords who were appeased was that of William de Redvers, earl of Devon. Earl William had succeeded his nephew in 1193. His wife was the daughter of Robert, count of Meulan, once a powerful figure on the borders of France and Normandy but who had lost most of his possessions in the wars between the Capetian and Plantagenet kings. He had had some sort of trouble with King Richard in 1196, had had his lands seized, and had paid 500 marks to get them back.[34] He apparently felt that he was obliged to buy John's good will. The earl had two daughters and no son. In the spring of 1200 both his daughters were affianced to royal favorites. The eldest daughter was to be the wife of Peter des Preaux. Peter had been a close friend of King Richard, and he and his brothers were powerful in Normandy. John felt the need of his active assistance in defending the duchy. Peter was to be earl of Devon and to have the castle and barony of Plympton.[35] The second daughter was affianced to John's chamberlain, Hubert de Burgh. She was

---

[30] Hovedon, IV, 117-118; *Curia regis rolls,* I, 380.
[31] Hovedon, IV, 118.
[32] *Pipe roll 9 John,* p. 82.
[33] Pipe roll 11 John, Public Record Office.
[34] *Pipe roll 8 Richard I,* p. 148.
[35] *Rot. chart.,* p. 33.

to have the Isle of Wight and the earl's lands in Hampshire with the castles of Christchurch and Carisbrooke. If the earl should have a son, Hubert and his wife were to have £60 a year in the earl's demesnes and 10 knights' fees.[36] Apparently neither of these marriages took place. Earl William's son, Baldwin de Redvers, must have been born about this time.[37] In all probability his birth shortly after the arrangements were made seriously reduced the attractiveness of his sisters.

In 1204 Earl William was once more in trouble with the crown. His castle of Plympton was seized by William Brewer, sheriff of Devonshire, whose son was eventually to marry the earl's younger daughter.[38] The reasons for John's suspicions of the earl are unknown. Perhaps they grew out of his relationship with Robert of Meulan. At any rate Earl William offered the king 500 marks for the return of his castle, the possession of certain estates he claimed, and the right to exercise his customary judicial privileges on the Isle of Wight.[39] This affair seems to have closed the difficulties between John and the earl of Devon.

Despite his stern treatment of Ranulf of Chester, William de Mowbray, and William de Redvers John's general policy toward the great barons was one of appeasement—sometimes abject appeasement. Perhaps the most striking illustration is found in the cases of two barons whose names were to be closely linked throughout John's reign—Robert fitz Walter and Saher de Quency. In the spring of 1200 Robert fitz Walter appeared before the king's court to claim the hereditary custody of the castle of Hertford.[40] In all probability his argument was that this right had once belonged to his wife's ancestors. While there is no evidence that John recognized Robert's claim to the custody of Hertford as a matter of right, in August 1202 he placed the castle in his care.[41] In December of the same year he freed Robert and his wife from all debts owed to Jews by themselves or their ancestors.[42]

At the beginning of John's reign Saher de Quency was not even

---

[36] *Ibid.*, pp. 52-53.
[37] Baldwin had married and had a son by 1216.
[38] *Rot. pat.*, p. 44.
[39] *Rot. oblatis*, pp. 235-236.
[40] *Curia regis rolls*, I, 116.
[41] *Rot. pat.*, p. 17.
[42] *Cartae antiquae rolls*, no. 308.

a baron much less a great one. In 1155 Henry II had granted Saher's grandfather the manor of Buckby in Northamptonshire, a demesne of the barony of Chokes then in the king's hand.[43] Saher's father, Robert de Quency, a crusading companion of Richard, died in 1196 in possession of Buckby and perhaps some other mesne fiefs. Saher himself had been a partisan of Henry the young king, eldest son of Henry II, in the revolt of 1172-3 and had also enjoyed Richard's favor.[44] Both he and his brother Robert had married magnificently. Saher married Margaret, sister of Robert of Leicester, and Robert married Hawise, sister of Ranulf of Chester. But while Saher's prospects were brilliant in 1199, his actual possessions were modest. In March 1203 John granted him the manors of Chinnor and Sydenham in Oxfordshire for the service of one-half knight's fee.[45] In May he forgave him a debt of 300 marks owed the Jews.[46] Perhaps this sudden interest in Saher was the result of the latter's relationship to Robert of Leicester, but it seems equally possible that John sought to secure the gratitude of an experienced warrior.

In the spring of 1203 John assigned Robert fitz Walter and Saher de Quency to a crucial command—the castle of Vaudreuil. Rouen was the heart of Normandy and the path to Rouen lay along the valley of the Seine. On the right bank stood the magnificent fortress of Chateau-Gaillard commanded by Roger de Lacy, constable of Chester. On the left bank a little farther down the river was Vaudreuil. No French king could hope to besiege Rouen in safety while these castles held out. John had picked their commanders carefully. They were Englishmen with no interests of any importance in Normandy, and they were experienced soldiers. But when in July 1203 King Philip laid siege to Vaudreuil, Robert and Saher surrendered the castle immediately. Coggeshall and Wendover seem to believe that this was pure cowardice, and the latter states that Philip was so disgusted that he threw them both into prison and exacted enormous ransoms for their

---

[43] *Ibid.*, no. 293.
[44] Benedict of Peterborough, *Gesta regis Henrici secundi* (ed. William Stubbs, Rolls series), I, 45-47.
[45] *Cartae antiquae rolls*, no. 238.
[46] *Rot. liberate*, p. 38.

release.[47] The *Historie de Gullaume le Maréchal* does not mention their names but gives a conversation between Philip Augustus and William Marshal that almost certainly refers to them. William asked Philip why he stooped so low as to encourage traitors. Philip replied that they were like torches to be used and then thrown into the latrine.[48] There are obviously a number of possibilities. The charge of cowardice seems improbable. Both Robert and Saher had long knightly records and were to continue to hold good military reputations. Moreover the stanch defender of a castle had little to fear beyond capture and the necessity of ransoming himself. Perhaps Philip, as his words to William Marshal imply, bribed them with promises and then cheerfully broke the promises. Yet when Robert fitz Walter was in trouble with John in 1212, he sought refuge in France. It is also possible that Saher and Robert were involved in a general baronial conspiracy against John. According to the *Histoire de Guillaume le Marèchal* the king believed such a plot existed later in the year.[49] On the whole this seems the most likely explanation of John's action when he learned of the surrender of Vaudreuil. On July 5 he issued letters patent stating that the castle had been surrendered at his command.[50] If the barons were plotting or even if the king only feared they were, it might seem worth while to attempt to buy the favor of Saher and Robert. To condemn them might serve to bring the conspiracy to a head.

Although John does not seem to have aided Saher and Robert to pay their ransoms beyond giving them permission to mortgage their lands, they were on reasonably good terms with the king for some years.[51] When Robert's uncle, Godfrey de Lucy, bishop of Winchester, died in 1204, Robert was given his share of the Lucy inheritance.[52] In 1207 he received the manor of Burton in Yorkshire that he claimed as part of his wife's inheritance.[53] In 1210

---

[47] Coggeshall, pp. 143-144; Wendover, I, 317-318.
[48] *Histoire de Guillaume le Maréchal*, lines 12687-12700.
[49] *Ibid.*, lines 12797-12804.
[50] *Rot. pat.*, p. 51.
[51] *Ibid.*, pp. 35, 37.
[52] *Rot. claus.*, I, 14.
[53] *Ibid.*, p. 99.

he was given the custody of the heir of Hubert de Anstey, an important tenant of the honor of Boulogne.[54] When Earl Robert of Leicester died in 1205, Saher de Quency was granted custody of all his lands except the castle of Mountsorrel. Apparently Saher offered the king 1,000 marks for the custody of the honor and 5,000 marks for full possession in right of his wife.[55] Unfortunately for Saher Earl Robert had had two sisters. One of them had married Simon de Montfort, a great lord whose lands lay on the borders of France and Normandy. His elder son Amauri de Montfort had married a daughter of Earl William of Gloucester and was recognized by John as earl of Gloucester though he had only a small part of the lands of the honor.[56] The younger son, Simon de Montfort, who was to become the leader of the crusade against the Albigensians, laid claim to the earldom of Leicester. In 1206 John recognized Simon as earl of Leicester.[57] On March 10, 1207, the honor of Leicester was divided between Saher de Quency and Simon de Montfort. Simon got the third penny of the shire, the town of Leicester, and the dignity of seneschal of England. The lands and fees were divided evenly. Saher was forgiven half the money he had promised for the custody and possession of the honor.[58] In addition John created him earl of Winchester and granted him £10 a year as the third penny of Hampshire.[59]

While the historian viewing the scene from a distance is obliged to conclude that John treated Robert fitz Walter and Saher de Quency fairly if not generously, it is not difficult to see how they might have felt otherwise. John did not help them pay their ransoms as he did other royal constables captured in his service. It seems likely that Robert fitz Walter felt that he had not received

[54] Pipe roll 12 John, Public Record Office.
[55] *Pipe roll 7 John,* p. 32; *Rot. oblatis,* pp. 268, 320; *Rot. claus.,* I, 25; *Pipe roll 9 John,* p. 197.
[56] *Pipe roll 2 John,* p. 119; *Memoranda roll 1 John,* pp. 89-90.
[57] *Rot. claus.,* I, 74; *Pipe roll 8 John,* p. 107.
[58] *Cartae antiquae rolls,* no. 300; *Rot. claus.,* I, 97; *Rot. oblatis,* pp. 416-417; *Pipe roll 9 John,* p. 197.
[59] *Cartae antiquae rolls,* no. 284; *Rot. claus.,* I, 97; *Pipe roll 9 John,* p. 138.

a fair share of the inheritance that descended from his grandfather, Richard de Lucy, justiciar of England under Henry II. An important part of the Lucy lands, the honor of Ongar in Essex and Cornwall, was given to Geoffrey fitz Peter, probably as custodian for an infant great-granddaughter of Richard de Lucy. Another royal favorite, William Brewer, got other lucrative custodies from the Lucy lands.[60] Robert may well have felt that these custodies should go to him. Then Simon de Montfort did not actually hold his share of the honor of Leicester very long, and it passed into the hands of royal custodians. Saher may have felt he should have had it in charge. Moreover the king seems to have kept the chief castle of Saher's share, Mountsorrel.[61]

John's early relations with Robert fitz Walter and Saher de Quency are peculiarly important because of the prominent part they were to play in the great baronial revolt. The king's efforts to appease other great lords must be reviewed more briefly. Earl Hamelin de Warren died in 1202 and was succeeded by his son William.[62] On April 19, 1205, Earl William was given the castle and borough of Stamford and the manor of Grantham in Lincolnshire to hold until he recovered his Norman lands.[63] Earl Robert of Leicester received a number of charters guaranteeing him the special privileges enjoyed by his ancestors, the custody of the barony of Fulbert of Dover with its castle of Chilham, and the grant of Richmondshire discussed above.[64] It is possible that the last was considered as compensation for his large Norman fiefs. Earl William of Arundel was freed from his debts to the Jews and given custody of the barony of Laigle with its castle of Pevensea. He was also given custody of his nephews, sons of William de Montchesney and the earl's sister, Aveline, and their lands with leave to marry his sister to whom he pleased.[65] He promptly

[60] *Rot. pat.*, p. 39; *Rot. oblatis*, p. 229.
[61] *Rot. claus.*, I, 13, 25; *Pipe roll 9 John*, p. 196.
[62] *Rot. pat.*, p. 10.
[63] *Ibid.*, p. 52; *Rot. claus.*, I, 28.
[64] *Rot. chart.*, p. 5; *Calendar of charter rolls* (Rolls series), I, 180; *Cartae antiquae rolls*, no. 299; J. H. Round, *Ancient charters* (Pipe roll society), no. 69; *Rot. pat.*, pp. 22, 34.
[65] *Ibid.*, p. 16; *Rot. claus.*, I, 10; *Rot. chart.*, p. 133.

strengthened his political position by marrying Aveline to Geoffrey fitz Peter.[66] David, earl of Huntingdon, was forgiven all the debts he had owed Henry II and Richard, including obligations to Jews.[67] Warin fitz Gerold was given free warren in all his lands and a manor that had belonged to a Norman, Ralph Taxon.[68] In 1204 Earl Aubrey de Vere offered 200 marks for the third penny of Oxfordshire. He does not seem to have made any effort to pay this fine and did not receive the third penny until 1208.[69]

One of the most interesting attempts of John to satisfy a baron was his agreement with Henry de Bohun. On April 28, 1200, John created Henry earl of Hereford and gave him £20 a year as the third penny of the shire. In return Henry promised that he would never make any claim against John or the legitimate heirs of his body on the basis of a charter given his great-uncle, Roger earl of Hereford, by King Henry II. The charter was to be deposited in the priory of Winchester. If John had a legitimate heir of his body, Godfrey de Lucy, bishop of Winchester, was to destroy the charter. If John died without an heir of his body, Henry would get his charter back and was free to make the most of it. As the charter of Henry II had granted Earl Roger the castle of Hereford and the hereditary constableship of the castle of Gloucester, overlordship over two minor barons, two royal forests, and eight manors, John made an excellent bargain.[70]

Let us now turn to the small group of great barons whom John favored and trusted during the early years of his reign but who were in no sense his creatures. The most powerful and most important members of this group were the two earls who had aided him to secure the crown—William Marshal and Geoffrey fitz Peter. Until after the loss of Normandy William Marshal had a

---

[66] *Calendar of ancient deeds* (Rolls series), II, Nos. A 2533, A 2548. It is interesting to note that Geoffrey fitz Peter's coat of arms combined the arms of Mandeville and Montchesney. Anthony R. Wagner, *Historical heraldry of Britain* (Oxford, 1939), pp. 38-39.

[67] *Rot. pat.*, p. 15.

[68] *Rot. claus.*, I, 6; *Rot. oblatis*, p. 254.

[69] *Pipe roll 6 John*, p. 34; *Pipe roll 9 John*, p. 95; *Pipe roll 10 John*, p. 134.

[70] *Rot. chart.*, pp. 53, 61.

unique position in the realm. When John was in his continental possessions, the earl was with him almost continually. He served as his most trusted deputy in military, administrative, and diplomatic affairs.[71] With the possible exception of William de Briouse he was the only great baron who could be called an intimate of the king. Considering his services the rewards received by Earl William were modest. The importance of the Marshal family before William's marriage to Isabel de Clare had rested on their office and some grants from the royal demesne. On April 20, 1200, John confirmed to Earl William the office of marshal and the demesne manors he held at fee farm. He also confirmed to him and his wife Richard's grant of half the barony of the Giffards who had been earls of Buckinghamshire and lords of Longueville in Normandy.[72] On August 16 of the same year William was given the patronage of the abbey of Nutley that had been founded by the Giffards.[73] During these years William was also sheriff of Gloucestershire and Sussex and had the custody of the royal castle of Cardigan that served as a defense for his shire of Pembroke.[74] Finally on April 1, 1204, John gave William Castle Goodrich on the river Wye for the service of two knights.[75] The spring of 1205 marked the beginning of an estrangement between William Marshal and the king that was to last until 1211. While on a diplomatic mission to the court of Philip Augustus, William made an arrangement with the French king by which he could keep his Norman lands. He performed to Philip "liege homage on this side of the sea." In short when in England he was John's liege man, but when he crossed to the continent, he was Philip's. As far as I can discover this was a form of homage unknown to feudal custom. John had apparently given William permission to do ordinary homage to Philip for his Norman fiefs, but this peculiar device annoyed him and aroused his ever-ready suspicions. These came to a head later in 1205 when William refused to accompany

---

[71] For a full account of John's relations with William Marshal see Sidney Painter, *William Marshal* (Baltimore, 1933).
[72] *Rot. chart.*, pp. 46-47.
[73] *Ibid.*, p. 74.
[74] *Rot. liberate*, pp. 27, 71; *Rot. claus.*, I, 54, 68.
[75] *Rot. chart.*, p. 124.

John to Poitou because of his new obligation to the French king.[76] Although the estrangement between Earl William and the king did not become acute until 1207, it began in this summer of 1205.

Until John left Normandy for the last time in December 1203, Geoffrey fitz Peter ruled England as viceroy. During these years the king was in England for less than ten months, and Geoffrey's visits to Normandy were confined to a few brief trips to consult his royal master. But Geoffrey seems to have made little personal profit out of these years of power. He did get John to confirm what looks like a dubious transaction. William de Tracy, lord of Bradninch in Devon, had been one of the murderers of Archbishop Becket and had lost his lands. Richard gave the barony to William's nephew, Hugh de Curterne.[77] Hugh gave Geoffrey fitz Peter one of the most valuable demesne manors of the barony for the service of one-half knight's fee.[78] When John came to the throne, Oliver de Tracy, lord of half the barony of Barnstaple and probably a relative of William, offered 1,000 marks for Bradninch. But in the same year William's son, Henry, offered 1,000 marks for the barony. Hugh de Curterne offered 2,000 marks to keep it, but apparently could not raise the money or find pledges.[79] At any rate Henry de Tracy was given possession. Henry granted the manor to Geoffrey for the service of one sore sparrowhawk. On June 20, 1199, Geoffrey obtained John's confirmation of Henry de Tracy's grant. Then in November 1200 he obtained a confirmation of Hugh's charter and had both entered on the charter roll.[80] Apparently he did not feel sure which claimant would end in possession. Both these confirmations have a common peculiarity. A charter of confirmation customarily ended with the phrase " as the charter of Joe Doe reasonably testifies." Under each of these charters there is a note " reasonably is omitted in this confirmation by special command of the lord king." Now

---

[76] Painter, *William Marshal*, pp. 138-144.
[77] *Pipe roll 6 Richard I*, p. 171; Round, *Calendar*, pp. 194-195.
[78] *Rot. chart.*, p. 79.
[79] *Pipe roll 1 John*, p. 198; *Pipe roll 2 John*, p. 234; *Rot. chart.*, p. 61.
[80] *Ibid.*, p. 79.

reasonably seems to have meant in these cases legally.[81] In short the confirmation bearing that word would be invalid if it could be shown that the donor had no right to make the grant. Presumably without the " reasonably " the confirmation was valid in all circumstances. When one considers Geoffrey's position in the government, it seems safe to conclude that the grants were bribes and that Geoffrey had doubts about Hugh and Henry's rights to the barony.

In April 1204 John gave Geoffrey the manor of Ailsbury at £60 fee farm with all the franchises he enjoyed in the Mandeville barony.[82] In May 1205 he received the honor of Berkhamsted with its castle and borough for a fee farm of £120 and the knight service owed the crown.[83] As this barony was yielding over £400 a year in 1214, the gift was a very valuable one.[84] But it is interesting to notice that despite his position as justiciar Geoffrey got no really lucrative custodies during this period. While it is possible that this was the result of his disinterestedness, it seems more likely that he was unable to compete with the most efficient custody grabber of the day, Hubert Walter, archbishop of Canterbury.

The third baron in this group, Roger de Lacy, constable of Chester, seems to have owed his favor with John entirely to his military capacity. John placed him in command of the meager garrison that held the chief fortress of Normandy, Chateau-Gaillard. While he was holding this castle he was given the English lands of Guy, lord of Laval, and the custody of the lands and heir of Richard de Montfichet.[85] After a prolonged and vigorous defense Roger was forced to surrender to Philip Augustus. John contributed £1000 toward paying his ransom.[86] On his release from captivity Roger became sheriff of Cumberland and Yorkshire. In May 1205 he was granted the manor of Snaith with its soke for the service of one knight.[87] Until 1210 Roger de Lacy

[81] *Ibid.*, p. 93.
[82] *Ibid.*, pp. 127-128.
[83] *Ibid.*, p. 151.
[84] Pipe roll 16 John, Public Record Office.
[85] *Rot. pat.*, p. 26; *Pipe roll 5 John*, p. 132.
[86] *Rot. liberate*, p. 103; *Rot. claus.*, I, 4.
[87] *Rot. chart.*, p. 152.

remained one of the men John relied on to protect northern England from the Scots.

Earl William of Salisbury was in a peculiar position. He was John's half-brother and apparently enjoyed intimate personal relations with him. The king used him freely as a soldier and occasionally as an emissary. He seems to have been at court for long periods. Yet though he was an important figure in England, his barony was comparatively small. He had only about 50 knights' fees and no castle. While the income from the fief is unknown, there is no reason to believe it was very large. Earl William was vigorous, proud, and ambitious. Two things rankled in his mind. His wife's great-great-grandfather, Edward of Salisbury, had given a large part of his lands with the castle of Trowbridge to his daughter Maud in marriage to Humphrey de Bohun, great-grandfather of Henry de Bohun, earl of Hereford. To have no castle himself and to see Henry de Bohun enjoying Trowbridge and the 30 fees attached to it must have annoyed Earl William intensely. Then William believed that his wife's ancestors had been hereditary custodians of Salisbury castle and hereditary sheriffs of Wiltshire. John gave the shrievalty to William and probably the custody of the castle as well, but he refused to acknowledge that he held them by hereditary right.[88] As a matter of fact I can find no evidence that such a right existed, but there is no doubt that William believed it did. The king gave Earl William an annual pension and was continually lending him money against it.[89] He also made him frequent gifts of wine. In short he was well treated as the king's brother and servant, but was not aided in building up his landed power.

The last of this group of moderately favored lords was Baldwin de Bethune, count of Aumale. By right of his wife Baldwin was lord of Holderness with its castle of Skipsea, of the castle and barony of Skipton-in-Craven, of the castle of Cockermouth and its fief, and of the scattered lands of the house of Aumale. In his own right he held three English manors given to him by King Richard. In November 1199 John confirmed this grant and a

---

[88] *Bracton's note book* (ed. F. W. Maitland, London, 1887), III, 248-249.
[89] *Rot. claus.*, I, 80.

month later gave Baldwin four more manors for the service of three knights.[90] In November 1203 the king confirmed a marriage agreement between Baldwin and his old friend and comrade-in-arms William Marshal. William's eldest son, also named William, was to marry Baldwin's oldest daughter, Alice, and receive with her all Baldwin's lands.[91] As the heir to the Aumale estates was a Poitevin, William de Fortibus, son of the countess of Aumale by a previous husband, there was always a chance that young William Marshal might get that vast barony as well. When William Marshal got into difficulties with John, Baldwin supported him as he had years earlier when he had been estranged from Henry the young king. While Baldwin and John were never openly at odds, their close relations ended soon after 1205.

We have now surveyed, perhaps in too much detail, John's relations during the early years of his reign with most of the great barons of England. They included men whom John considered his foes and was determined to weaken, men whom he believed discontented and tried to appease, and men whom he trusted and favored to a reasonable extent. We must now glance at a man whose power John built up or at least aided in building up, William de Briouse.

The house of Briouse had never been backward in advancing its wealth and power. William the Conqueror had given William I de Briouse the castle and rape of Bramber in Sussex. William married the daughter of Judhael, lord of Totnes in Devonshire.[92] His son and heir, Philip, was given or conquered the Marcher barony of Radnor.[93] Philip's son, William II, married Bertha, daughter of Miles of Gloucester, earl of Hereford. At the death without issue of the last of Miles' sons, William and his wife inherited the baronies of Abergavenny and Brecon.[94] Meanwhile Judhael of Totnes and his son Alured had been having a turbulent history that is known to us only in the barest outline. King Wil-

[90] *Rot. chart.*, pp. 31, 62.
[91] *Ibid.*, pp. 112-113.
[92] Round, *Calendar*, p. 460.
[93] *Ibid.*, p. 401.
[94] William Dugdale, *Monasticon Anglicanum* (ed. J. Caley, H. Ellis, and B. Bandinel, London, 1817-1830), IV, 615.

liam II deprived Judhael of the barony of Totnes and gave it to Roger de Nonant.[95] But the king seems to have compensated Judhael by granting him the barony of Barnstaple that had belonged to the bishop of Coutance.[96] Throughout the reign of Henry I Judhael and Alured in turn held Barnstaple while the Nonants ruled in Totnes.[97] Then early in the reign of Stephen Alured joined Baldwin de Redvers in his revolt. As a result he lost Barnstaple and it was given to one of Stephen's Norman knights, Henry de Tracy.[98] But when Henry II ascended the throne, William II de Briouse laid claim to the barony of Barnstaple as the grand-nephew and heir of Alured. The result was a compromise by which the barony was divided between William and Henry de Tracy.[99] Later in Henry's reign William's brother, Philip, was granted Limerick in Ireland, but it is improbable that he ever really conquered it.[100] Thus when William III de Briouse succeeded his father he found himself lord of Bramber, of half the barony of Barnstaple, and of a large and compact territory in the Marches of Wales. From Abergavenny the Briouse fiefs of Abergavenny, Brecon, and Radnor stretched for some thirty miles to the north-west along the very edge of the English settlements. These baronies could hardly be called English. William de Briouse and his vassals dominated, ruled, and exploited the Welsh inhabitants from their castles in the river valleys. It required rough and ready warriors to hold this wild borderland, and the males of the house of Briouse were well suited for the task.

[95] *Ibid.*, IV, 630; VI, 53-54.
[96] *Monasticon diocesis Exoniensis* (ed. Oliver, 1845-1854), pp. 198-199. The fact that the barony of Barnstaple belonged to the bishop of Coutance is established by tracing its manors in *Domesday book*.
[97] *Monasticon Exoniensis*, pp. 198-199; J. H. Round, *Feudal England* (London, 1895), pp. 483, 486; *Pipe roll 31 Henry I* (Record commission), pp. 153-154.
[98] *Monasticon Exoniensis*, pp. 199-200; *Gesta Stephani regis Anglorum* (ed. Richard Howlett in *Chronicles of the reign of Stephen, Henry II, and Richard I*, Rolls series, III), pp. 24, 52.
[99] *Red book of the exchequer*, I, 255, 259; *The great rolls of the pipe for the second, third, and fourth years of the reign of King Henry II* (ed. Joseph Hunter, Record commission), p. 183.
[100] R. W. Eyton, *Court, household, and itinerary of King Henry II* (London, 1878), p. 215.

William de Briouse was not a man who would leave claims, no matter how vague, unexploited. In 1195 he sued Henry de Tracy's son, Oliver, for his half of the barony of Barnstaple. The result was a compromise. Oliver recognized William as lord of the whole barony. As long as Oliver lived he would hold his half as William's vassal and would receive from William £20 a year. If Oliver should die without heirs of his body, his lands went to William. If Oliver should have an heir of his body, William would receive a demesne manor and the service of five knights from Oliver's half of the barony.[101] Thus Oliver for £20 a year disinherited his own relatives of the house of Tracy and reduced the inheritance of any future heir of his body. While the money may have been the only consideration involved, one cannot help wondering if a little bullying backed by the royal favor did not have some part in persuading Oliver.

I have discussed in the previous chapter the possibility that William de Briouse played an important part in securing the throne for John. It is also possible that the king considered William a loyal baron whose power should be increased. The lord of Barnstaple was well fitted to serve as a check on a distrusted earl of Devon. Moreover the master of Abergavenny, Brecon and Radnor if his position was somewhat improved by additional lands and castles might become as great a power in the southern Marches of Wales as Ranulf of Chester was in the northern. Then the interests of Earl Ranulf and William in Wales made them extremely likely to be foes. The natural Welsh enemy of Earl Ranulf was Llywelyn, prince of North Wales. William's foes were the lords of Powis and the princes of South Wales. He was inclined to form an alliance with Llywelyn and his son Reginald eventually married the Welsh prince's daughter. Thus policy as well as friendship and gratitude may well have influenced John's favor to William de Briouse.

In June 1200 the king granted William all the lands he could conquer from the Welsh enemies of the crown to increase the extent of his barony of Radnor.[102] In January 1201 John accepted

---

[101] *Pipe roll 7 Richard I*, pp. 111-112.
[102] *Rot. chart.*, p. 66.

a fine of 5,000 marks from William for a grant of all Limerick except the city and the service of William de Burgh, the brother of John's chamberlain, for the service of 60 knights. William departed for Ireland at once to take possession.[103] During the year 1202 William was given custody of the land of William de Beauchamp, lord of Castle Elmley in Worcestershire, and of the Marcher lordships of Glamorgan and Gower.[104] The Beauchamp custody was a rich financial plum being worth over £300 a year.[105] The custody of Glamorgan and Gower gave William control of the border country between the Bristol Channel and Brecon and Radnor. John also forgave William all his debts to Henry II and Richard.[106] Thus at the end of 1202 William de Brıouse ruled all the major baronies in the southern marches except Netherwent and Pembroke, the fiefs of Earl William Marshal. Moreover in 1200 William's son Giles had become bishop of Hereford. This gave the Briouse family a block of knights' fees and the great Shropshire fortress of Bishop's Castle.

Whether or not William de Briouse actually participated in the murder of Arthur of Brittany in the spring of 1203, he was certainly one of the small group who knew the young prince's fate.[107] He had no objection to profiting from this knowledge. In February while Arthur was still alive, John had given William the Marcher fief of Gower with its castle of Swansea.[108] In June he was forgiven £50 of debts to the Jews, and given custody of the Devonshire barony of Torrington.[109] In July he received the custody of the city of Limerick.[110] In addition during the course of 1203 he was granted the barony of Kington in Herefordshire with its 22 fees and its castle lying on the eastern border of Radnor

---

[103] *Rot. oblatis*, p. 99; *Rot. chart.*, pp. 84, 99-100.
[104] *Pipe roll 4 John*, p. 20; *Rot. pat.*, p. 19.
[105] Pipe roll 13 John, Public Record Office.
[106] *Rot. pat.*, p. 18.
[107] Powicke, *Loss of Normandy*, pp. 469-470.
[108] *Calendar of charter rolls*, III, 46. Years later an earl of Warwick charged that William had extorted Gower from John by blackmail. Powicke, *Loss of Normandy*, p. 470.
[109] *Rot. pat.*, p. 30; *Rot. liberate*, p. 39.
[110] *Rot. chart.*, p. 107.

for the service of one-half a knight's fee.[111] The same year found him in actual control of the great Lacy barony in Herefordshire, Shropshire, and Gloucestershire.[112] Walter de Lacy had married William's daughter, Margaret. As Walter spent most of his time in his Irish lordship of Meath, he seems to have allowed William what amounted to custody of his English barony.[113] Finally sometime in 1203 John gave William's son John de Briouse Amabile de Limesi, widow of Hugh Bardolf, for a fine of £1000.[114]

John did, however, take some steps to prevent William's power from growing too great. Except for the first half of 1199 William was sheriff of Herefordshire from 1192 to 1200. But late in the latter year John entrusted this office to Hubert de Burgh. Then in July 1201 the king gave Hubert custody of the castles of Grosmont, Skenfrith, and Llantilio that lay just to the north-east of Abergavenny.[115] One wonders if John's idea was to use the Burghs to check the Briouses. William de Burgh, the chief lord of the Limerick region, would keep William de Briouse from getting out of hand in Ireland while his brother Hubert would watch the Briouse Marcher lordships.

William devoted the year 1204 to his war with Gwenwynwyn of Powis and received only a few minor favors from John. But in 1205 he was on his way once more. In the spring of that year Hubert de Burgh was captured at Chinon by Philip Augustus. While the shrievalty of Herefordshire went to the seneschal of the royal household, William de Cantilupe, John granted William de Briouse the castles of Grosmont, Skenfrith, and Llantilio as a fief to be held for the service of two knights' fees.[116]

In 1205 William de Briouse sued Henry de Nonant for the barony of Totnes. If I am correct in my belief that William's ancestor, Judhael, had received Barnstaple in compensation for Totnes, his claim was not very strong, but Henry de Nonant could not resist John's favorite. William de Briouse was recognized as

[111] *Pipe roll 5 John,* p. 58.
[112] *Ibid.,* p. 70.
[113] *Rot. chart.,* p. 80.
[114] *Pipe roll 5 John,* p. 197.
[115] *Rot. liberate,* p. 19.
[116] *Rot. pat.,* pp. 46, 57; *Rot. chart.,* p. 160.

lord of the whole barony and received the castle, port, and town of Totnes worth £24 a year. Henry was to hold the rest of the barony for life as William's vassal. After Henry's death William would have half the demesnes and knights' fees.[117] Thus William acquired a castle and overlordship at once and had the prospect of gaining £45 a year in revenue and the service of some thirty knights' fees.

The year 1206 saw William de Briouse at the height of his power. He held as fiefs or in custody 352 knights' fees and some 16 castles in England and Wales. His income from these lands was certainly over £800 and may have approached £1,000. This landed power was buttressed by marriage alliances. Earl William de Ferrers was his nephew, Adam de Port, lord of Basing in Hampshire, his brother-in-law, and Hugh de Mortimer, heir to the Marcher barony of Wigmore, and Walter de Lacy his sons-in-law.[118] His eldest son William was married to a daughter of Earl Richard de Clare. Only the title of earl was needed to place William in the forefront of the English baronage in wealth, power, dignity, and prestige. Whether his motive was policy, gratitude, or fear of blackmail, John had aided William to become a truly formidable figure in English politics.

While William de Briouse waited hopefully for the comtal dignity, the wildest of his Marcher associates attained it. The English settlements on the eastern coast of Ulster in Ireland were ruled by a certain John de Courcy who for some reason had a very low place in King John's favor.[119] Walter de Lacy, lord of Meath, and his younger brother Hugh had long eyed his lands greedily. In 1201 they captured him by treachery but were forced by his vassals to let him go.[120] In 1204 King John came to the aid of the Lacys. He summoned John de Courcy to England. If he did not

---

[117] *Fines sive pedes finium* (ed. Joseph Hunter, Record commission), II, 65-66.

[118] Rymer, *Foedera*, I, 107-108; *Rot. chart.*, p. 80; *Rot. pat.*, p. 122.

[119] John was clearly a member of the family of Courcy of Stogursey in Somerset. J. P. Migne, *Patrologiae, series Latina,* ccxv, 370; *Rot. claus.,* I, 33.

[120] Hovedon, IV, 176; Walter of Coventry, *Memoriale* (ed. W. Stubbs, Rolls series), II, 190-191.

obey, the Lacy brothers could seize his lands.[121] John was caught in a trap. If he obeyed the summons, the Lacys could conquer his lands illegally in his absence. If he did not, they could take them legally. John chose to defend his lands, but he was defeated and captured by the Lacys. On May 29, 1205, King John created Hugh de Lacy earl of Ulster and gave him all the Irish lands of John de Courcy.[122] Not even a papal letter could shake the Lacy grip on the district.[123] Why John created Hugh an earl while leaving his brother Walter and William de Briouse simple barons is a complete mystery. Perhaps the king could not resist the temptation to annoy every one to some extent.

While it is comparatively easy to describe King John's relations with the great barons of England as individuals during the early years of his reign, it is extremely difficult to form a coherent picture of his relations with the English baronage as a whole. The remarks of the chroniclers are vague, and the supplementary material is scanty and hard to interpret. Gervase of Canterbury states that after John concluded a short-lived peace with Philip Augustus in May 1200 " he by peace or war subdued all who before the peace with the king of France wanted to revolt." [124] This reference may allude chiefly to the barons of John's continental lands. When John crossed to England in October of that year, he took with him one of his mercenary captains and a considerable body of hired troops, but there is no evidence that he actually used them against the English barons.[125] In fact his visit was primarily devoted to conciliation of his vassals. Then on April 30, 1201, the king summoned his English tenants to gather at Portsmouth on May 13 prepared to cross to Normandy.[126] According to Hovedon the earls of England replied to this summons by meeting at Leicester and announcing that they would not cross until John gave them their rights. The chronicler goes on to tell us that the

---

[121] *Rot. pat.*, p. 45.
[122] *Rot. chart.*, p. 151; *Chronica de Mailros* (Bannatyne Club), p. 105.
[123] Migne, *Patrologia*, ccxv, 681.
[124] Gervase of Canterbury, *Gesta regum* (ed. William Stubbs, Rolls series), II, 92.
[125] *Rot. liberate*, pp. 2, 6.
[126] Wendover, I, 311.

king then demanded that the barons surrender their castles to him. When William de Albini was asked to give up his castle of Belvoir, he gave his son as a hostage instead.[127] While it is possible that a son of William de Albini became a hostage this time, none of Hovedon's statements can be confirmed from other sources. Certainly John did not take any baronial castles into his hands. When he crossed to Normandy, he was followed by the vast majority of his baronage.[128] Nor is there any evidence of any extensive concessions made to the dissident lords.

Although there is no evidence to support Hovedon's story of John's troubles with his barons in the spring of 1201, the king had some reason for disquiet over the state of England. In Normandy and Poitou his officials were already at war with the members of the house of Lusignan who were enraged because John had married the fiancée of their chief, Hugh de Lusignan, count of La Marche.[129] Ralph de Lusignan, count of Eu, was lord of the barony of Hastings in England. His seneschal of Hastings was imprisoned by the English government, but it is not clear whether this was the result of actual hostile actions or of mere suspicion.[130] Then at least two small armed bands were defying the king's authority. William Marsh, a Somersetshire knight, was using the island of Lundy in the Bristol Channel off Bideford Bay on the coast of Devon as a center for raids on the coasts around. Fulk fitz Warin, who was to become a hero of romance, was ranging the country from Shropshire to Wiltshire at the head of his band. There may have been some connection between these two groups, and Fulk probably had some understanding with Llywelyn, prince of North Wales. Hovedon states that when John crossed to Normandy, he left his chamberlain Hubert de Burgh with 100 knights to hold the Welsh Marches.[131] This may be the basis for the story in the romance *Fouke fitz Warin* that John ordered 100 knights

---

[127] Hovedon, IV, 161.
[128] This can be ascertained from the lists of those freed from paying scutage. These lists appear on the pipe roll.
[129] Fred A. Cazel and Sidney Painter "The marriage of Isabelle of Angoulême" *English historical review*, LXIII (1948), pp. 85-86.
[130] *Pipe roll 3 John*, p. 226.
[131] Hovedon, IV, 163.

to hunt down Fulk.[132] And the legend sounds as plausible as the chronicle.

In landed estate Fulk fitz Warin was a very minor personage. He held one or two knights' fees in chief, £10 a year in the manor of Alveston in Gloucestershire, and two small mesne fiefs.[133] Through his mother, Hawise de Dinan, he held half the lands of her father Joyce de Dinan the most important of which was the manor of Lambourn in Berkshire.[134] Fulk's favorite residence was the manor of Alburbury in Shropshire that he held of the Corbets, lords of Cause.[135] He was a turbulent and ambitious knight with many friends and relatives among the fierce Shropshire Marchers. Fulk claimed, on what grounds is far from clear, the important Shropshire castle of Whittington. The Fitz Warins had been given a fief in Cambridgeshire by William Peverel, lord of Bourn, who also was lord of Whittington, and the claim must have grown in some way out of that connection.[136] King Henry II gave Whittington to the lords of Powis.[137] In 1195 the father of Fulk offered King Richard 40 marks " for having the castle of Whittington as it was adjudged to him in the king's court," but the fine remained unpaid, and it seems unlikely that the Fitz Warins actually got possession of the fortress.[138] When John came to the throne Fulk raised his bid to £100.[139] But Maurice, lord of Powis, offered 50 marks to be confirmed in possession, and John was anxious to gain his friendship. On April 11, 1200, the king granted Whittington to Maurice of Powis for the service that his father and uncle had performed to Henry II. When Maurice died a few months later, John issued a similar charter for his sons.[140] According to the romance *Fouke fitz Warin* Fulk re-

---

[132] *Fouke fitz Warin* (ed. Louis Brandin, *Les classiques français du moyen âge*), p. 35.
[133] *Pipe roll 1 John*, pp. 21, 34, 74, 254; *Book of fees*, II, 922, 964.
[134] *Pipe roll 1 John*, p. 255; *Book of fees*, I, 106.
[135] *Fouke fitz Warin*, pp. 33, 34, 44, 53, 83; *Book of fees*, II, 964.
[136] For a full discussion of this question see R. W. Eyton, *Antiquities of Shropshire* (London, 1854-1860), XI, 29-42.
[137] *Rot. chart.*, p. 43.
[138] *Pipe roll 7 Richard I*, p. 246; *Pipe roll 1 John*, p. 74.
[139] *Pipe roll 2 John*, p. 175; *Fouke fitz Warin*, p. 32.
[140] *Rot. oblatis*, p. 58; *Rot. chart.*, pp. 43, 74.

nounced his homage to John immediately after the grant to Maurice on the ground that the king had denied him justice.[141]

The romance *Fouke fitz Warin* gives a long and detailed account of the activities of Fulk and his band during their revolt. It is a weird mixture of accurate information, plausible stories that lack confirmation, and magnificent flights of pure imagination. The author knew how much money Fulk offered John for Whittington, and it seems probable that only a scribal error conceals his knowledge of the place where the grant to Maurice was made.[142] He knew that Fulk and his men once took refuge in an abbey, but he had no idea where the abbey was.[143] His story that Fulk killed Maurice of Powis is plausible.[144] The claim that John detached the 100 knights to hunt down Fulk is not impossible—he was the chief source of trouble in the Marches in early 1201. But the historian cannot separate fact from fiction in a work of this sort with sufficient certainty to use it effectively.[145]

It seems very likely that the romance is correct in placing the beginning of Fulk's revolt immediately after the grant of Whittington to Maurice of Powis in April 1200.[146] If Fulk killed Maurice as the romance asserts, that event took place before August 1200.[147] In the spring of 1201 the most important baron of Shropshire, William fitz Alan, was removed from the office of sheriff and his place taken by the justiciar himself—undoubtedly acting through his sub-sheriff Henry Furnel. As a goodly proportion of Fulk's friends mentioned in the romance were Fitz Alan tenants, this change of sheriffs may well have been connected with his activities. During 1201 the bereaved son of Maurice of Powis received 100 shillings of the king's gift by order of Geoffrey fitz

[141] *Fouke fitz Warin*, p. 33.
[142] The text says "Wyncestre" but the author states that John was on his way to the Welsh Marches and the names Winchester and Worcester are easily confused by a careless scribe. *Fouke fitz Warin*, pp. 31-35.
[143] *Ibid.*, pp. 37-40.
[144] *Ibid.*, p. 45.
[145] See historical notes in *Fulk fitz Warine* (ed. Thomas Wright, London, 1844) and Sidney Painter, "The sources of Fouke fitz Warin," *Modern language notes* (January, 1935), pp. 13-15.
[146] *Fouke fitz Warin*, p. 33.
[147] *Rot. chart.*, p. 74.

Peter, and a Simon de Lenz received four marks to support him while hunting outlaws.[148] These facts indicate that the romance is correct in stating that Fulk was active in Shropshire during 1200 and 1201. But the first actual reference in official records to Fulk as a rebel comes in the spring of 1202. On April 30 John pardoned a man named Eustace de Kivelly who had incurred outlawry by being a companion of Fulk.[149] Then in July 1202 came the only incident of Fulk's revolt that is mentioned by a source other than the romance. He and his men took refuge in the abbey of Stanley in Wiltshire and were besieged there for two weeks by the men of the province—presumably the *posse committatus*.[150] As Fulk's maternal relatives had been generous benefactors of Stanley, he may not have been an entirely unwelcome guest.[151] And the fact that the sheriff of Wiltshire, William, earl of Salisbury, was one of those who procured his pardon from the king a year later suggests that the siege may not have been pressed too energetically by the sheriff's men. Earl William himself was in Normandy with the king.

There is no evidence as to what Fulk and his men did between July 1202 and the summer of 1203. The romance tells of a series of voyages on the seas. Fulk had a reputation as a ship-captain and a ship of his was captured by royal officials during this period.[152] Hence the romance may well be on sound ground when it puts him afloat—improbable as the adventures described may be. At any rate during August, September, and October 1203 three safe conducts were issued to Fulk and his men.[153] On November 11 they were formally pardoned at the request of Earl William of Salisbury and John de Grey, bishop of Norwich. Thirty-eight men who had been outlawed because of Fulk were pardoned and seven more were included who had been outlaws before they joined his band.[154] Two of these were Fulk's brothers

---

[148] *Pipe roll 3 John*, pp. 276-277.
[149] *Rot. pat.*, p. 10.
[150] William of Newburgh, II, 506-507.
[151] *Calendar of charter rolls*, I, 38.
[152] *Rot. claus.*, I, 136; *Pipe roll 6 John*, p. 218.
[153] *Rot. pat.*, pp. 33-34.
[154] *Ibid.*, p. 36.

and two more his cousins. The rest were minor figures unknown to history. A year later in October 1204 Fulk was given Whittington castle as " his right and inheritance." [155] In 1207 he was granted in return for a fine of 1,200 marks a rather valuable lady, Matilda, widow of Theobald Walter, an important baron in Lancashire and the chief vassal of William Marshal in Leinster.[156]

The whole affair of Fulk fitz Warin is extremely curious. A simple knight of meagre landed power defies the king, rises in revolt, gathers a band of outlaws, and wanders about the realm for three years. Then he is pardoned at the request of two of the king's most intimate friends, given what he had originally wanted, and later allowed to marry a rich widow. The romance *Fouke fitz Warin* says that Fulk as a boy had lived at Henry II's court with the king's sons and had quarreled bitterly with John. That is the reason given for John's grant of Whittington to Maurice of Powis.[157] There were certainly other reasons for the grant to Maurice, but the tale may be true and account for the interest of Earl William and John de Grey in Fulk. But it is important to remember that fierce and able soldiers were a valuable asset to a feudal monarch. John may well have felt that any one capable of defying his government for three years was too good a man to lose. Slightly reformed outlaws made excellent servants.

The affair of William Marsh was not unlike that of Fulk fitz Warin. Henry II granted the island of Lundy off the north coast of Devonshire to the Templars.[158] It seems likely that John as ruler of Devonshire during Richard's absence on the crusade disseised the Templars and gave the island to William Marsh. At any rate in 1194 William offered Richard 300 marks for custody of Lundy.[159] But when John came to the throne, he confirmed his father's grant of Lundy to the Templars.[160] The king apparently attempted to mollify William by giving him a pension of £20 a year.[161] Unfortunately William was an ambitious, hardy, and war-

---

[155] *Ibid.*, p. 46.
[156] *Pipe roll 9 John*, p. 110; *Rot. oblatis*, pp. 405-406.
[157] *Fouke fitz Warin*, pp. 30, 32.   [159] *Pipe roll 6 Richard I*, p. 190.
[158] *Rot. chart.*, p. 4.   [160] *Rot. chart.*, p. 4.
[161] *Rot. claus.*, I, 14; *Pipe roll 7 John*, pp. 18-19; *Rot. oblatis*, p. 230.

like seaman with piratical tendencies, and Lundy exactly suited him as a base of operations. He refused to give it up. In 1200 the Templars offered 50 marks and a palfrey for William's land in Somersetshire as long as he held Lundy, and John granted it to them in January 1201.[162] In March of that year the king gave a license to Alan de Dinan, lord of Hartland in Devon, to build a castle and garrison it to protect his lands from William's forays.[163] In 1201 or 1202 a special tax was assessed in Devon and Cornwall to reduce Lundy, but there is no indication as to whether or not anything effective was done.[164] On February 10, 1204, John issued letters patent saying that he had forgiven William Marsh and received his homage.[165] In April he was given £20 a year in the royal demesne in Devon in exchange for his pension.[166] In 1205 he was one of the admirals of the king's war galleys.[167] He still held Lundy in May 1204 and it was in the possession of his heirs in the 1220's.[168]

The indications that there may have been some connection between William Marsh and Fulk fitz Warin are slight but interesting. A Eustace de Kivelly was pardoned the outlawry incurred as a companion of Fulk—a Nicholas de Kivelly had some connection with William Marsh.[169] Alan de Dinan who received permission to build a castle to check William's raids was a cousin of Fulk, and Fulk's mother and aunt were suing Alan for the barony of Hartland on the ground that it had once belonged to their father Joyce de Dinan.[170] One cannot but wonder if Fulk did not sail to Lundy in his ship and amuse himself plundering Alan's lands. Whether or not there was any relationship between these bandit captains, their stories certainly pointed the same moral—it paid to defy John's government. The rebel got what he wanted.

[162] *Ibid.*, p. 101; *Rot. chart.* p. 101.
[163] *Ibid.*, p. 103.
[164] *Pipe roll 4 John*, p. 129.
[165] *Rot. pat.*, p. 38.
[166] *Rot. liberate*, p. 90.
[167] *Pipe roll 7 John*, p. 133; *Rot. claus.*, I, 16.
[168] *Rot. liberate*, pp. 97-98; F. M. Powicke, *King Henry III and the Lord Edward* (Oxford, 1947), II, 748-749.
[169] *Rot. pat.*, p. 10; *Rot. oblatis*, p. 101; *Rot. chart.*, p. 101.
[170] *Rot. oblatis*, p. 221; *Curia regis rolls*, III, 318.

Although neither Fulk fitz Warin nor William Marsh can have been a serious menace to the safety of the English government, it is clear that by the winter of 1201-1202 John had grave doubts about the loyalty of his barons. In fact he was so disturbed that he wrote to the pope to seek his support. On March 7, 1202, Innocent III ordered the archbishop of Rouen to force any rebels against John to return to their allegiance. Similar instructions were sent to Archbishop Hubert Walter.[171] On March 27 the pope wrote to John. The archbishop of Canterbury had informed the pope that the king had confessed and desired to give full satisfaction to the church. Innocent assured John that no one could avoid sin and that God rejoiced over a repentent sinner. The king was to support 100 knights in the Holy Land for a year and found a Cistercian monastery.[172] It seems unlikely that anything short of serious fears for his position would have moved the king to this sudden burst of piety. Moreover while nothing more is heard of the 100 knights, John actually founded the abbey—Beaulieu in Hampshire. Finally years later Innocent reminded John that he had saved him when he was in grave trouble.[173] It seems clear that in the eyes of both John and the pope a serious situation existed early in 1202.

John's fears and suspicions probably reached their climax in the spring of 1203. It may well have been this growing distrust of his barons that moved him to commit his most frightful crime— the murder of his nephew Arthur. Soon after that came his short-lived suspicion of Ranulf of Chester and Fulk Painel. The fear of provoking a general baronial revolt if he was severe toward Robert fitz Walter and Saher de Quency seems the best explanation for his attitude toward their treason or poltroonery. The *Histoire de Guillaume le Maréchal* assures us that in the autumn of 1203 John believed that there was a baronial plot to capture him and surrender him to King Philip. The king's departure from Normandy in December resembled a secret flight.[174] When he reached

---

[171] Migne, *Patrologia*, ccxiv, 984-985.
[172] *Ibid.*, columns 972-973.
[173] *Ibid.*, ccxv, 1208-1210.
[174] *Histoire de Guillaume le Maréchal*, lines 12800-12804, 12808-12828.

England, he accused his barons of deserting him.[175] There is no evidence to support this charge. All the English earls except Aubrey de Vere, Richard de Clare, and Geoffrey fitz Peter were in Normandy during the last months of John's sojourn there and the barons were well represented.[176] John's fearful mood persisted. It probably accounts for his extremely vigorous action against Ranulf of Chester late in 1204 and the ease with which his suspicions of William Marshal were aroused in the spring of 1205. In November 1204 in a letter begging Innocent III to allow Geoffrey fitz Peter to delay making the crusading expedition to which he was sworn John told the pope that day by day his men were leaving his service and rising in revolt.[177] Only when in 1207 and 1208 his suspicions became centered on William de Briouse and his friends and relatives did John abandon for a time his distrust of the baronage as a whole.

The earls and barons of England had stayed in Normandy as long as the king did, but they clearly had no enthusiasm for a prolonged struggle to save John's continental possessions. Very few English barons of importance had extensive lands in Normandy. The two who were most deeply interested, William Marshal and Robert of Leicester, had come to private arrangements with Philip Augustus by which they could keep their Norman fiefs.[178] Others had solved the problem by leaving a younger son in Normandy. But there was a difference of opinion among the English magnates as to what course John should follow. William Marshal and others in a similar position wanted a formal peace with Philip so that their private arrangements could operate freely. Those with no interests in Normandy saw no point in making peace. That would involve abandonment of John's claim that might be useful in the future. This group was led by Archbishop Hubert Walter. In the spring of 1205 the two groups joined to dissuade John from leading a fresh army to Normandy, but Hubert sabotaged William's efforts to make a formal peace.[179]

---

[175] Wendover, I, 318.
[176] This can be seen by examining the lists of witnesses to John's acts during this period.
[177] Rymer, *Foedera*, I, 91.
[178] Painter, *William Marshal*, p. 138.
[179] *Ibid.*, pp. 137-139; Wendover, II, 9-10; Coggeshall, p. 152.

One incident of this spring of 1205 shows that John despite his many faults and weaknesses was a man of imagination. As a prelude to his projected expedition to recover Normandy he summoned a great council to meet at Northampton.[180] Gerard de Canville, sheriff of Lincolnshire, and Reginald de Cornhill, sheriff of Kent, were directed to send fifteen tuns of wine to Northampton. Reginald was to send two tuns to the king at Windsor—presumably to sustain him till the meeting. Moreover Reginald was to send to the king a " Romancium Historia Anglie."[181] The obvious translation of this would be " a romance of the history of England," but I suspect it could have meant a history of England in French. There was apparently no need for a more accurate description—Reginald would know what was wanted. But it is hard to escape the conclusion that John planned to give his barons enough wine to make them amenable and then ply them with tales of the great deeds of their ancestors. The picture of John sitting in Windsor castle preparing for the council with two tuns of wine and a book on English history is thoroughly entrancing.

[180] *Ibid.*
[181] *Rot. claus.*, I, 29.

Chapter III

THE KING'S SERVANTS

AS a feudal monarch could not rule without the acquiescence, however unenthusiastic, of his barons, his relations with them were his chief political concern. But given this acquiescence his power depended very largely on the efficiency of the royal government, the extent of the king's control over it, and his success in obtaining the funds necessary for its support. Hence John desired an administrative staff that was both efficient and devoted to him, an effective governmental organization, and a military force adequate to maintain the extent of his domains and his authority within them. If he could attain this, his dependence on his barons would be greatly reduced. The English baronage fully realized this. Moreover the funds required to support the royal government and its professional army would have to come, to some extent, from them. The offices that would be filled by men devoted to the king's interests were ones that they desired for themselves, their friends, and their relatives. In short, while clarity and order demand that John's relations with his barons and his governmental policy be discussed in separate chapters, both were in reality closely interrelated aspects of the same problem.

A realistic discussion of the government of England in John's reign from the point of view of personnel is extremely complicated for a number of reasons. The early kings of England like other feudal monarchs obtained much of the assistance they needed in carrying on their government by granting hereditary offices to their vassals. As the business to be done grew greater, the actual functions of these offices were more and more performed by other men who might or might not be the appointed deputies of the titular holders of the dignities. The question as to whether or not the men who did the work for an official whose position had become largely honorary were his appointees was extremely important because of the contemporary conceptions of the fidelity owed by a vassal to his lord and by an ecclesiastic to his superior. If the honorary officer appointed deputies to perform his duties, he could exercise control over their actions and thus enjoy political authority. Otherwise his position had little practical importance. This consideration was, of course, of equal weight in the case of non-hereditary offices that were held by men who clearly did not perform the functions in person.

The three chief hereditary officers of the English crown were the seneschal, the constable, and the master marshal. The seneschalship was in a most peculiar position—it was an office without functions to perform. In most feudal states the seneschal was the head of the administration, the king or lord's immediate deputy, but in England this function belonged to the non-hereditary justiciar. Thus the seneschalship had no real meaning except when the seneschal was also justiciar as Earl Robert of Leicester had been in the early years of Henry II. There is no evidence that Earl Robert's grandson, the Earl Robert of Leicester of John's reign, performed any governmental functions. Certainly none were entrusted to his titular successor, Simon de Montfort. Many years later when the justiciarship had decayed, Simon's son was to make the seneschalship into an important office. Under John it was purely honorary. The seneschals of the royal household were the king's appointees. As to the constableship and the marshalship there is no evidence that either Henry de Bohun, earl of Hereford, or William Marshal, earl of Pembroke, performed the functions of these offices during John's reign. But here an argument from silence is dangerous. In the latter part of the thirteenth century we find the constable and marshal inspecting the feudal levy gathered at the king's summons and accepting or rejecting the contingents offered. Henry de Bohun and William Marshal could have done this in John's time without any evidence of it having survived. I am, however, inclined to doubt that they did. While there is some reason for believing that William Marshal appointed the marshal of the exchequer, there is no indication that Earl Henry appointed the constables of that body.[1] In

[1] The marshal of the exchequer, Jocelin Marshal, had close connections with Earl William and his brother, Henry, bishop of Exeter. H. G. Richardson, " William of Ely, the king's treasurer," *Transactions of the royal historical society*, fourth series, XV, 85-86.

short Henry de Bohun seems to have had no connection with John's government. While William Marshal did at times play an active part in both civil and military administration, there seems no ground for maintaining that he owed his position to his hereditary office.

In striking contrast to these three great offices that had become largely honorary were two whose holders at times performed their functions in person and at other times were represented by their own deputies—the two chamberlainships of the exchequer. These were held in John's reign by a great baron, Warin fitz Gerold, and a minor one, Robert Mauduit. The fact that all writs ordering the payment of money out of the royal treasury were addressed to the treasurer and the two chamberlains by name seems to indicate that the latter or their men were carrying out the duties of their office.[2] In addition there is clear evidence of Robert Mauduit's active interest in the exchequer and its affairs.[3]

Little need be said about the minor hereditary offices. Two hereditary constableships of royal castles, those of the Beauchamps at Bedford and of the Canvilles at Lincoln, were consistently recognized during John's reign.[4] Several other claims were briefly accepted under strong pressure from the claimants.[5] The only claimant to a hereditary shrievalty who held office during John's reign was William, earl of Salisbury, in Wiltshire, and the king refused to recognize his hereditary right to the office.[6] There were a number of hereditary chamberlains holding lands by right of their offices, but there is no evidence that they performed other

---

[2] See all writs ordering payments from exchequer in *Rot. liberate* and *Rot. claus.*
[3] Richardson, "William of Ely," p. 63 and appendix IV.
[4] King Richard confirmed the constableship of Lincoln to Gerard de Canville and Nichola de la Haye his wife in 1189. Round, *Ancient charters*, p. 91. Nichola held it during the revolt against John in 1215-1216. In 1190 Simon de Beauchamp paid £100 for possession of Bedford castle. *Pipe roll 2 Richard 1*, p. 144. His son William held it at the outbreak of the civil war. Wendover II, 116, 163.
[5] William de Lanvalay in Colchester, *Rot. oblatis*, p. 89. Robert fitz Walter in Hertford, *Rot. pat.*, p. 17b. Robert Mauduit in Rockingham, *Rot. oblatis*, p. 9. William de Mowbray in York, *Rot. pat.*, p. 143b.
[6] *Bracton's note book*, III, 248-249.

than ceremonial functions.[7] The same can be said of the minor marshals.[8] On the other hand the majority of the hereditary foresters or foresters-in-fee as they were called seem to have carried out the duties of their offices or at least to have been expected to.[9]

The central government of England was headed by four non-hereditary active officials: the justiciar, the chancellor, the treasurer, and the chief forester. Below them was a group of important royal servants whose functions were varied. They sat at the exchequer as barons of the exchequer, performed judicial duties as royal justices, acted as household officers, and served as sheriffs and constables of castles. In short they were men whom the king used as he saw fit in many different capacities often simultaneously. They held no great office but numerous minor ones. As a body they were the backbone of the king's government. Below them were men who were more, though by no means completely, specialized in their functions such as the clerks of the chancery and exchequer. These men performed routine functions and were of comparatively little importance politically. All these royal servants made their living to a greater or lesser extent from the king's service. The higher ones could aspire to build up a landed position—even to become barons. The lesser men had to be content with smaller and less permanent fortunes. But in general the king's service was profitable and was the best means by which a man of ability and modest fortune could rise in the world.

As we have seen, the justiciar, Geoffrey fitz Peter, was an old and tried servant of the Plantagenet kings. He had used his position as a protégé of Ranulf de Glanvill to obtain a minor heiress whom fortune and Geoffrey's political influence made into a major one. When Hubert Walter resigned the office of justiciar, King Richard gave it to Geoffrey. The power of the justiciar varied greatly according to whether the king was in England or absent from the realm. In the king's absence he ruled as viceroy. While the king would send him orders on major questions, the whole routine of government was in his hands. His writs bearing his

---

[7] *Rot. claus.*, I, 216; *Rot. chart.*, p. 107; *Book of fees*, I, 89, 260.
[8] *Rot. claus.*, I, 77, 116; *Rot. chart.*, p. 160.
[9] *Ibid.*, pp. 52, 80, 112, 123, 132; *Rot. claus.*, I, 93. *Book of fees*, I, 6. *Pipe roll 3 John*, p. 267.

seal had the full authority of the king's writs.[10] When the king was in England his power was more limited, and it is extremely difficult to discover its real extent. He was the king's deputy as head of the entire administration. But as all orders were issued in the king's name over the royal seal, there is little clear evidence as to what the justiciar was doing.[11] Many members of the king's entourage issued executive writs in his name. While there is some reason for believing that Geoffrey occasionally issued such writs when absent from court, it is difficult to prove conclusively.[12] It seems probable that he authorized the more important writs controlling the conduct of judicial business, but again there is no clear proof. The justiciar often, perhaps usually, presided over the sessions of the exchequer and the court of common pleas. He went on eyre with his fellow justices. But in general his functions were so closely related to those of the king that no clear line can be drawn between them. When Geoffrey died, John is reported to have remarked, " When he comes to hell, may he greet Hubert archbishop of Canterbury whom he will without doubt find there. By the feet of God now for the first time am I king and lord of England." [13] While this may indicate that Geoffrey had the power and inclination to interfere with John's desires, it may simply represent John's jealousy of any powerful subject. There is no shred of evidence that Geoffrey ever differed from his master on questions of policy or failed to carry out his will. I am inclined to believe that Geoffrey was an efficient, loyal, industrious, and unimaginative servant who carried out John's policy with singular fidelity. While he profited to a reasonable extent from his royal master's generosity as we have seen in the last chapter, when one considers the possibilities of his office he does not appear as inordinately greedy.

[10] For an excellent discussion of this subject see Richardson's introduction to *Memoranda roll 1 John*, pp. lxv-lxxxvii. The index under Geoffrey fitz Peter will show many of his writs.

[11] In 1210 the abbot of St. Albans objected to being summoned by Geoffrey's writ when the king was in England. *Curia regis rolls*, VI, 80-81.

[12] For instance on October 22, 1204, Geoffrey appears to have issued letters close at Dunstaple while John was at Brill. *Rot. claus.*, I, 12. There are other similar cases, but all may be simply errors on the roll.

[13] Matthew Paris, *Chronica maiora* (ed. H. R. Luard, Rolls series), II, 559.

One thing, of course, must be remembered in connection with Geoffrey—his possession of the great Mandeville barony was never entirely secure. His rival, Geoffrey de Say, never gave up his claim, and after the justiciar's death, pressed it against his son.[14] Hence John always had one weapon he could use against his chief servant.

Geoffrey fitz Peter died on October 14, 1213.[15] John may well have wanted to rule without a justiciar, but his prospective expedition against Philip Augustus made it necessary to provide a viceroy for England during the king's absence. On February 1, 1214, Peter des Roches, bishop of Winchester, was appointed justiciar.[16] Peter's origins are unknown. He was probably a relative of William des Roches who was seneschal of Anjou for both John and Philip. He had become a prime favorite of King Richard and may have been his chamberlain. While Peter seems to have held no court office during John's early years, he was one of the king's intimates and took an active part in the business of both the chamber and the exchequer.[17] He was made precentor of Lincoln and later bishop of Winchester. Peter was avid for both money and power, but he was an able and devoted royal servant. His greed and arrogance added to his foreign birth and his close connection with John's policy made him unpopular with the barons. On the day Magna Carta was issued, he was replaced by Hubert de Burgh who will be discussed in connection with his earlier office of chamberlain.[18] Hubert clearly was a compromise between king and barons. The activities of both these men as justiciar belong to a later chapter.

King John had three chancellors. On the day of his coronation he gave this great office to Hubert Walter, archbishop of Canterbury.[19] As long as Hubert lived, he was a dominant figure in English politics, but it is difficult to say whether he owed his power to his personal influence, his office, or his position as primate.

---

[14] Migne, *Patrologia*, ccxv, 745-746; *Curia regis rolls*, VII, 110-111.
[15] Wendover, II, 91.
[16] *Rot. pat.*, p. 110.
[17] *Rot. liberate*, pp. 78-79, 86, 109-112, 116-120, 122, 134.
[18] Matthew Paris, *Chronica maiora*, VI, 65.
[19] Hovedon, IV, 90.

Hubert had started his career as a clerk of Ranulf de Glanvill. He and Geoffrey fitz Peter worked closely together, and there is no evidence of any conflict between them. One finds Geoffrey postponing important cases until he can have Hubert's advice.[20] Moreover the primate of England was by tradition the chief adviser of the king in all matters remotely connected with religion. Hence even without the chancellorship Hubert would have had immense power and prestige. It is extremely difficult to assess the actual power of the chancellor. The chancellor was the king's chief spiritual adviser and also the bearer of the royal seal and responsible for the writing of royal letters. But by John's time these functions were performed by well-staffed departments. The king had an almoner and several chaplains to perform the chancellor's spiritual duties.[21] All that remained to the chancellor of his former duties as almoner was an income of £33 a year consisting of payments due on every important church holiday.[22] While Hubert acted as John's private spiritual adviser on important occasions, it is hard to say whether he did so as chancellor or as primate.[23] The chancery proper, the secretarial branch of the government, had a large staff of clerks. For the first few months of John's reign Hubert Walter bore the royal seal and personally directed the operations of the chancery, but in September 1199 he relinquished the seal to the senior clerks of the chancery and from then on only on rare occasions did he act in person.[24] Now the actual bearer of the seal had the opportunity to exercise enormous influence on royal policy. He was always closely associated with the king and supervised the drawing up of all documents issued by the court. Giraldus Cambrensis accused Hubert Walter of persuading the senior clerks of the chancery to alter royal letters for his benefit.[25] Be that as it may,

---

[20] Richardson, Introduction to *Memoranda roll 1 John*, p. lxxxix.
[21] " *Rotulus misae 14 John* " in *Documents illustrative of English history in the thirteenth and fourteenth centuries* (ed. Henry Cole, Record Commission), pp. 230, 234, 235, 240, 244; Pipe roll 13 John, Public Record Office, *Rot. liberate*, p. 1; *Rot. claus.*, I, 75; *Rot. chart.*, pp. 33, 75, 109, 171.
[22] *Rot. claus.*, I, 34, 85, 100.
[23] Migne, *Patrologia*, ccxiv, 972-973.
[24] *Rot. chart.*, pp. 1-22.
[25] Giraldus Cambrensis, *Opera*, III, 302.

the office was clearly an important one. The chancellor shared with the justiciar the duty of supervising the functions of the adminstration as a whole. A copy of the pipe roll was provided for his use.

Hubert Walter was thoroughly secular in his interests. His ecclesiastical interests were limited almost entirely to a deep affection for the Cistercian order.[26] He loved wealth and power and was a past master at acquiring both.[27] The lushest custodies in England were nearly always in his hands.[28] His particular delight was to rival if not to surpass the king in lavishness of entertainment and magnificence of life.[29] This did not increase his popularity with his jealous master. Gervase of Canterbury suggests that his departure from court in 1199 was the result of a quarrel with John, but I can find no other evidence for this.[30] Whatever John's real feelings toward Hubert may have been, the two men seem to have worked together effectively as long as the archbishop lived.

Hubert Walter died on July 13, 1205.[31] Early in October Walter de Grey offered the king 5,000 marks for the grant of the office for life.[32] Walter was a nephew of John's favorite, John de Grey, bishop of Norwich.[33] He seems to have had no experience in the government service, and he rarely acted in person during his tenure of the office. While Walter de Gray was active as a royal emissary and general agent, there is little indication that he was active in the duties properly belonging to the chancellor's office. He seems to have bought it as a business matter. The chancellor received ten marks for every new charter issued by the king, one mark for every confirmation without additions, and two shillings for every letter patent of protection.[34] The income from this source obviously

---

[26] Coggeshall, p. 106. *Rot. chart.*, p. 153. Dugdale, *Monasticon*, VI, 900.
[27] Gervase of Canterbury, *Actus pontificum Cantuariensis ecclesiae* (ed. William Stubbs, Rolls series), p. 411.
[28] He had six at the time of his death. *Rot. claus.*, I, 42-43.
[29] *Histoire des ducs de Normandie et des rois d'Angleterre* (ed. F. Michel, Société de l'histoire de France), pp. 106-107.
[30] Gervase of Canterbury, *Actus pontificum*, p. 410.
[31] *Ibid.*, p. 413.
[32] Rymer, *Foedera*, I, 93; *Rot. chart.*, p. 159; *Rot. oblatis*, p. 368.
[33] *Cartulary of Oseney abbey* (ed. H. E. Salter, Oxford historical society, Oxford, 1934), IV, 332.
[34] Rymer, *Foedera*, I, 75-76.

would vary greatly—it must have been very large during the first two years of the reign when everyone was seeking the new king's confirmation of charters. We have a figure for the chancellor's income from this source for the three months of 1205 that the office was vacant. If this be taken as representative, the chancellor had an income of about £350 a year from fees in addition to the £33 a year from royal alms.[35] In short it would take something over eight years for this revenue to equal the 5,000 marks that Walter de Grey paid for the office. But in all probability an ingenious chancellor could find other sources of profit, and the prestige, dignity, and power attached to the office could not be entirely neglected even by one whose chief interest in it was financial.

Another strong attraction of the chancellorship to a man who was not a bishop was that it practically gave him his choice of mitres as they fell vacant. While Walter's activities in this respect are rather confusing, there is no doubt of his enthusiasm for ecclesiastical preferment. Geoffrey Muscamp, bishop of Chester, died in October 1208. By 1210 Walter is called bishop-elect.[36] But as a royal favorite at the very height of John's contest with the papacy he could not be consecrated, and his election may well have been dubious. At any rate he was apparently elected again in August 1213.[37] But by this time Walter had sighted a more attractive plum. In January 1214 he was elected bishop of Worcester and was consecrated on October 5 of that year.[38] Shortly after his consecration he resigned the chancellorship. His later activities belong in another chapter.

Walter de Grey was succeeded as chancellor by Richard Marsh.[39] Richard had started his career as a clerk of the chamber.[40] By 1209 he was a senior clerk of the chancery acting as keeper of the seal.[41] He was one of John's most trusted private agents with apparently an unusual capacity for extorting money from monastic establish-

[35] *Rot. pat.*, p. 70.
[36] Pipe roll 12 John, Public Record Office.
[37] *Rot. pat.*, p. 103.
[38] *Ibid.*, p. 109.
[39] *Rot. chart.*, p. 202.
[40] *Rot. claus.*, I, 111; *Rot. pat.*, p. 74.
[41] *Calendar of charter rolls*, I, 281-282.

ments. By the time he became chancellor he was archdeacon of Northumberland and Richmond, a canon in several cathedral chapters, and had a number of other benefices.[42] His activities as chancellor belong to the latter part of the reign.

Since the reign of Henry I the office of treasurer had been in the same family. In 1166 Nigel, bishop of Ely, who had worked out the complicated financial system that we know through the pipe roll of 31 Henry I and those of the early years of his grandson's reign, was replaced as treasurer by his illegitimate son, Richard fitz Nigel. Richard improved and refined the system and described its operations in his *Dialogue of the exchequer*.[43] Sometime before August 1197 Richard, who had been elevated to the dignity of bishop of London, was succeeded by William of Ely. All that is known about William is that he was a relative of Richard and hence presumably a descendant of bishop Nigel.[44]

As the chief professional official of the exchequer the treasurer was responsible for the mechanical details of the financial system. He worked out the accounting system that is reflected in the pipe rolls, directed the drawing up of these rolls, and controlled the procedures by which money was paid out of the treasury. He arranged for the transportation of the king's treasure from place to place. He must have formulated with the chancellor and the chamberlains of the household the methods of liaison between chancery, chamber, and exchequer. But he can have had little independent authority beyond mechanical details. The chancellor kept a close eye on the whole financial administration. His clerk sat at the sessions of the exchequer and made a copy of the pipe roll for his use. Then a number of royal servants attended the meetings as barons of the exchequer and supervised the drawing up of the accounts. In short in the formal sessions of the exchequer the treasurer was simply the secretary of a large committee of which the chairman was the justiciar or even the king. Then in the operation of the exchequer between formal sessions the treasurer was under

---

[42] *Rot. pat.*, pp. 86, 87, 93, 103, 105.

[43] *Dialogus de scaccario* (ed. Hughes, Crump, and Johnson, Oxford, 1902).

[44] I owe my material on William of Ely to Richardson's excellent article "William of Ely."

the supervision of the two hereditary chamberlains or their deputies. The chancellor, the royal servants who sat as barons of the exchequer, and the two chamberlains were all men of greater power and prestige than the treasurer. He was the man of business—the chief clerk. But as the financial business of the realm was a matter of prime importance, the chief clerk who ran it was a great official of the realm.

Like most of the officials of the Plantagenet kings William of Ely was well paid for his services. About the time he became treasurer he was made a canon of St. Paul's.[45] When John came to the throne, William was given the Hertfordshire manors of Essendon and Bayford that had been held by Richard fitz Nigel.[46] In 1201 he was made archdeacon of Cleveland. This office had been vacated the year before by the elevation of John de Grey to the bishopric of Norwich and had been the subject of a fierce dispute between Geoffrey Plantagenet, archbishop of York, and his chapter. Apparently when Geoffrey was unable to install his first choice, Ralph de Kyme, because of the opposition of the chapter, he chose as his second nominee a man who was sure to have the support of the crown. In a letter entered on the pipe roll of 1201 the archbishop assured Geoffrey fitz Peter then ruling as viceroy that William of Ely was the rightful archdeacon of Cleveland.[47] Then in 1207 when the see of Lincoln was vacant, John gave William the prebend of Leighton Buzzard.[48] William of Ely served as treasurer until the exchequer suspended operations during the baronial revolt.[49] He was a partisan of the rebels, but his activities in the revolt belong to another chapter.

A strong argument could be advanced for the thesis that the royal official who wielded the most actual power during John's reign was the chief forester, Hugh de Neville. Hugh's uncle, Alan de Neville, had been chief forester in the reign of Henry II. Hugh himself had been custodian of the baronies of Wark and Muscamp

---

[45] Richardson, "William of Ely," p. 47.
[46] *Pipe roll 1 John*, p. 58.
[47] Hovedon, IV, 158; *Pipe roll 3 John*, p. 243.
[48] *Rot. pat.*, p. 73.
[49] Richardson, "William of Ely," pp. 55-58.

in Northumberland before Henry's death.[50] He was a companion of King Richard on the crusade and received the office of forester.[51] Richard also gave him an heiress, Joan daughter of Henry de Cornhill, who would eventually share the barony of Courcy with her younger sister.[52] Actually for the time being Hugh got only the modest possessions of Henry de Cornhill. His wife's mother, Alice de Courcy, married Warin fitz Gerold the chamberlain and carried her extensive fiefs to him.[53] When John came to the throne, Hugh retained his office of forester and received numerous marks of the king's good will. In 1199 he was given custody of the Wac barony of Bourn and in 1203 that of the lands of Hamo de Valognes.[54] In 1204 he was granted two royal manors with extensive franchises.[55] He was one of John's most intimate companions. He gambled freely with the king, and as we shall see there is some reason for believing that his wife was even more intimate with John.[56]

As chief forester Hugh was practically the absolute master of all lands included in the bounds of the royal forests. Alone or with a colleague he held the forest courts and punished offenders against the forest laws.[57] He had the power to permit or to forbid clearing of new farm land.[58] When anyone wanted to buy a privilege connected with the forest such as to enclose a deer park, keep hunting dogs, or build a fence, he usually negotiated the arrangement with Hugh. Even when such deals were made directly with the king, Hugh collected the fines offered.[59] The hereditary foresters were responsible to him, and he appointed the non-hereditary forest of-

[50] *Pipe roll 33 Henry II*, p. 20.
[51] Landon, *Itinerary*, p. 68; *Pipe roll 10 Richard I*, pp. 16, 63, 72, 104, 136, 149, 159, 164, 186, 222, 227.
[52] *Pipe roll 7 Richard I*, pp. 252-253.
[53] Farrer, *Honours and knights' fees*, I, 108.
[54] *Memoranda roll 1 John*, p. 33; *Rot. chart.*, pp. 27, 104; *Pipe roll 5 John*, p. 132.
[55] *Rot. chart.*, p. 128.
[56] See below, p. 231.
[57] See under heading *Placita foresta* in Pipe rolls.
[58] *The earliest Northamptonshire assize rolls* (ed. Doris M. Stenton, Northamptonshire Record Society, 1930), p. 125; *Rot. pat.*, p. 31.
[59] *Rot. oblatis*, pp. 183, 221, 224, 326.

ficials.⁶⁰ Except for a few cases where the revenues from particular forests were paid directly into the exchequer, Hugh collected them. He usually had in his care a number of the king's hunting lodges. The great castle of Rockingham was essentially a hunting lodge, and Hugh had its custody whenever it was not in the possession of the baron who claimed to be its hereditary constable, Robert Mauduit.⁶¹ Except for the penalties assessed in the forest courts and a few other items, the revenues of the forest were not accounted for at the exchequer. Hugh had his own exchequer of the forest and accounted directly to the king.⁶² As a matter of fact he seems to have rendered no accounts whatever before 1207.⁶³ Thus he was entirely free from the meticulous supervision that the barons of the exchequer exercised over most royal officials. Occasionally the king would intervene in forest affairs, usually to punish a forester for poor administration, but in general Hugh was entirely independent.⁶⁴ The large sums he sent the king from the forest revenues show clearly the importance of his office.⁶⁵

As in the case of most of John's servants it is hard to say when Hugh was acting as chief forester and when as a general royal agent. From 1199 to 1200 and again in 1203-1204 he was sheriff of Essex and Hertfordshire and in 1210-1213 he held the same office in Cumberland. Until the latter part of the reign he was custodian of the castles of Marlborough and Ludgershall and of the town and manor of Marlborough. As his uncle Alan had held Marlborough while he was chief forester, it may have been considered an appurtenance of the office. John fitz Gilbert Marshal, father of the earl of Pembroke, had held Marlborough and Ludgershall in Stephen's reign, and while there is no evidence that William Marshal ever pressed a claim against Hugh, he took posses-

---

[60] *Ibid.*, p. 437; *Rot. pat.*, pp. 72, 88.

[61] *Pipe roll 1 John*, p. 174; *Pipe roll 7 John*, p. 170; *Pipe roll 8 John*, p. 171; *Pipe roll 9 John*, p. 130.

[62] *Rot. oblatis*, pp. 183, 221, 224, 326; *Rot. pat.*, p. 70.

[63] *Cartae antiquae rolls*, no. 286; *Rot. pat.*, p. 78. An account of Hugh de Neville for forest revenues appears on the memoranda roll 10 John.

[64] *Rot. oblatis*, p. 437.

[65] *Rot. liberate*, p. 23; *Rot. pat.*, pp. 13, 18, 22, 27, 29, 35; *Rot. claus.*, I, 15, 19, 35, 38, 71. Hugh's account in 1208 seems to indicate a revenue from the forests of over £2,000 a year.

sion of it when it was recovered from Louis of France in 1217.[66] Besides holding shrievalties and the custody of royal fortresses, Hugh was often called on to act for the king. When Ruald fitz Alan, hereditary constable of Richmond castle fell into disfavor in 1207, Hugh was directed to seize Richmond.[67] In 1212 John's suspicion of the loyalty of David, earl of Huntingdon, brought an order to Hugh to take over by force if necessary his castle of Fotheringay.[68] A man of power and prestige who controlled a large organization Hugh was a very useful man for tasks that might be beyond the powers of the local sheriff.

Thus when John came to the throne he found the offices of justiciar, treasurer, and chief forester filled by men who had served his father and brother and who were devoted to the crown rather than to him personally. He had felt obliged to appoint as chancellor another man of the same stamp. Only one of these four officials, Hugh de Neville, seems to have become a personal intimate of the king though Geoffrey fitz Peter's duties kept him at court a large part of the time. When Hubert Walter and Geoffrey fitz Peter died, they were replaced by favorites of John. Hugh de Neville and William of Ely remained in office until they joined the baronial revolt against their master. Whatever one may think of John's policy as a king and however convinced one may be that these tried servants of the crown had better judgment than their master, it is hard to blame a king for chafing at finding the chief offices of his realm filled by men who were not essentially of his choice.

Below the four great administrative officials came a small group of men who were almost their equals in importance in John's government. They were the king's trusted agents and were employed by him in many varied capacities. The two most influential of these men during the early years of the reign, William Marshal and William de Briouse, have already been discussed at some length. While both were men of the sword rather than of the pen, William Marshal had at some time in his career served in most of

---

[66] Painter, *William Marshal*, p. 270.
[67] *Rot. pat.*, p. 72.
[68] *Rot. claus.*, I, 122.

the offices of the Angevin government. He had been baron of the exchequer, sheriff, royal justice, and associate justiciar. In John's early years he was sheriff of two shires, custodian of a number of royal castles, and an intimate counselor and agent of the king. William de Briouse's political experience was much more limited, but he was a highly trusted royal agent and a regular member of John's entourage. A third member of this group was Peter des Roches who succeeded Geoffrey fitz Peter as justiciar. He was apparently one of John's most trusted financial agents. He is regularly found at the exchequer, and while he seems never to have held the office of chamberlain under John, he performed the functions of that position.

The two other members of this group, Hugh Bardolf and William Brewer, deserve more extensive discussion here because neither ever held any high office. Both of them started their careers under Henry II. William Brewer was sheriff of Devonshire for the last ten years of Henry's reign, and Hugh Bardolf appeared in 1187 as custodian of the great honor of Gloucester. Both were members of the group of associate justiciars that played so important a part in the government of England during Richard's absence in Palestine.[69] Both are excellent examples of men who found the royal service highly profitable. Henry II gave Hugh Bardolf the barony of Bampton in Devonshire and Somersetshire, but later allowed another claimant to offer a large fine for the fief. Richard gave Hugh the valuable manor of Ho in Kent as an exchange.[70] He also gave Hugh one of the sisters and heirs of John de Limesi and thus half of that barony. As the other sister was apparently unmarried, Hugh seems actually to have had all the Limesi lands. He also had custody of his young relative, Doun Bardolf, and his lands.[71] John gave him two royal manors at fee farm.[72] Hugh died toward the end of 1203.[73] Between the beginning of John's reign and his own death he was sheriff of Cornwall,

---

[69] Painter, *William Marshal*, p. 83.
[70] Cartae antiquae rolls, Pubic Record Office; *Pipe roll 26 Henry II*, p. 94.
[71] *Memoranda roll 1 John*, pp. 53-54.
[72] *Rot. chart.*, p. 55; *Rot. oblatis*, p. 68.
[73] *Pipe roll 5 John*, pp. 103, 197.

Devon, and Westmoreland for one year each, of Cumberland and Northumberland for one and a half years each, and of Nottinghamshire and Derbyshire for three and a half years. While he was sheriff of these last two counties, he was also custodian of the honor of Peverel of Nottingham. When Hugh died, a distinguished group of ecclesiastics and laymen owed him considerable sums of money.[74] There is no evidence to indicate whether Hugh was a man of unusual generosity or one who had no objection to a little usury on the side. Certainly at his death he was an important figure in English politics.

Death cut short Hugh Bardolf's career as a servant of John, but William Brewer was active throughout the entire reign. He was sheriff of Berkshire for a year, of Cornwall twice for a total of a year and a half, of Devonshire twice for a total of seven and a half years, of Dorset and Somerset for two years, of Hampshire three times for a total of four years, of Nottinghamshire and Derbyshire twice for a total of three years, of Oxfordshire for one year, of Sussex for two years, and of Wiltshire for two years. He was clearly not beloved by the people of the shires that he administered. At Michaelmas 1209 he was sheriff of six counties. He was deprived of one at that time. Then early in 1210 he was removed from the shrievalties of Dorset and Somerset, Hampshire, and Wiltshire. The men of Dorset and Somerset paid 1,200 marks to get rid of him.[75] With rare delicacy John ordered that William's daughter should not be obliged to contribute toward this fine.[76] It is possible that the other shires made similar offers. In addition to his services as sheriff William was in regular attendance at the exchequer, but he seems to have considered this duty an unwelcome burden. William's son was captured while taking part in the defense of John's continental lands. On June 21, 1204, the king loaned William 1,000 marks to pay his son's ransom on condition that he sit at the exchequer for two weeks every year.[77] In July he added 700 marks to the loan. These loans were soon transformed into gifts. During 1206 and 1207 William was forgiven 2,000

---

[74] *Rot. pat.*, pp. 50-51.
[75] Pipe roll 12 John, Public Record Office.
[76] *Rot. claus.*, I, 204.
[77] *Rot. pat.*, p. 55.

marks of debts due to the crown.[78] But William continued to be a prominent figure at the sessions of the exchequer.

The dearest ambition of most lay servants of the crown was to build up a barony that would enable them and their descendants to take their places among the magnates of the realm. It was comparatively easy for an influential official to acquire extensive temporary landed power through custodies, but it was far more difficult to raise one's family to permanent baronial rank. The easiest way was to marry the heiress to a barony. William Marshal and Geoffrey fitz Peter had placed themselves among the great lords of the realm by this means. Henry I's justiciar, Ralph Basset, Hugh Bardolf, Robert de Turnham, and Hugh de Neville had married the heiresses to smaller baronies. But the supply of heiresses was limited, and many ambitious officials were obliged to undertake the extremely difficult task of creating a new barony. Henry II's justiciar, Richard de Lucy, had done this very successfully. William Brewer was to be equally successful. It required consistent loyalty and usefulness to the crown combined with a lack of squeamishness in acquiring demesnes and fees. William Brewer was well supplied with these qualifications.

While William Brewer was clearly not popular with the men of his shires, he was apparently deeply beloved by various barons—at least they showed great enthusiasm for giving him estates. On October 18, 1199, John confirmed to William a manor in Cornwall given him by Godfrey de Lucy, bishop of Winchester, one in Northamptonshire given by Earl William de Ferrers, and one in Somersetshire given by Fulk Painel, lord of Bampton.[79] The grant by Godfrey de Lucy may have been motivated simply by good will, but the other two look very much like bribes. Blisworth in Northamptonshire was attached to Higham Ferrers that Earl William had acquired by John's gift. One cannot help suspecting that the grant to William Brewer who was sheriff of Nottinghamshire and Derbyshire and custodian of the honor of Peverel of which Higham Ferrers and Blisworth were a part had something to do with John's generosity to Earl William. In the early twelfth century William

---

[78] *Rot. claus.*, I, 2, 3, 78; *Rot. pat.*, p. 62.
[79] *Rot. chart.*, p. 28.

Painel who belonged to one of the branches of that fecund Norman house married Juliana, heiress of Bampton. The history of the barony during Henry II's reign is obscure, but in 1180 William's son Fulk offered 1,000 marks for its possession.[80] In 1194 an entry on the pipe roll stated that Fulk Painel owed £359 8s. 9d. of his fine for the barony of Bampton, but that he had fled and William Brewer held the fief, presumably as custodian.[81] As the counties in which the barony of Bampton lay formed part of the region ruled by John during Richard's crusade, it seems likely that Fulk fled because he had been involved in John's revolt. At any rate when John came to the throne, he accepted Fulk's offer of 1,000 marks for the barony.[82] But about this time Fulk gave the important demesne manor of Bridgewater with the service of several knights to William Brewer. Once more a generous gift was required to shake loose lands that William had in his custody. Then on March 28, 1200, the king confirmed another series of gifts to William Brewer.[83] One of these seems to have been essentially a purchase. In 1198 Henry de Pomeroy, an important baron in Devon and Cornwall, granted William a demesne manor and the service of four and one-half knights' fees to hold for the service of one fee. William gave Henry 70 marks for the grant. Another looks like a bribe.[84] We have seen that King Richard gave the escheated barony of Bradninch in Devonshire to a Hugh de Curterne and that Hugh made a generous gift to Geoffrey fitz Peter. Apparently Hugh also felt obligated to William Brewer for he gave him too a manor from his demesne.

Probably William Brewer's most profitable venture was the custody of the barony of Dover. Fulbert of Dover, lord of a barony of some fourteen fees centering in the castle of Chilham in Kent, died in 1202 leaving young children. In January 1203 Earl Robert of Leicester was given custody of the fief and at his death it passed to William Brewer for a fine of £800.[85] But of far greater interest to William than the young heirs of Fulbert was their grandmother,

---

[80] This Fulk Painel should not be confused with his relative Fulk Painel, lord of Hambye in Normandy and Drax in England.
[81] *Pipe roll 6 Richard I*, p. 167.   [83] *Rot. chart.*, p. 42.
[82] *Pipe roll 1 John*, p. 191.   [84] *Fines sive pedes finium*, II, 68-69.
[85] *Curia regis rolls*, II, 223; *Rot. pat.*, p. 22; *Rot. oblatis*, p. 229.

The King's Servants

Rohese, daughter of Geoffrey, eldest son of the justiciar, Richard de Lucy. According to the usual customs of feudal inheritance Rohese and her sister were the rightful possessors of the Lucy barony. Richard de Lucy had held some thirteen fees in chief in the counties of Kent, Norfolk, Suffolk, and Devon, the castle and barony of Ongar in Essex consisting of twenty fees held of the honors of Boulogne and Gloucester, and nineteen fees and some demesne manors held of the earls of Cornwall.[86] In the early years of Richard's reign Godfrey de Lucy, bishop of Winchester, held the barony presumably as custodian for his young nephew Herbert who was Rohese's brother. In 1194 he lost the lands.[87] Probably Herbert died, and Richard I took the barony into his own hands. Rohese offered the king £700 for permission to choose her own second husband and to have her half of the Lucy lands.[88] By 1199 she had paid all but £250 of this fine, but it is not clear whether or not she got possession of any of the lands.[89] In 1195 the barony of Ongar and nine of the Cornish fees came into the possession of a Geoffrey de Lacelles who was probably Rohese's brother-in-law.[90] Then in 1201 Godfrey de Lucy is found in possession of the other eleven Cornish fees and some other Lucy lands.[91] In short it seems that during the early years of John's reign the barony of Lucy was divided between Geoffrey de Lacelles and the bishop of Winchester.

Rohese made no payments on her fine after 1199. Sometime during these first years of John's reign she committed a major indiscretion. Although she had not paid the fine she had offered to marry whom she pleased, she chose a second husband without the king's leave, and her dower in the barony of Dover was seized into the king's hands. Hence when William Brewer received the custody of this barony it included Rohese's dower.[92] Then on September 11, 1204, Godfrey de Lucy died, and William was given possession

[86] *Red book of the exchequer*, I, 261, 351; II, 611-612.
[87] *Pipe roll 2 Richard I*, pp. 91, 104; *Pipe roll 6 Richard I*, pp. 24, 28, 45.
[88] *Ibid.*, p. 250.
[89] *Pipe roll 1 John*, p. 62.
[90] *Pipe roll 7 Richard I*, p. 217; *Pipe roll 1 John*, p. 186.
[91] *Pipe roll 3 John*, p. 191; *Rot. claus*, I, 14; *Rot. chart.*, p. 137.
[92] *Rot. oblatis*, p. 229; *Pipe roll 7 John*, pp. 117, 195.

of the lands belonging to Rohese that he had held.[93] But he found that he had a formidable competitor. Robert fitz Walter, cousin of Rohese and nephew of Godfrey, asked John for the lands of the late bishop of Winchester. As John was then bent on appeasing Robert he gave him the lands.[94] Rohese offered 100 marks for John's forgiveness for her marriage, and she and William bided their time.[95] In 1207 Rohese offered £100 in addition to the £250 she already owed for one-half the Lucy lands except those held by Robert fitz Walter. William Brewer was her pledge for the payment of this sum.[96] It is difficult to discover what these lands were. Geoffrey de Lacelles had either died or stayed in France in 1204, and Ongar with nine Cornish fees had passed into the custody of Geoffrey fitz Peter.[97] Robert fitz Walter had eleven Cornish fees and some other lands. It looks as if William Brewer had made an alliance with Rohese and hoped that the time would come when he could get the best of Robert fitz Walter. He did not have to wait too long. Late in 1210 John who was beginning his famous quarrel with Robert took away from him the Lucy lands.[98] On November 12, 1212, the king solemnly gave Rohese her half of the Lucy barony. On that same day Rohese granted William Brewer five demesne manors in Cornwall, one in Devon, and one in Kent with the service of eleven knights' fees to hold of her for eleven fees.[99] Thus Rohese recovered her inheritance at the price of giving most of it to William Brewer as a fief.

While William Brewer was extracting demesnes and fees from his fellow barons, John was not niggardly in showing his appreciation for William's services. On April 3, 1200, he gave him the custody of five heirs and the privilege of marrying them to whom he chose.[100] In 1203 he granted William the services of fourteen knights' fees previously held in chief from the crown.[101] In 1204

[93] *Rot. claus.*, I, 8.
[94] *Ibid.*, p. 14.
[95] *Pipe roll 7 John*, p. 195.
[96] *Rot. oblatis*, p. 414.
[97] *Rot. pat.*, p. 39.
[98] Pipe roll 13 John, Public Record Office.
[99] *Rot. claus.*, I, 127; *Rot. chart.*, p. 189.
[100] *Ibid.*, p. 48.
[101] *Ibid.*, p. 110.

the king gave William the escheated barony of Buron except for the castle of Horsley that he kept in his own hands.[102] Later in the same year he granted William the manor of Chesterfield in Derbyshire with two attached manors and the wapentake of Scarsdale, the manor of Sneinton in Nottinghamshire, the manor of Axminster in Devon, and a fishery in Somersetshire to hold for a fee farm of £112 and the service of one knight. Later the fee farm was dropped, and William held these lands for the service of three knights.[103] This extensive grant included special privileges. Chesterfield was made a borough and its burghers were given the same privileges as those of the royal towns of Nottingham and Derby. William was to have at Chesterfield an annual fair to last eight days and a bi-weekly market. He was also granted a weekly market at Axminster. As John had previously granted William permission to create a borough on his manor of Bridgewater in Somerset, he was well supplied with towns, fairs, and markets.[104]

Demesne manors, knights' fees, boroughs, fairs, and markets were all important elements of a barony, but no one could feel that he was really a baron unless he had a castle. Here too John came to William's aid. In 1200 he gave him license to build three castles —one at Bridgewater, one in Hampshire and one in Devonshire.[105] William had a castle at Bridgewater, but I can find no evidence that he actually built the other two. Another mark of baronial status was the patronage of monastic foundations. Whether his motive was pride, piety, or repentance, William dealt generously with the regular clergy. The earliest monastic foundation ascribed to William, that of the Benedictine nunnery of Polsloe in Devonshire before 1169, may have been made by his father.[106] In 1196 William founded a house of Premonstratensian canons at Torre in Devonshire.[107] In 1201 he made two foundations—a Cistercian

---

[102] *Ibid.*, p. 123.
[103] *Ibid.*, pp. 139, 217.
[104] *Ibid.*, p. 73.
[105] *Ibid.*, p. 70.
[106] Eileen Power, *Medieval English nunneries* (Cambridge, 1922), p. 690.
[107] David Knowles, *The religious houses of medieval England* (London, 1940), p. 97; *Rot. chart.*, p. 70.

abbey at Dunkeswell in Devonshire and a house of Augustinian canons at Mottisfont in Hampshire.[108] He also endowed a hospital at Bridgewater.

In addition to building up his own barony William Brewer devoted his energy and influence to caring for his children. He married his daughter Isabel to Baldwin Wac, lord of Bourn.[109] An Alice Brewer who was either his daughter or his sister, was married to a Somersetshire baron named Roger de la Poole.[110] His eldest son William was married before 1201 to Joan, younger daughter of the earl of Devon who had previously been affianced to Hubert de Burgh.[111] But William's true talents came into play in the search for a barony for his second son, Richard. Walter Brito, lord of a barony of fifteen fees, died in 1199. Soon two claimants were quarreling over the barony.[112] By the end of 1200 one of the claimants had transferred his rights to Richard Brewer.[113] The other claimant simply disappeared from the case and Richard Brewer emerged as lord of the whole fief. While it is clear that William Brewer paid the cost of the litigation over the barony, it is hard to believe that money alone eliminated the two claimants.

The men in the next lower grade of John's administration whose work was pretty well confined to specific departments need not detain us long, but they cannot be entirely neglected. Probably the most important members of this group were the senior clerks who ran the chancery when the chancellor was absent from court. Richard's custom was to have a vice-chancellor and in his absence to appoint a clerk to act as vice-chancellor. A charter issued by John as lord of England was sealed by Master Roscelin "*tunc agentis vices cancellarii nostri.*" Roscelin had borne Richard's seal at Chaluz. But after his coronation John never appointed a vice-

---

[108] Knowles, *Religious houses,* pp. 74, 86; *Rot. chart.,* pp. 139, 164; *Annals of Margam,* p. 26.
[109] *Rot. claus.,* I, 146; *Rot. chart.,* p. 194.
[110] *Curia regis rolls,* I, 85.
[111] William had 8 fees of the barony of Plympton in his hands in 1201. *Pipe roll 3 John,* p. 224.
[112] *Pipe roll 1 John,* pp. 128, 238; *Rot. oblatis,* p. 23.
[113] *Pipe roll 2 John,* p. 99; *Curia regis rolls,* I, 239.

chancellor and the title was never used in his reign. Charters and royal letters were sealed by the senior clerks.[114] When Hubert Walter left court in September 1199, two clerks took over the custody of the seal—John de Grey and Simon, archdeacon of Welles.[115] John de Grey probably had some connection with John as early as Richard's absence on the crusade. In 1196 he pledged one of the men who had been penalized for joining John's revolt.[116] By 1198 he was bearing John's seal and sealing at least some of his charters.[117] John de Grey rose rapidly in his master's affections and confidence and as a result his wordly advance was rapid. By March 4, 1200, he was archdeacon of Cleveland, by April 10 archdeacon of Gloucester, and on September 3 he was styled bishop-elect of Norwich.[118] He bore the seal for the last time on June 28. We shall hear a great deal more of John de Grey. He was probably the only man whom John trusted absolutely and without reservation for the entire period of their association.

Simon, archdeacon of Welles, had been a fairly constant member of Richard's entourage during the last two years of his reign, but seems never to have borne his seal.[119] From June 1200 to June 1204 he shared the duties of senior clerk with Hugh de Welles and John de Branchester, archdeacon of Worcester, who had acted as vice-chancellor in Richard's reign.[120] By May 1203 Simon had been made provost of Beverley and by April 9, 1204, he was bishop-elect of Chichester.[121] From July 1203 to May 1206 the chancery was in the hands of two brothers, Hugh and Jocelin de Welles.[122] Hugh de Welles had become archdeacon of Welles when Simon vacated that office on his elevation to the bishopric of Chichester. By April 4, 1206, Jocelin de Welles was bishop-elect

---

[114] Richardson, Introduction to *Memoranda roll 1 John*, p. xxxviii; Round, *Calendar*, p. 36; Landon, *Itinerary*, p. 145.
[115] *Rot. chart.*, pp. 21-73.
[116] *Pipe roll 8 Richard I*, p. 75.
[117] *Calendar of charter rolls*, II, 387.
[118] *Rot. chart.*, pp. 37, 48, 75.
[119] See Landon, *Itinerary*.
[120] *Ibid.; Rot. chart.*, pp. 73-135.
[121] *Ibid.*, pp. 104, 125.
[122] *Ibid.*, pp. 135-163.

of Bath and Welles.[123] Hugh de Welles was styled bishop-elect of Lincoln by April 14, 1209.[124] Thus all the three senior clerks had passed from the chancery to the episcopate.

Hugh de Welles was succeeded in his office by Richard Marsh, the future chancellor.[125] Richard bore the seal from June 1209 to October 1213.[126] From then until John's departure for Poitou the king's charters were sealed by no less a dignitary than Peter des Roches.[127] While the king was in Poitou, his chancery was headed by Ralph de Neville, another future chancellor.[128] When Richard Marsh became chancellor in October 1214, the day of the senior clerks was over for a time. Richard himself performed the functions of his office. It is interesting to notice that all the clerks who sealed John's charters except John de Branchester became eventually bishops. High office in the chancery was the one sure path to ecclesiastical preferment. While you served you had an archdeaconry or two, and eventually you were rewarded with a bishopric. Hugh de Welles was also granted secular benefits—two royal manors with their attached hundreds and a number of valuable custodies, but the others seem to have been satisfied with ecclesiastical pluralities.[129]

It is extremely difficult to describe the judicial personnel of John's government because specialization of duties was less pronounced in the courts than in the chancery or the exchequer. It was a litigious age and most men of position had a fair knowledge of the law. Joseph Hunter lists some eighty men who were called justices in final concords concluded during John's reign.[130] These included four earls, fifteen barons, twenty-three knights, and four high ecclesiastics. Then there were four who can best be classified as professional servants of the crown, William Brewer, William de

[123] *Ibid.*, p. 163.
[124] *Ibid.*, p. 185. In a number of charters Hugh appears as a witness as elect of Lincoln and seals them as archdeacon of Welles.
[125] *Calendar of charter rolls,* I, 281-282.
[126] *Rot. pat.,* p. 105.
[127] *Rot. chart.,* pp. 195-196.
[128] *Ibid.,* pp. 196-201.
[129] *Ibid.,* pp. 99, 129.
[130] *Fines sive pedes finium,* pp. lx-lxvi.

Wrotham, archdeacon of Taunton, Reginald de Cornhill, and John fitz Hugh. Four more were officials of the chancery—Jocelin de Welles, Hugh de Welles, Walter de Grey, and Richard Marsh. The treasurer, William of Ely, and William de Cornhill, archdeacon of Huntingdon, can best be described as exchequer officials. Finally there were about a score of men whose chief occupation in the government was to serve as justices. But about half of these served for only a year or two. The men who sat in the courts regularly over an extended period and hence can properly be called professional justices number but twelve.

While in theory Angevin England had only one royal court, the *curia regis,* that court had several branches.[131] The king's justices sat at Westminster as the court of common pleas. Then groups of justices rode through the shires on judicial eyres. Finally there was the court that followed the king, the court *coram rege* that was later to be known as the king's bench. When the court of common pleas held its sessions at Westminster, exchequer officials and other royal servants often sat with the professional justices. Quite frequently a group of justices on eyre or justices itinerant as they were usually called would be headed by a lay or ecclesiastical dignitary who had no particular training in the law. Thus in the fourth year of John's reign a group was headed by John de Grey, bishop of Norwich, in the eighth year one by William de Wrotham, archdeacon of Taunton, and one by Robert de Vieuxpont, and in the tenth year one by Adam de Port, lord of Basing, and one by Gerard de Canville.[132] The justices that followed the king on his travels found themselves reinforced by household officials and anyone else who might be in the king's entourage. A few generalizations seem valid. All sessions of the *curia regis* whether at Westminster, on eyre, or with the king included some professional justices. Moreover every group of itinerant justices included at least one man who was not a professional justice—usually a baron or knight with little or no connection with the royal administration.

---

[131] For an excellent general discussion of the courts in John's reign see Sir Cyril T. Flower, *Introduction to the curia regis rolls* (Selden Society, vol. LXII).

[132] *Fines sive pedes finium,* pp. xlix-lix.

Seven of the twelve professional justices had served King Richard in the same capacity. One of these was the justiciar, Geoffrey fitz Peter. Another was Simon de Pattishall who served continually as a royal justice from the seventh year of King Richard to the end of John's reign. In knowledge of and experience in the law he was second only to Geoffrey. A third was Geoffrey de Buckland who was the brother of Geoffrey fitz Peter's brother-in-law, William de Buckland. While Geoffrey fitz Peter was ruling as viceroy in John's early years, Geoffrey de Buckland seems to have acted as his representative at exchequer sessions.[133] Of the five professional justices who started their careers under John the most notable was Eustace de Fauconberg who eventually succeeded William of Ely as treasurer. Except for James de Poterna who served for a short time as sheriff of Wiltshire, the other eight professional justices are known only for their judicial services. It is also interesting to notice that neither of the two men who served as justiciar after the death of Geoffrey fitz Peter had extensive judicial experience. Peter des Roches sat occasionally in the *curia regis,* but Hubert de Burgh does not appear on Mr. Hunter's list.

While the professional jurists who carried on the work of the *curia regis* probably wielded less political power than the senior clerks of the chancery and exchequer, they had a far greater influence on the development of English institutions. The practices of chancery and exchequer were important at the moment but essentially ephemeral. They affected only a tiny segment of the English people. But Geoffrey fitz Peter and his colleagues were molding the common law of England as described by Glanvill into the form known to us in Bracton. Geoffrey had a favorite clerk, Martin de Pattishall, who was to be the justice most admired and most frequently quoted by Bracton.[134] Geoffrey himself had been the clerk of Ranulf de Glanvill. These three generations of jurists constructed the common law of England. Every man, woman, and child in the realm from the king on his throne to

---

[133] *Pipe roll 1 John,* p. 264; *Memoranda roll 1 John,* pp. 17, 67.
[134] Martin served both Geoffrey fitz Peter and Simon de Pattishall, *Earliest Northamptonshire assize rolls,* pp. xviii-xix; *Rot. claus.,* I, 106.

the homeless wanderer in their own day and for centuries thereafter were affected by their work.

Below these officials whom we have discussed there were, of course, a host of minor civil servants. There were the chancery clerks who wrote the charters, letters patent, and letters close and the innumerable writs required in carrying on the business of the exchequer and the courts of justice. There were chancery and exchequer clerks who made the rolls that supply so much of our information about John's reign.[135] There was a spigurnel who saw to the wax for sealing writs and messengers who bore them to their destinations.[136] The exchequer had its constable, its usher, its weigher, and the serjeants who were responsible for transporting treasure around the country.[137] The justices had clerks like Martin de Pattishall who wrote their rolls.[138] But while all these men were important cogs in the wheels of John's government, they require no individual discussion.

The center of the government of England was the king. The chancery and the chief branch of the *curia regis*, the *coram rege*, followed him in his travels. Thus the king's entourage formed both a domestic household and an important segment of the administrative machinery of the realm. The two are extremely difficult to separate. While the senior clerks of the chancery were clearly government officials and the keeper of the king's bath very clearly was not, between them lay many officers who cannot be definitely classified. Most important of these were the officials of the chamber. The chamber administered King John's private purse. While its chief source of funds was payments made to it out of the treasury, it could collect money directly from the king's debtors. As the court moved about the country, people who owed the king money paid it into the chamber. The chamber also paid the king's daily expenses. Obviously it had to keep in close contact with the exchequer. When a debtor paid his money into the chamber,

---

[135] Richardson, Introduction to *Memoranda roll 1 John* and " William of Ely."
[136] See the *misae* and *prestito* rolls in *Rot. liberate*.
[137] Richardson, " William of Ely," pp. 68-79.
[138] Flower, *Introduction to curia regis rolls,* pp. 8-10.

the exchequer had to be notified. But in many cases the chamber received funds that never appeared on the pipe roll—such as sums extorted from the Jews and the church. Although most of the time its payments were confined to buying articles for the king's use, paying the costs of transporting and feeding the court and the vast packs of hunting dogs that accompanied it, and making small gifts and loans at the king's order, in times of emergency its functions expanded greatly. When the king was engaged in a military expedition, the pay and provisioning of the troops was the task of the chamber.

In theory the chief officer of the chamber was the chamberlain, but neither of the two men who bore this title during John's reign seems to have spent much time performing the functions of his office. Hubert de Burgh had been Count John's chamberlain during the last years of King Richard's reign.[139] He bore the title until 1205, but only occasionally is he found at court acting as head of the chamber.[140] Only five of the men who are known to have served John as count of Mortain had positions in the English government during the early years of his reign. Gerard de Canville was sheriff of Lincolnshire from 1199 to 1204. Richard Fleming was sheriff of Cornwall for two years. William de Cantilupe who had been seneschal for John as count of Mortain became seneschal of the royal household and sheriff of Worcestershire. John de Grey was senior clerk of the chancery until his elevation to the see of Norwich. Hubert de Burgh was employed far more extensively by his royal master. He was sheriff of Herefordshire and of Dorsetshire and Somersetshire from 1201 to 1204 and sheriff of Berkshire from 1202 to 1204. When John crossed to Normandy in the spring of 1201, he left Hubert with 100 knights to watch the Welsh and perhaps to suppress Fulk fitz Warin and William Marsh. In 1202 he made him custodian of the great fortress of Dover and warden of the Cinque Ports.[141] We have

---

[139] Round, *Ancient charters*, no. 67.

[140] *Rot. liberate*, p. 14; *Rot. oblatis*, p. 73; *Pipe roll 2 John*, p. 241; *Rotuli Normanniae* (ed. T. D. Hardy, Record commission), pp. 23, 35, 36, 65, 66, 67. I owe many of these references to Mr. Fred Cazel who is writing a biography of Hubert de Burgh.

[141] *Rot. pat.*, pp. 7, 9.

already seen that during these years the king was apparently using Hubert and his brother William to contain the ambitions of William de Briouse. In the summer of 1202 John decided that he needed Hubert in Normandy. After the battle of Mirabeau he became the chief custodian of the valuable prisoners taken there. Arthur and the Lusignan brothers were guarded under his own eye in the castle of Falaise while many lesser captives were distributed in the castles of Hubert's English shires—Corfe, Sherborne, and Wallingford. Contemporary chroniclers carry a dramatic tale of Hubert refusing to mutilate Arthur despite John's express command.[142] Be that as it may the king apparently decided that Hubert was more useful as a captain than as an executioner. Hubert was given command of the castle of Chinon while John himself saw to Arthur.[143]

Hubert de Burgh was generously rewarded for his services. Early in 1200 he was affianced to the younger daughter of the earl of Devon. If the earl died without a son, Hubert was to have the Isle of Wight and the barony of Christchurch in Hampshire. If the earl had a son, he would receive land worth £60 a year and the service of ten knights' fees.[144] Presumably Hubert lost interest in the lady when her brother was born, and she married William Brewer the younger. About this same time Hubert was given the Roumar lands in southern England. In 1201 he received the Welsh castles of Grosmont, Skenfrith, and Llantilio and the royal manor of Causton in Norfolk.[145] During these years he was custodian of three baronies—Beauchamp of Somersetshire, Dunster, and that of Walter de Windsor.[146] In 1205 he fell out of favor temporarily. Perhaps John was troubled by his disobedience in connection with Arthur and the king may have felt that his defense of Chinon was not sufficiently determined. Hubert's lands were seized into the king's lands, his shrievalties were given to others, and he lost his office as chamberlain. While he

[142] *Ibid.*, pp. 16, 17; *Pipe roll 4 John*, p. 85; Coggeshall, pp. 139-141.
[143] *Rot. pat.*, p. 24.
[144] *Rot. chart.*, pp. 52-53; *Rot. oblatis*, p. 68; *Pipe roll 3 John*, p. 37.
[145] *Rot. liberate*, pp. 11, 19; *Pipe roll 3 John*, p. 200.
[146] *Rot. liberate*, p. 23; *Pipe roll 3 John*, pp. 38, 126; *Pipe roll 4 John*, p. 6.

never regained that dignity, his eclipse was brief and we shall hear much about him in later chapters.

Hubert's successor as titular chamberlain was Geoffrey de Neville.[147] While the Neville genealogy is too confused to allow one to expound it with any conviction, it seems likely that Geoffrey was the uncle of Hugh de Neville. Geoffrey held important posts during the latter half of John's reign. During the baronial revolt he commanded the great fortress of Scarborough and was John's chief lieutenant in Yorkshire. He also served for a time as seneschal of Poitou and Gascony.[148] But there is no indication that he ever performed the functions of chamberlain for any considerable period.

After Hubert de Burgh gave up all pretense of fulfilling the duties of chamberlain by taking command of Chinon, the functions of the office seem to have been performed by a series of John's intimates. Peter des Roches was obviously serving as an official of the chamber while Hubert still held the office and he continued to do so after Hubert's dismissal. His position is particularly noticeable in the *rotulus de prestito* for 1209-1210.[149] Later in the reign Peter de Maulay and William de Cornhill archdeacon of Huntingdon, clearly acted in this capacity.[150] But as in other departments the routine work throughout the reign was done by clerks. Early in the reign there are references to Thomas and Bartholomew, clerks of the chamber.[151] It seems likely that for some years prior to 1207 Philip de Lucy was the senior clerk in actual charge of the chamber.[152] Richard Marsh was a chamber clerk before he became the bearer of the seal.[153] John used his clerks of the chamber for various confidential tasks but except for Richard Marsh and William de Cornhill none of them seems to have been advanced to a position of great importance.

[147] *Rot. claus.*, I, 93.
[148] *Rot. pat.*, pp. 102, 103, 115, 131, 152, 159, 164, 165; *Rot. claus.*, 171, 192, 194, 214.
[149] *Rot. liberate*, pp. 78-79, 86, 109-112, 116-120, 122, 134.
[150] P. de Maulay was serving by 1210. *Ibid.*, pp. 111, 113, 141.
[151] *Rot. claus.*, I, 2, 3, 23, 35.
[152] *Rot. pat.*, p. 74.
[153] *Ibid.*

It seems very likely that King John did not want a resident chamberlain who would be a permanent intermediary between him and the clerks of the chamber. In the absence of such an official the king could deal directly with the minor clerks or act through any of his intimates who might be on hand. No one man of high position would know all that passed through the chamber. Various entries on the rolls indicate the confidential nature of some of the chamber's business. Thus in 1210 a clerk wrote "to a certain messenger going on an errand for the king five marks delivered to Hugh de Neville to give to the messenger whose name we dare not know nor place in this writing."[154] Hugh de Neville clearly knew about this mission, but next time the man entrusted with the confidential information could be Peter des Roches, Peter de Maulay, William Brewer, or anyone else whom the king trusted.

In addition to the chamberlainship there was one other domestic office that conferred on its holder enough power and prestige to make him an important figure in the realm—the seneschalship of the household. Apparently this office could be held by several men at once. While William de Cantilupe was seneschal of the household throughout the entire reign, others bore the title at various times.[155] Peter de Stoke served from 1201 until his death in 1206.[156] During 1207 Geoffrey de Neville, the future chamberlain, appeared several times as seneschal.[157] From 1208 to 1213 William de Harcourt held the office.[158] During the last three years of the reign Brian de Lisle and Fawkes de Bréauté bore the title.[159] All these men with the possible exception of Peter de Stoke were important royal servants with other administrative responsibilities—shrievalties, custodianships, and constableships. Hence it seems certain that they had deputies to

---

[154] *Rot. liberate*, p. 157.
[155] *Ibid.*, pp. 1, 128; "Rotulus misae 14 John," pp. 232, 266; *Rot. pat.*, 45; *Rot. claus.*, I, 85, 100.
[156] *Rot. liberate*, p. 1; *Rot. claus.*, I. 35, 62.
[157] *Ibid.*, p. 85; *Cartae antiquae rolls*, no. 138.
[158] *Rot. liberate*, p. 212; "Rotulus misae 14 John," p. 266; *Rot. claus.*, 141.
[159] *Ibid.*, p. 139.

serve in their absence. Unfortunately we have little precise information on the seneschal's duties, but it is probable that he was the executive head of the royal household. We find him authorizing writs of liberate to pay for supplying and transporting the court and he apparently was responsible for the discipline of those attached to the household.[160]

If the seneschal of the household was actually the administrative head of the king's entourage, his office cannot have been a sinecure. The household was large and was continually moving about the country. There were carters and pack-horse men to transport the king's wardrobe from place to place, falconers, huntsmen, and keepers of the hunting dogs, squires and grooms who cared for the horses, laundresses, messengers, watchmen, cooks and a host of other servants.[161] In addition to those who had actual duties in the royal household the court was apparently followed about by a miscellaneous rabble. There were merchants of the court—probably purveyors for its daily needs.[162] Henry de la Mare held three estates by serjeantry—one for guarding the door of the king's hall and two for supervising the prostitutes who followed the court.[163] While I can find no evidence that Henry performed his duties in John's reign, the existence of his office is most illuminating.

One more office that was closely connected with the household should be mentioned—the chamberlainship of London. The holder of this post was the chief purchasing agent for the court. As the royal household was undoubtedly the largest single market for luxury goods of all sorts, the chamberlain of London must have had tremendous power over the merchants of the realm. While the title of chamberlain of London is rarely mentioned during John's reign, it is clear that the office was held for most of the period by Reginald de Cornhill, sheriff of Kent.[164] As the head of

[160] *Ibid.*, pp. 84, 85, 87, 89, 91, 93, 101; *Curia regis rolls,* VI, 27.
[161] See " Rotulus misae 14 John " for a general view of the household.
[162] *Curia regis rolls,* VI, 27.
[163] *Book of fees,* I, 103, 251, 253.
[164] Reginald purchased extensively for the household. *Rot. claus.,* I, 21 22, 27, 52, 55, 87, 88, 91, 109, 128, 157, 193. His son and William de Cornhill shared the office in 1213. *Rot. pat.,* p. 96.

the greatest of London merchant families Reginald was peculiarly fitted for the post.

The chief local representatives of the royal government were the sheriffs. The sheriff was primarily a financial officer. The regular royal revenues in a county were valued at a certain sum that was called the farm of the county, and the sheriff was responsible for paying this amount into the exchequer. The items that made up the farm varied from county to county. In every shire there were royal manors and boroughs that contributed to it. In all counties there were the revenues from the shire and hundred courts. Then in some counties the sheriff collected an annual tax called sheriff's aid at a fixed sum per hide. In the counties where the frankpledge system existed the sheriff collected fees when he toured the shire to inspect the functioning of the system —the view of frankpledge. The amounts of the county farms had been set in Henry II's reign and did not vary throughout the reigns of Richard and John. When the king granted a royal manor that had contributed to the farm, the sheriff was credited for it. In theory the same principle applied to royal grants of exemption from sheriff's aid and view of frankpledge, but in practice these seem usually to have been credited for a few years and then forgotten. Thus as time went on there appeared items in the farm that the sheriff could not collect. At the same time the general rise in prices and in the returns from agriculture increased the revenues from the royal manors. In John's reign the value assigned to a manor in the county farm was usually far less than its real value. Both Richard and John realized this and demanded extra payments or increments from some sheriffs.[165] They also sold the office of sheriff for considerable sums.[166] Moreover in addition to paying the farm and increments into the exchequer, the sheriff had to bear certain regular expenses. When he repaired the king's castles and hunting lodges, hired troops to hold the castles and keep order in the countryside in time of trouble, bought supplies for the court, or made any other unusual payments at the

---

[165] See under *crementum* in indices to the pipe rolls.
[166] *Pipe roll 6 John*, p. 32; *Pipe roll 8 John*, p. 103; *Pipe roll 9 John*, p. 214; *Rot. oblatis*, p. 109.

king's order, he received credit for it on his account. But the ordinary costs of his administration and the peace-time custody of the castles were his responsibility. In short the man who took office as sheriff was engaging in a financial speculation of considerable magnitude. This system had two obvious faults. The sheriff could profit largely from money that should have gone to the crown. The evidence available indicates that Yorkshire could be made to yield between £600 and £700 beyond its farm of £440. Buckinghamshire and Bedfordshire were worth between £200 and £300 more than the farm of £477. Staffordshire and Shropshire showed a profit of over £300 for the sheriff. While the possibilities were more moderate in the other shires, they were generally fairly substantial. The other deficiency of the system was that it encouraged the sheriff to make use of the numerous opportunities he had to extort money from the people of the shire. While precise evidence on this subject is naturally hard to find, there is enough to suggest that the sheriffs were not negligent in the matter but made full use of their power.[167] One of John's most interesting governmental experiments was an attempt to abolish the system of farms. It will be discussed at some length in the next chapter.

In addition to conducting his own financial relations with the exchequer the sheriff was responsible for seeing that the people in his shire who owed money to the crown paid or at least appeared at the exchequer sessions. When the debts were small, the sheriff might collect them himself and pay them into the exchequer. But all major debtors were obliged to appear at Westminster either in person or in the case of a baron through his seneschal. Then the sheriff and his men had to serve the writs of summons sent out by the exchequer to all debtors and the mass of judicial writs issued in connection with the business of the courts. He was the official errand boy for the central administration. He collected the juries needed for the possessory assizes and other purposes, arrested criminals, kept the prison, and collected the penalties imposed by the courts. When a criminal fled or was

[167] *The earliest Lincolnshire assize rolls* (ed. Doris Stenton, Lincoln Record Society), pp. 146-147.

hanged, it was the sheriff's duty to see that the crown got the value of his chattels. When a man was killed falling from his horse, drowned by falling out of a boat, or smothered in a vat of new ale, he seized the article responsible, the horse, boat, or vat of ale, for the king's use. In short it was the sheriff's duty to see that the crown received every penny due it from every conceivable source. In addition to his financial and police duties he had some judicial ones. When a vassal complained that his lord had seized his cattle for default of service without good cause, the sheriff heard the case as a justice. He presided over the courts of the shire and hundred. When he toured his county in what was called his "tourn," he acted as a police court judge for minor cases. Finally he was usually the custodian of the royal castles in his shire and often had charge of escheated lands and those in the custody of the crown.

The power of the sheriff was rather inadequately controlled in several ways. There were independent officers called coroners who supervised his administration of criminal justice. As the coroners kept a record of all crimes committed that were of interest to the crown, it was difficult for the sheriff to accept money for immunity from prosecution. Then the justices itinerant had a view of his conduct of the business of interest to them. Moreover they were frequently commissioned to conduct special inquiries into all sorts of questions dealing with the king's interests. Finally the king himself was continually on the move about his realm and John had a vigilant eye. But actually none of these checks can have made much difference. Most of the time the sheriff was free to do as he pleased and the people of his shire were at his mercy. The only real checks on his power were the great barons and his fellow royal agents such as constables of castles and custodians of escheated baronies.

As John's attempt to abolish the sheriff's farm resulted technically at least in the abolition of the office of sheriff during the middle years of his reign, we shall here discuss only those sheriffs who held office before 1205. Of the forty-six men who held the office during this period seventeen were barons, twelve knights, and eleven professional royal officials such as Geoffrey fitz Peter,

William Brewer, Hubert de Burgh, Hugh Bardolf, and Hugh de Neville. Seven were minor figures who may have been either knights or clerks. Two belonged to a newly rising class—professional administrators who served whoever hired them. Thus in 1199 John de Cornard was the seneschal of the earl de Clare, but in 1204 he was sheriff of Norfolk and Suffolk. Obviously most of the barons and royal officials did not actually perform their duties as sheriff—the work was done by the under-sheriff. In fact one finds the king's justices calling the under-sheriff sheriff as he was to all practical purposes. Yet if the under-sheriff was the man of the titular sheriff, the latter had full control if he wished to exercise it. This is made clear in an arrangement between John and William de Stutville. William promised to pay 1,500 marks for the shrievalty of Yorkshire, but John was to appoint two under-sheriffs and the constables of the royal castles.[168] In short William was taking the office as a financial speculation while leaving the king the military and political authority. Similar arrangements may have been made in other cases, but they were probably rare. Most sheriffs were fully as much interested in the power as they were in the revenue.

---

[168] *Rot. oblatis*, p. 109.

CHAPTER IV

THE ROYAL ADMINISTRATION

FROM THE point of view of governmental policies, methods, and procedures the early years of John's reign were a time of innovations and experiments. As rapidly changing economic conditions and the political and social developments that grew out of them presented the royal government with new problems, the king and his servants devised expedients to solve them. The fact that many of these innovations were largely abortive does not detract either from their interest or their importance to the historian. Some experiments failed because they were attempts to patch up institutions that were essentially dead—others because the time for them had not yet arrived. The royal government twisted and wrenched the traditional system of feudal knight service in the hope that it could be made to meet the military needs of the crown, but it also experimented with customs duties and income and property taxes. The effort to mold the government of England to fit new needs was bound to be unpopular and it gave rise to a fair part of the complicated maze of grievances that led to the baronial revolt and the formulation of Magna Carta.

Any attempt to ascribe these innovations and experiments to individuals is essentially futile—there is no evidence on which such conclusions can be based. The Victorian historians were inclined to give the monarch credit for the developments made during his reign. Recently it has become fashionable to ascribe changes to the chief of the department concerned. Thus the inauguration of the great series of chancery rolls, the charter, patent, liberate, and close rolls, is generally stated to be the work of Hubert Walter. The only evidence for this is the fact that Hubert became chancellor just before the series began. But John became king on the same day that Hubert assumed the chancellor's office. Hubert's service as active head of the chancery, as the actual bearer of the seal, lasted only five months. Throughout the period in which these rolls began to appear the chancery was directed by its senior clerks. It is, of course, perfectly possible that Hubert Walter was responsible for the inauguration of the rolls, but as strong a case can be made for the hypothesis that the idea was John's and was put into effect by his chancery clerks. There is no evidence to support either view. While it seems unnecessary to attempt to ascribe governmental developments to particular men, if one feels the need of doing so, the monarch seems the wisest choice. Certainly no innovation could be made without his consent, and few could be carried out without his active support. John's preference for having his chancery and chamber run by clerks rather than by the chancellor and the chamberlain and his inclination to center judicial business in the court that followed his person indicate his desire to maintain close personal control over his administration. He had an active, ingenious, and inventive mind. In short while I cannot prove that John himself was responsible for the majority of the innovations and experiments made during his reign, a better case can be made for him than for his servants.

On the first day that John used his new great seal, June 7, 1199, he issued a charter setting the fees that the chancery was to receive for preparing and sealing charters and letters patent.[1] In this solemn "constitution" John announced that these fees had been exorbitant under Richard and that he was restoring the scale of Henry II's day. Richard's chancery had charged twelve marks and five shillings for a charter of confirmation while the just fee was but eighteen shillings four pence. Henceforth the rate for a new grant was to be twelve marks and five shillings— ten marks for the chancellor, a mark each for the vice-chancellor and prothonotary, and five shillings for the serjeants who applied the wax. A simple charter of confirmation with no additions should yield eighteen shillings four pence—a mark for the chancellor, a bezant, or two shillings, for the vice-chancellor and prothontary and twelve pence for the wax. Ordinary letters patent of protection should bring two shillings. Anyone who violated this ordinance was to suffer from the indignation of both God and the king. The bishops who assisted at the king's consecration would

[1] Rymer, *Foedera*, I, 75-76.

excommunicate such offenders. This solemn pronouncement was witnessed by thirteen bishops, ten earls, and seven barons.

This is a truly fascinating document. The newly annointed king made a magnificent gesture at reform—the brand new royal broom erased a fly-speck. Moreover the fly-speck was skilfully chosen. Charters and letters patent were bought by prelates, barons, towns, and guilds. They were people of importance whose favor was worth gaining. While the fees paid to the chancery were insignificant compared to the lordly fines demanded by the king, they were undoubtedly annoying. A return to the rates of Henry II's day was a pleasant gesture toward the virtuous past that could be expected to be well received. Best of all except for the rare occasions when the chancery was vacant and the chancellor's fees came to the king the reform cost John nothing. The burden fell on the chancellor and his subordinates. The document states that it was issued at Hubert Walter's request, and it may well be true. Men were saying that the primate of all England debased himself by accepting a royal office. Chancellors had become archbishops, but never before had an archbishop become a chancellor.[2] Hubert may well have felt that some public self-denial was in order. And he could well afford it. The difference between the old fees and the new could mean little to the master of the vast archepiscopal barony who was besides the most successful gatherer of rich custodies in the realm.

Despite the reference to a vice-chancellor and prothonotary, these offices, as we have seen, never existed under John. The chancellor got his fee and the clerks and waxers or spigurnels divided the rest.[3] Mr. Richardson has shown that while there were clearly special fees for extraordinary documents, the general scale set by this charter was maintained throughout John's reign.[4] If one remembers the archdeaconries and church livings that were showered on the chancery clerks and the short time it took for most of them to reach the episcopal dignity, one will feel no great sympathy for these victims of John's great reform.

[2] Hovedon, IV, 90-91.
[3] *Rot. claus.*, I, 48; *Rot. chart.*, p. 201.
[4] Richardson, Introduction to *Memoranda roll 1 John*, pp. xxxvi-xxxviii.

Shortly after reducing the fees of the chancellor and his clerks John took steps to secure for himself the largest possible revenue from fines for the renewal of charters. While most charters were in the form of perpetual grants binding on the grantor and his heirs for the benefit of the grantee and his heirs, it had always been considered prudent to secure confirmations from time to time. The general practice was to ask a newly crowned king to confirm the grants made by his predecessors. But there is no evidence that any king went so far as to declare the grants of his predecessors invalid unless they had been confirmed by him. John took this step. Sometime during the first year of his reign he instructed the justices in his courts to refuse to accept charters or letters patent issued by his ancestors unless they had been confirmed by him.[5] The oblate rolls and the pipe rolls show clearly how profitable the confirmation of grants was to the royal treasury.

The most interesting feature of the history of the chancery during this period was the development of the system of chancery enrollments. Whether the initiative came from the king or the chancellor, the details must have been worked out by the chancery clerks. Mr. Richardson has shown conclusively that some rolls were kept in the chancery in King Richard's time and the practice may well go back to the reign of Henry II.[6] These early rolls were connected with the relations between the royal household and the exchequer. As the king wandered about his English and continental lands, he made agreements with his subjects involving payments into the exchequer. It is clear that in Richard's reign fines arranged by the king were entered on a roll kept by the chancery clerks and called variously a fine or oblate roll. At intervals the fines were copied from this roll to form an originalia roll that was sent to the exchequer. The exchequer could then issue summonses to those who had offered the fines and enter the debts and payments made on the pipe roll. But while all fines were in theory made with the king, his high officials often made the actual arrangements and in Richard's reign sent their own lists of fines to the exchequer. Perhaps late in the reign of King Richard and certainly at the

[5] *Curia regis rolls*, I, 331.
[6] Richardson, Introduction to *Memoranda roll 1 John*, pp. xxi-xxvii.

beginning of John's these rolls were consolidated. When a royal official arranged for a fine, he notified the chancery, and it was entered on the fine or oblate roll with the proper notation. Thus an entry on the oblate roll of the first year of John states that William Brewer offered 250 marks for two custodies and bears the notation "per the lord of Canterbury."[7] The fine had been negotiated with Hubert Walter who notified the chancery clerks. This centralized system had obvious advantages. The king could supervise closely the financial bargains made by his officials in his name and could keep track of the revenue that might be expected from fines. Occasional totals entered on the rolls show that this last item was of particular interest to him.[8]

As the king roamed about his domain, he arranged to spend money as well as to receive it. When a royal manor the revenues of which had formed part of a county farm was granted by charter, the exchequer had to be directed to credit the sheriff with its value. When a newly created earl was given the third penny of the pleas of a county, the sheriff had to be ordered to make the payment and the exchequer to be instructed to credit the sheriff. If a royal castle needed repairs, the constable received an authorization to make them. Sometimes separate orders were issued, but more often the exchequer was notified of the king's orders that affected its business by a copy of the writ—a *contra brevia*. Writs ordering the expenditure of the king's money or a reduction in his sources of revenue were generally called writs of liberate. Early in John's reign the chancery began to enter these writs on a roll called the liberate roll. As a matter of fact there were for a time two liberate rolls, one dealing with matters of interest to the English and the other to those concerning the Norman exchequer.[9]

From the very beginning of John's reign the chancery clerks kept a record of the charters and letters patent issued by them. During the first two years there was but one roll. In the third year of the reign a separate roll was kept for the letters patent and

[7] *Rot. oblatis*, p. 10.
[8] *Ibid.*, pp. 4, 8, 12, 15, 19, 28, 32, 35, 38, 40, 51, 90.
[9] For a full discussion of this subject see Richardson, Introduction to *Memoranda roll 1 John*, pp. xxxiii-xxxv.

this practice was continued. The official distinction between charters and letters patent lay in their form. A charter was a solemn document drawn up according to a precise formula. It usually had a fairly long list of witnesses, gave the name of the clerk who sealed it, and stated the place, day, month, and regnal year of issue. Letters patent were far more informal. After a prescribed form of greeting the business of the letter was stated briefly. It rarely bore more than one attestation and usually did not state the regnal year of its issue. No mention was made of the clerk who sealed it. Despite their marked difference in form, it is not easy to draw a clear line between the uses made of the two types of document. One can say in general that charters were used for grants in perpetuity while letters patent were temporary in their nature. Thus a hereditary earldom would be created by charter and the appointment of a sheriff to serve at the king's pleasure would by made by letters patent. But exceptions can be found to both statements. Temporary grants of custodies and life appointments to offices were made by charter, and grants in perpetuity were made by letters patent.

The bulkiest and in many ways the most interesting of the chancery rolls, the close rolls, made their appearance in the sixth year of John's reign. It has long been recognized that the close rolls were a development of the liberate rolls. The roll that is called a close roll for the sixth year of John is in reality a transitionary form between the early liberate rolls and the later close rolls. But from the beginning the close rolls contained entries that had no connection with the royal revenue, and as time went on the proportion of such entries increased enormously. In the reign of Henry III the liberate roll was revived for the material that was of interest to the exchequer, and the close roll was left free for the enrollment of other writs.

In order to understand this development of the liberate rolls into the close rolls one must consider once more the practices of the chancery. From the point of view of form the chancery issued two types of document—charters and letters. But the letters were sealed in different ways. Letters patent had the seal attached to it by ribbons as did a charter. The other type, letters close, were folded and the seal placed over the fold so that it would be broken when they were opened. Letters patent were intended to be carried open and shown to all concerned while letters close were private directions to individuals. The difference can best be shown by examples. On September 9, 1204, John issued letters patent addressed to all free tenants and all men of the manor of Sturminster. They were to obey Earl William Marshal as their lord and do him the homage and service owed by their fees as the count of Meulan, their former lord, had ordered them to do by his letters. These letters were undoubtedly given to the earl to show to the men. Then letters close were despatched to the sheriff of Dorset and Somerset directing him to accompany William Marshal to Sturminster to see that the king's orders were obeyed.[10] Again on June 27, 1213, John addressed letters patent to the knights and free tenants of the barony of Barnstaple notifying them that he had given the barony to Henry de Tracy and directing them to obey him as their lord. Letters close informed the sheriff of Devon of the king's action and ordered him to give Henry formal seisin.[11] While many similar cases can be found in the rolls, it was by no means general practice to issue both types of letters in connection with a single matter. Usually one was made to suffice, and there seems no clear rule to govern the type used. Letters of protection that were meant to be carried as a sort of passport and letters of appointment to office were always letters patent, but orders addressed to individuals could be either patent or close. While I am convinced that the chief distinction was the way the letters were to be used, I cannot prove it conclusively.

The vast majority of letters dealing with the king's financial affairs were letters close. Hence when the liberate rolls were started a fair proportion of the letters close issued by the chancery were enrolled on them. By the sixth year of John's reign it was decided to extend the liberate rolls to form a general register of all letters close that were issued. Thus by 1204 all documents issued by the chancery clerks that accompanied the king's court were sup-

---

[10] *Rot. pat.*, p. 45; *Rot. claus.*, I, 7.
[11] *Rot. pat.*, p. 101; *Rot. claus.*, I, 137.

posed to be enrolled on one of the three chancery rolls—charter, patent, or close.[12]

No serious discussion of the inauguration of the chancery rolls can ignore the obvious question as to the purposes the rolls were intended to serve. Mr. Richardson has dealt with this subject at some length.[13] He is clearly correct in his belief that the oblate, originalia, and liberate rolls were intended to control the financial relations between the ambulant court and the exchequer at Westminster. He does not attempt to furnish any explanation for the enlargement of the scope of the liberate rolls when they became the close rolls. His chief attention is devoted to a discusion of the purpose served by the charter and patent rolls. Mr. Richardson argues that the sole purpose of these rolls was to record the fees that were due to the chancellor and his clerks.[14] In support of this argument he points out various notations on the rolls that had to do with those fees. Now there can be no doubt that the chancellor and his clerks were interested in their fees and wanted a record of those due them. The rolls were certainly used for this purpose. But it seems highly improbable that this was either the sole purpose or even the chief purpose of keeping the rolls.

Let us glance first at the charter rolls. Mr. Richardson recognizes one objection to his theory. The charters issued by the king are reproduced in full on the roll—many of them take up a column or more in the Record Commission's edition. Mr. Richardson argues that the clerks needed enough of the document to show its nature for the purpose of charging fees and were too stupid to know where to draw the line. It is difficult to prove that Mr. Richardson is mistaken, but his explanation seems to me utterly incredible. For one thing why would the clerk laboriously copy out a long charter and then, as was usual in the charter roll, abbreviate the list of witnesses? And why if fees were the only subject of interest should the witnesses be mentioned at all? Then there are some notations on the charter roll that cannot be connected with

---

[12] An exception to this statement would be the writs issued by the chancery for the justices accompanying the king—purely routine judicial writs.
[13] Richardson, Introduction to *Memoranda roll 1 John*.
[14] *Ibid.*, pp. xxxv-xlvii.

chancery fees. Thus on page 17 is a note saying "Be it remembered that this land is assigned to him [Robert de Harcourt] until £100 as a marriage portion is given his son and that the charter was extorted because of the war."[15] In short the grant was temporary and was squeezed out of John by a great Norman lord whose support he needed. In the last chapter when discussing the activities of Geoffrey fitz Peter reference was made to a note on the charter rolls explaining the unusual form of a confirmation charter issued for him.[16] Then in two cases at least notes indicate where a charter that is enrolled out of its proper place can be found.[17]

In attempting to show that the charter rolls could not be meant for any purpose other than collecting fees, Mr. Richardson shows clearly that there was one purpose for which they were not used. They were not intended to be a public record in the sense that they could be used by a grantee who had lost or mislaid his original charter. When anyone wanted a charter registered in such a way that it could be used for this purpose, he either had it entered on the pipe roll or on the *cartae antiquae* rolls. Not only was the charter roll a chancery record and hence not readily available to the courts at Westminster, but the charters as enrolled on it often differed from the original documents. Moreover if an enrollment was to be a legal record, a full list of witnesses was most important. But the fact that the charter rolls were not available to the king's subjects does not mean that they could not be a useful record for his officials. Occasions must frequently have arisen when it was useful for the king and his officers to know just what had been granted to someone. And the clerk who wrote the two unusual charters for Geoffrey fitz Peter was anxious to register the fact that it had been done "by special order of the lord king" rather than by his negligence or misconduct. The charter roll supplied the king's officers with a reasonably accurate text and the chief witnesses to all the charters issued. The mere fact that one cannot produce clear evidence that they used it for purposes of general reference seems to me to be of slight importance.[18]

[15] *Rot. chart.*, p. 17. [16] *Ibid.*, p. 79. [17] *Ibid.*, pp. 166, 185.
[18] A possible case is found in 1201 when John made inquiry as to the terms of a charter *per registrum suum*. Jocelin de Brakelond, *Chronica de*

When one turns to the patent rolls, Mr. Richardson's theory seems even less tenable. There is no doubt that when letters patent were issued at the request of an individual and for his benefit, he paid fees to the chancery for them. But if Mr. Richardson's theory is to be accepted, all the letters enrolled on the patent rolls should fall into this class or should bear a notation showing that no fees were due for them. As a matter of fact a large number of letters patent clearly dealt with the king's business alone and were of no interest to any individual. Perhaps a man would pay a fee for letters patent appointing him sheriff or constable, but it is hard to believe that the king of Scotland or a Welsh chieftain paid fees for their letters of safe-conduct to meet John. And who would pay the fees for letters that assured men who had rebelled against John and joined Philip Augustus that arrangements to return to John's service made with certain of his officials would be recognized by him? Mr. Richardson makes his distinction between letters patent and letters close on the basis that the former were for the benefit of individuals while the latter dealt with the king's business. This statement is probably true for the bulk of the documents on the two sets of rolls, but the fact that many of the entries on the patent rolls clearly deal with the king's business would appear to make the rolls of little use as a register of fees. The purpose of the patent rolls seems to me to be essentially the same as that of the charter rolls. They supply the texts of the letters patent issued by the chancery and show who ordered the clerks to draw them up and seal them. Thus *teste me ipso* or *teste rege* means that the king in person ordered the letters sealed. *Teste Geoffrey fitz Peter* means that the order was given by the justiciar. Information as to what the king's orders had been and who was responsible for their issuance must have been frequently of value to the royal government.

The value of the chancery rolls for purposes of general reference becomes particularly clear when one examines the close rolls. There are found the great mass of letters issued by the chancery. Charters were solemn documents that were sealed only on the king's personal order. While the actual command to the clerks to

rebus gestis Samsonis abbatis monasteri Sancti Edmundi (ed. John L. Rokewood, Camden society, xiii, London, 1840), p. 98.

draw up and seal letters patent could come from a servant of the crown, it seems probable that the king always knew they were being issued. But the king could not attend in person to all the details of his business that gave rise to letters close. Sometimes he authorized the issuance of letters and had someone else carry the order to the clerks and presumably dictate the letter. Thus in November 1205 he ordered letters close sent to the sheriff of Hampshire directing him to supply various articles to William de Cornhill. As the king gave the original order, the letters bear the phrase *teste me ipso*. But a note under them *per W. de Cornhill* shows that the actual order to the clerk was given by him.[19] At times a high official would carry through the whole transaction. On November 15, 1205, letters close to Robert de Vieuxpont directed him to return some pigs, or their meat, to Jocelin de Neville. Hugh de Neville, the chief forester, issued this order himself and directed the clerks to seal it—the form is *teste H. de Neville per eundem*.[20] The king may never have heard of the order. As a rule the writs dealing with the king's business were issued at the direction of the officer whose department was concerned. If the king had given his approval, the form would be *teste me ipso* and *per* the official. If the king knew nothing about it, the form would be "teste so and so—per eundem." In the early years of John's reign it is impossible to prove conclusively that more than a very occasional letter close was issued when the king was not in the vicinity. Later in the reign such cases became fairly common. A concrete example may be useful to show how this system worked. On October 27, 1207, letters close were issued directing the barons of the exchequer to credit Henry of London, archdeacon of Stafford, for a sum of money paid into the chamber from the revenues of the see of Exeter that was in his custody. The letters were attested by Geoffrey de Neville, the chamberlain, and the order for drawing them up and sealing them was given the clerks of the chancery by Richard Marsh, the clerk of the chamber.[21] Thus the chamberlain had re-

---

[19] *Rot. claus.*, I, 56. The later use of *per breve de parvu sigillo* and *per os domini regis* seems to demonstrate the meaning of *per* in these notations. *Ibid.*, pp. 116, 125-126.
[20] *Ibid.*, p. 57.   [21] *Ibid.*, p. 94.

ceived the money and ordered his chief clerk to see that the chancery issued letters to the exchequer.

Now it seems clear that when letters could be issued in the king's name without his knowledge and when most letters close were drawn up and sealed by the chancery clerks without any direct command from the king, a record showing who was responsible for the letters was of great importance. The attesting clause in the letters themselves showed whether the king or someone else had given the original command, but only the notations on the roll showed who had transmitted the order to the clerks. While it is impossible to prove that the rolls were actually used to discover who had authorized various letters, their presumptive value for the purpose is clear.

In summary one can say that the charter, patent, and close rolls served a number of purposes. The charter and patent rolls were undoubtedly an aid to the chancery clerks in keeping track of the fees due them. The close rolls were an important part of the financial system. All the rolls were used for memoranda of various kinds. Charters and letters patent given to the king by private individuals, papal letters, notes concerning judicial business, the summary of the decrees made by a church council held in France— in short any document of interest to the king and his government— might be entered on whichever roll offered a convenient blank space.[22] But all the rolls seem basically designed to serve a single chief end—effective control of the operations of the government. Through them the king and his ministers could discover what the government had ordered and who was responsible for it. The idea of supplying such records can well have come from an experienced and careful administrator like Hubert Walter. It could also have been conceived by a suspicious minded monarch who wanted to keep close supervision of the operations of his government.[23] In

[22] *Ibid.*, pp. 33, 69, 70, 114, 164, 202, 203, 269. *Rot. pat.*, pp. 42, 55, 82, 83, 115, 139, 181. *Rot. chart.*, pp. 58 59, 60, 61, 96, 97, 191, 207, 208, 221.

[23] While the statement of Giraldus Cambrensis that the clerks of the chancery changed royal letters to favor Hubert Walter may well be untrue, it indicates that such behavior was not inconceivable and so justifies to some extent the suspicions I ascribe to John. Giraldus Cambrensis, *Opera*, III, 302.

either case the working out of the details must have fallen on such clerks as the Welles brothers.

There was obviously one extremely vital step in the procedure of the chancery—the process by which the king's command reached the clerks who drew up and sealed his letters. As we have seen orders dealing with routine royal business did not have to be issued by the king in person. When such orders were given by members of his entourage and sealed by the clerks attending the court, abuses of this power would be difficult. It was sufficient to have the name of the official who gave the command appear as the attestant. In the early years of the reign all the letters enrolled on the patent and close rolls apparently were issued by the chancery clerks who were in immediate attendance on the king. It is, of course, important to notice that this statement is restricted to writs that were enrolled. Vast numbers of writs in the king's name were issued by the justiciar and sealed by chancery clerks in his household. These were the writs that kept the judicial system in operation. Again the summonses of the exchequer went forth in the king's name. Both these classes of writs dealt with purely routine business and were sealed with the seal kept at the exchequer. They were not expressions of the king's will in the same sense as the writs enrolled on the patent and close rolls. In the case of charters there is no evidence that any royal charter was issued during these years except at the express oral command of the king to the clerks of the chancery. But precedent existed for a different practice. In the first year of King Richard's reign his chancellor, William de Longchamp, bishop of Ely, had issued a number of charters in England while the king was in his continental fiefs.[24]

Prior to the inauguration of the chancery rolls there is little information available on the practices of the English chancery beyond the final form taken by the documents it issued. Hence it is impossible to say how much of the system outlined above in discussing the rolls was new. As the form of John's documents was the same as those of King Richard, it seems likely that the system that produced them was little different. The only striking variation between the two reigns was John's practice of having his seal

[24] Landon, *Itinerary*, pp. 173-174.

borne by clerks who had no official title—who were not even called acting vice-chancellors. Occasionally John would seal his documents himself, or at least take the responsibility for the action by directing the clerks to use the phrase *datum per manum nostram*.[25] At times some entirely non-clerical member of his entourage such as Robert de Vieuxpont would seal a charter.[26] But there is no evidence that the early years of John's reign brought any essential change in chancery practice.

Unfortunately for the historian time has dealt harshly with the chancery rolls of John's reign. The charter rolls are missing for the third, fourth, and eighth years. Worse yet the charter, patent, and close rolls have all been lost for three years of the reign, the eleventh, twelfth, and thirteenth—from May 1209 to May 1212. There is no close roll for the tenth year—1208-1209. Hence for three years it is impossible to trace chancery practice in detail. When the evidence is available once more in the charter, patent, and close rolls of 1212-1213, an interesting innovation has appeared. The bearer of the great seal is no longer in constant attendance on the king. Letters patent, letters close, and even charters were issued at Westminster while the king was wandering about his realm. Thus from May 8 to 13, 1212, letters patent and close were issued at Westminster attested by William de Cornhill, archdeacon of Huntingdon, Earl William of Salisbury, and Earl Saher de Quency while John was in Hampshire.[27] Then on June 5 King John started on a trip through the northern part of his kingdom, but his seal stayed in Westminster with its keeper, Richard Marsh.[28] Again from October 6 to 16, the king was in the west of England, and his seal was once more in Westminster.[29] During November the king was in London only one day, but Richard Marsh and the seal were there most of the month.[30] On June 24 a royal charter was sealed at Westminster while the king was at Carlisle.[31] Char-

---

[25] *Rot. chart.*, pp. 140, 142, 157, 169.
[26] *Cartae antiquae rolls*, no. 234.
[27] *Rot. claus.*, I, 117, 118; *Rot. pat.*, p. 92.
[28] *Rot. claus.*, I, 118, 119; *Rot. pat.*, p. 93; *Rot. chart.*, p. 187.
[29] *Rot. claus.*, I, 125, 126; *Rot. pat.*, p 95.
[30] *Rot. claus.*, I, 126, 127; *Rot. pat.*, p. 95; *Rot. chart.*, p. 189.
[31] *Ibid.*, p. 187.

ters were issued at Westminster on November 12 and December 2.[32] John was at Canford on the first date and Northampton on the second.

Thus for considerable periods in 1212 the bearer of the seal and presumably the majority of his staff stayed at Westminster while the king roamed over his realm. During these periods John made use of a new device—a privy seal. With it he issued some letters patent and close that were despatched directly to their destinations. But more often he sent letters under his privy seal to his keeper directing him to issue letters under the great seal. Notations on many of the documents sealed at Westminster in the king's absence indicate that they were authorized by royal writs under the privy or small seal.[33] On at least one occasion John used the seal of William Brewer to convey his orders to the chancery.[34] Thus the procedure was devised that was to become the regular practice in later years when the chancery became permanently sedentary. For the rest of John's reign it remained an occasional expedient.[35]

I have suggested that one of the reasons, perhaps the chief one, for the inauguration of the chancery rolls was the king's desire to have the facilities for close supervision of the use of his seal. There is fairly ample evidence that the possibility of its misuse worried John throughout his reign. The most striking indication of the king's suspicion was his practice of arranging complicated countersigns that were to be included in letters ordering certain courses of action. The earliest case I have found, a very simple one, appears on the first page of the patent rolls. Robert de Vieuxpont had been instructed not to free a prisoner, Guy de Chatillon, unless the letters ordering it were borne by Thomas de Burgh. We learn of the arrangement because the king is sending Peter des Roches instead.[36] A case about a year later shows one of the hazards of the system. John had ordered his chamberlain, Hubert de Burgh, who was guarding the more important prisoners taken at Mirabeau,

[32] *Ibid.*, p. 189.
[33] *Rot. pat.*, pp. 92, 93, 95; *Rot. claus.*, I, 116-119, 127; *Rot. chart.*, p. 187.
[34] *Rot. claus.*, I, 116.
[35] See for instance *ibid.*, pp. 176-177.
[36] *Rot. pat.*, p. 1.

not to allow any one to speak with Guy de Lusignan unless he was escorted by one of three members of the king's household. Unfortunately John had forgotten who the three were. He sent Thomas, the clerk of the chamber. If Thomas was not one of the three, he was nevertheless to be allowed to take the man he was escorting to Guy de Lusignan.[37] Then in 1206 while he was campaigning in Poitou John had entrusted a number of important prisoners to Robert de Vieuxpont. One of them was the king's niece, Eleanor, *de jure* duchess of Brittany. John had instructed Robert to do nothing in regard to Eleanor unless the messenger bearing the order showed him a certain ring. He had also directed Robert not to free another prisoner, Chalon de Rochefort, the first time he was ordered to. But the king became anxious to get Chalon freed at once. Hence the letters ordering it mention the countersign arranged in regard to the king's niece.[38] In short a reference to the existence of one of these secret countersigns, even if it did not apply to the matter in question or if the king had forgotten the exact countersign, showed the recipient of the letters that they had been dictated by the king in person. Although these examples are all from the early years of the reign, John continued to use this device.[39] It is most often found in connection with the freeing of prisoners or the transferring of the command of a royal castle. If money was paid out or lands given on the authority of improperly authorized letters, they could be recovered fairly easily. But the freeing of a captive or the transfer of a castle might involve serious consequences. Prisoners could move fast and castles are hard to take.

It is in connection with royal castles that another method of avoiding the danger of the misuse of the royal seal appears. Apparently John established a general rule that a constable was not to deliver the command of the castle entrusted to him to anyone else simply on the basis of royal letters ordering him to do so.[40] When the king was reasonably near at hand, the constable was

[37] *Ibid.*, p. 17.   [38] *Ibid.*, p. 66.
[39] See for instance *ibid.*, pp. 193, 195, and Painter, *William Marshal*, pp. 188-189.
[40] *Rot. pat.*, pp. 10, 12, 81, 83, 116, 150, 193.

expected upon receipt of letters relieving him to turn the castle over to a deputy and go to the king to receive direct confirmation of the order.[41] When the king was far away, the constable was directed to obey the order of a great dignitary such as Geoffrey fitz Peter or Richard Marsh.[42] We learn of this system through the difficulties John had in making it work. A constable who liked his job could use the rule as an excuse for long delay in surrendering a castle to his successor.

It seems likely that another cause of worry to John was the seal kept at the exchequer for sealing writs of summons and those dealing with the business of the courts. When in use it was in the care of a deputy of the chancellor, the forerunner of the later chancellor of the exchequer. But such a clerk could offer little resistance to the high officials of the exchequer. I suspect that one of the chief tasks of the royal intimates such as William Brewer who took part in the sessions of the exchequer was to supervise the use of this seal. This possibility that John feared the misuse of the exchequer seal gives rise to an interesting speculation. As we have seen the only times in John's reign when we know that the keeper of his seal was away from court for a considerable period were in the spring and autumn of 1212 and the autumn of 1214. These times correspond roughly with the exchequer sessions. In both these years John had strong reason to suspect baronial plots against him. Canons of St. Paul's who were intimates of the exchequer officials were involved in the conspiracy of Robert fitz Walter.[43] Geoffrey de Norwich, justiciar of the Jews, was put to death by John for complicity in this plot.[44] One cannot but wonder if the presence of Richard Marsh, whom John trusted beyond all others, at these exchequer sessions was caused by his suspicions of the exchequer officials and the use they might make of the royal seal entrusted to them. Such misuse could be effectively prevented by having the keeper of the seal perform in person the functions of his deputy at the exchequer.

[41] *Ibid.*, pp. 10, 12, 150.   [42] *Ibid.*, pp. 12, 116.
[43] H. G. Richardson, " Letters of the legate Guala," *English historical review*, CLXXXIX (1933), 252-253.
[44] See below, pp. 270-272.

Another interesting development in the use of the royal seals is connected with the relations between the chamber and the exchequer. In its financial aspects the chamber was the king's privy purse. Whenever the king's current needs for paying the expenses of his household, making gifts or loans to individuals, paying the wages of troops accompanying him, or for any other purpose could not be met by orders drawn on the exchequer, cash payments were made by the chamber. The chamber obtained the major part of its funds by drafts on the royal treasury.[45] But it also received large sums directly from the crown's debtors. In such cases letters close were issued, usually attested by a chamber official, directing the barons of the exchequer to credit the payment on the pipe roll.[46] On May 2, 1208, the king ordered the immediate collection of various debts due him. The letters close carrying the orders contained an interesting clause—"and because we want these debts paid into the chamber these letters have been sealed with the privy seal. If the payment were to be made to the exchequer, the letters would be sealed with the great seal."[47] While this is phrased as a statement of established practice, it seems likely that it was a recent innovation. Established practice does not have to be explained.

While no one with an interest in administrative history can resist the fascination of the innovations made by John's government in the practices of the chancery, it is important to remember that the basic problem facing the king was financial. Since the reign of Henry II, the cost of government had increased enormously and the regular, assured revenue of the crown had actually decreased. Laying aside special taxes such as scutages and tallages the income of the English crown when John ascended the throne was derived from two sources. There were the farms of the counties and royal boroughs and the revenue from the king's lands that did not form part of the county farms. To these should be added the income from mines, especially the tin mines of Devon and Cornwall, the profits of the coining and exchanging of money, and

---

[45] *Rot. claus.*, I, 1, 4, 12, 16, 37, 120.

[46] *Ibid.*, pp. 3, 16, 94, 101. Similar writs occur on almost every page of the rolls.

[47] *Ibid.*, p. 115.

the small fixed sums yielded by various royal forests. These sources were regular and reliable—they furnished what one might call budgetable income. Then there were the fines and penalties of various sorts. Many of the fines represented well recognized feudal obligations such as the payment of relief, but the majority were sums offered for various favors. As a matter of fact the line between fines and amercements was very thin. Fines could be offered to obtain forgiveness for offenses and to regain the king's good will. The actual amercements, penalties levied by the royal courts, were great in number but the total revenue did not compare with that from fines. These sources were obviously variable. They could within certain limits be increased or decreased by chance and by royal policy. Two factors prevented the increase of the income from fines to any very great extent. There was a limit to the favors the king could afford to sell—almost every grant reduced the power or the income of the crown. Then an exorbitant increase in fines, especially in those representing regular feudal obligations, was certain to lead to strong protests by the barons.

Had the English kings maintained intact the vast lands reserved for himself by William the Conqueror and conserved the escheats that had fallen into their hands, the financial position of the crown in the early thirteenth century would have been far better than it was. Henry I endowed his illegitimate son Robert and his favorite knight, Richard de Redvers, with large grants from the royal demesne. William de Warren received extensive lands in Surrey with the comtal title of that shire. William de Albini was given the great escheated barony of Arundel. All these grants were made before the county farms were set and do not appear in the pipe rolls. But after the farms were fixed the list of *terrae datae* for which the sheriffs were given credit was steadily enlarged. At the beginning of the reign of Henry II the total stood at £2,450.[48] By the end of the reign it had increased to £3,372.[49] This figure King Richard doubled to bring the total to £6,816 early in John's reign.[50]

---

[48] Sir James H. Ramsay, *A history of the revenues of the kings of England, 1066-1399* (Oxford, 1925), I, 65.
[49] *Ibid.*, p. 185.
[50] *Ibid.*, p. 233.

As the total sum of the county farms came to about £10,000, these grants diminished the revenue from this source by over 50 per cent. The same royal policy had gravely reduced the demesnes of the escheated baronies that were in the king's hands.

In contrast to the actual reduction in the king's income there was a great increase in the cost of government. Part of this was the result of a general rise in prices. One of the chief items of expense to a mediæval king as to a modern one was soldiers, and between the reign of Henry II and John the daily wage of a knight had risen from eight pence to two shillings. But probably of more importance was a general change in standards. The greater availability of luxury goods—silks, sugar, spices, jewels—made John's court more costly than his father's had been. In Henry II's day a number of royal castles were still made of wood, but by John's time stone was the only really acceptable material. John kept a standing army that was tiny by our measurements but very large by those of his day. He also built and maintained a navy. Moreover the rapid increase in the resources of John's enemies, the Capetian kings of France, demanded greater expenditures to keep them in check. While it is far from proved that John lost Normandy, Maine, and Anjou because he had less money than Philip Augustus, it is clear that far more would be needed to fight an effective war against Philip than had been required to do so against his predecessors.[51] John poured vast sums into his unsuccessful defense of Normandy. After its loss one of his chief preoccupations became the gathering of funds to enable him to reconquer his lost possessions and take vengeance on King Philip.

The observable results of the economic changes of the day must have been extremely exasperating to John. The steady growth of the market for the products of agriculture and the general rise in prices that went with it was increasing the income of everyone who drew revenue directly from the exploitation of the land. Most manors in England were increasing in annual value at an astound-

[51] Ferdinand Lot and Robert Fawtier, *Le premier budget de la monarchie française* (Bibliotheque de l'école des hautes études, Paris, 1932), pp. 135-139.

ing rate.[52] Progressive lords like William de Stutville were drawing large sums from clearing forests and turning wastelands into sheep pastures.[53] But the generosity of his predecessors had deprived John of the revenues of a large part of the royal lands. Moreover most of the demesnes he still possessed were let at fixed farms to the sheriffs or others, and the income they yielded the crown could be increased only with great difficulty. The same was true to a considerable extent of the revenues from commerce and industry. The borough farms had also become fixed and their increase was always met with resistance. Trade was flourishing as well as agriculture, but it was extremely difficult for the king to get his share of the profits. Hence John may well have felt that everyone in his realm was growing richer except himself.[54]

There were two obvious lines of approach to the problem of enlarging the royal income. One was through the use of the traditional types of special levies—scutages, tallages, hidages and carucages—and the development of new types. The other was by increasing the regular revenues of the crown in every possible way. John followed both these lines with energy. Although he worked them simultaneously, for purposes of convenience I shall discuss the two courses separately. We shall first examine his efforts to increase the regular revenues of the crown and then his experiments in taxation.

The earliest of John's moves to improve the efficiency of his financial administration has received less attention than it deserves from historians. It illustrates both the king's interest and the new problems that he faced. From at least the time of King Henry I barons had had the right to conduct their relations with the royal government through their seneschals. A baron could not be ex-

[52] Sidney Painter, *Studies in the history of the English feudal barony*, The Johns Hopkins University studies in historical and political science, vol. LXI, no. 3, pp. 152-161.
[53] *Ibid.*, pp. 163, 164.
[54] " The pipe roll of 1204 is a document of altogether exceptional interest, but the dominant note is financial urgency and it suggests a land of ever increasing resources which the government is only in the process of learning how to exploit." Doris M. Stenton, Introduction to *Pipe roll 6 John*, p. xlv.

pected to attend the local courts, appear before the king's justices, or journey to sessions of the exchequer. In the eleventh and twelfth centuries the seneschalship was in most, perhaps all, baronies an important hereditary office held by one of the baron's chief vassals. Such seneschals were responsible men of substance who could be amerced if they failed in their obligations to the crown. But in John's time the hereditary seneschal was rapidly disappearing. The barons were replacing them with hired administrators. They might be men of neither substance nor position who were simply efficient servants. A certain Osmund de Devereals appeared at the exchequer at Michaelmas 1199 as seneschal of Earl William Marshal.[55] Earl William's household and men are fairly well known and nothing is heard again of Osmund. He can have been little more than a manorial bailiff. Such men could not be effectively amerced and their imprisonment by the king would not trouble their lords greatly.

In the spring of 1200 or 1201 King John issued a decree that the sheriffs should not accept anyone as a baron's seneschal who was not a man of sufficient substance to pay any amercement he might incur. The seneschal was to swear that he would satisfy the exchequer in respect to his lord's debts. If he failed to satisfy the barons of the exchequer, he would be put in prison and the debts collected by seizing his lord's chattels. If the seneschal did not appear at the exchequer session or left before he received leave to do so, he should be imprisoned until the king saw fit to release him. Moreover the seneschal who failed to carry out his obligations should never again be allowed to pledge his faith at the exchequer for the payment of a debt—in short any future dealings he had with the exchequer must be on a cash down basis. To all practical purposes this meant that he could not again serve as a seneschal as few barons were able to pay their debts on the spot in cash.

The decree had one more provision. If a lord had offered the king a fine for his relief or for a grant of land and failed to maintain his payments, the king could seize the land until the fine was paid. In the case of most debts only the debtor's chattels

---

[55] *Memoranda roll 1 John,* p. 62.

could be seized to satisfy the debt, but John was anxious to make easier the collection of fines offered for the possession of lands.[56] As the largest fines were ordinarily those offered for this purpose, improved collection would be a decided benefit to the king's revenue.

This statute also stated that the seneschal's lord could not pledge his faith for the payment of the particular debt on which the seneschal had defaulted. No reference is made to what would happen if the lord was under these circumstances unable to pay in cash. It is clear that later in John's reign barons were being imprisoned for failure to pay the debts they owed the crown.[57] Whether this practice was based on this decree or a later one that we know nothing of must remain an interesting subject for speculation.

As we have seen when John lost Normandy, Maine, and Anjou, he immediately set to work to build up a war chest for their recovery. While much the largest sums were raised by special levies, the king did not neglect the regular revenues of the crown. He was convinced that the royal demesne manors had increased greatly in value since the farms had been fixed in the reign of Henry II and that the sheriffs were making handsome profits. This was no new idea in the royal mind—it had occurred to King Richard. When Richard died twelve English sheriffs were paying increments in addition to their regular farms. The sheriff of Bedfordshire and Buckinghamshire paid £10 and four marks, the sheriff of Cambridge and Huntingdon £20, the sheriffs of Northamptonshire and Worcestershire about £53 each, the sheriff of Essex and Hertfordshire £33, the sheriffs of Dorset and Somerset, Gloucester, Hampshire, and Lancashire £66 each, the sheriff of Lincolnshire £133, the sheriff of Warwick and Leicester £140, and the sheriff of Norfolk and Suffolk £166. With a few exceptions these increments were collected in the first years of John's reign. The sheriff of Dorset and Somerset disputed the justice of the increment and did not pay until some years later.[58] William

[56] Hovedon, IV, 152.
[57] *Rot. pat.*, p. 85; Painter, *Feudal barony*, p. 60.
[58] *Pipe roll 9 John*, p. 56.

Marshal persuaded John to grant him Gloucestershire at the farm alone.[59] When the barons of the exchequer tried to collect an increment on two manors, the king in person told them that William did not have to pay.[60]

In addition to forcing the sheriff to pay an increment there was another way that the king could lay hands on part of his supposed profits—he could make him offer a fine for appointment to the office. If the office of sheriff had been purely financial, this would not have been a bad system. The future sheriff would have offered a share of the profits he anticipated. But the office was also of great political importance. The sheriff usually controlled the royal castles of his shire. He was chief of police and police magistrate. He represented the crown's interests in his shire. Hence often someone would bid high to get the office for political rather than financial reasons, but once in possession he naturally tried to recover the money he had paid or promised. I suspect that completely honest sheriffs were few and far between, but their improper exactions must certainly have grown greater when they saw themselves losing money.

The only real solution was to get rid of the system of farms and make the sheriff render account of the various revenues collected by him, pay the proceeds into the exchequer, and accept a salary for his work. The farm was essentially a relic of the twelfth century when the revenues from land were comparatively stable. It had the obvious advantage that the lord received a fixed, regular return that was not affected by minor variations in the yield of the land and did not have to worry about the honesty or efficiency of the farmer. But when prices and income rose, the farmer made the profit. It seems clear that by John's time most of the barons had given up letting their demesne manors at farm and were exploiting them directly through hired custodians. The crown followed the same system for baronies that were in its custody. Only on the royal demesne and in the old escheats did the system of farms remain in full force. But it is important to remember that direct exploitation required a far more complicated administrative

---

[59] *Memoranda roll 1 John*, p. 38.   [60] *Pipe roll 6 John*, p. 147.

system than the older practice. A baron who let his manors at farm needed only an official to negotiate the annual rent and collect it. Direct exploitation required comprehensive accounts from manorial bailiffs, and if the lord was not to be continually cheated, an efficient auditing system. The lord or his chief agent had to have a pretty good idea of what the yield of a manor could be in order to judge of the efficiency with which it was being managed. Hence along with the trend from letting at farm to direct exploitation went a rapid increase in baronial administrative staffs and the development of methods of making extents or estimates of what an estate should yield.

To put an end to the system of farming the shrievalties would entail major changes in the financial administration of the realm. The revenues collected by the sheriffs were of many types and varied from shire to shire. There was the sheriff's aid—an annual levy of two shillings per hide. There were the fees paid at the view of frankpledge. While these and the yield of the demesne manors and boroughs were the chief sources of the sheriff's income, many other dues are found. The sheriff sometimes collected fees from those who were obliged to appear before him in his tourn and from the suitors at the courts held by him. Then in every county there were lands that were exempt from certain of these dues either by royal grant or by ancient custom. Moreover the liability for their payment was not distributed by any logical system. This too was a matter of ancient custom. Thus the lord of five knights' fees might assign the entire service due from them at the shire court to one of the fees. In short even in those counties where we know just what the sheriff's dues were and how they were assessed in theory, it is impossible to estimate with any confidence the liability of a particular estate. The central government had little idea of what the sheriff's revenues consisted of in any particular county. The compiler of the *Red book of the exchequer* was interested in the subject and included in his work such meagre records as he could find in the exchequer's archives. Thus he has a memorandum drawn up by one sheriff showing the distribution of his income between the various types of dues.⁶¹ But if the exchequer were to obtain sufficient information to audit the accounts of these dues presented by the sheriffs, an inquest far more complicated than Domesday would be required. In addition local auditors would have to check the accuracy of the sheriff's accounts. I suspect that the problem would have proved too complex for any thirteenth-century administration. Clearly John did not dare to try to tackle it directly. He preferred a cautious experiment.

At Michaelmas 1204 King John placed sixteen shrievalties on a new basis. The sheriff became a custodian instead of a farmer.⁶² He would account for the regular farm of the county and the established increments and then he would report the amount of his profit. In short the custodian sheriff was expected to account for and pay into the exchequer all the money he received. He would be given credit for the expenses formerly borne by the farmer sheriff. The king seems to have realized how difficult it would be to persuade the sheriffs to report their profits with any reasonable accuracy. Apparently his scheme for solving this problem was to place the office in commission. In ten of the fifteen shrievalties he appointed two joint custodians in the hope that they would check each other. In three cases these custodians were men of neither position nor administrative experience—men who could be supposed to be free from the traditions of the office. But in general there was no great revolution in personnel. Three of the commissions were headed by the former under-sheriff and two more under-sheriffs continued as sole custodians. In three more the former sheriff became head of the commission or sole custodian. There were eight shrievalties in which neither the sheriff nor under-sheriff remained in office. In five of these barons and royal servants were simply replaced by other barons and royal servant as custodians. The remaining three were those mentioned above where commissions of unknown and inexperienced men were appointed. These men clearly found the task beyond their powers. In Northamptonshire they lasted a half year, in Norfolk and Suffolk for three-quarters of a year, and in Surrey for a year. The

---

⁶¹ *Red book of the exchequer*, II, 774-777.
⁶² The material for this discussion comes from the pipe rolls.

The Royal Administration 119

were replaced by the former sheriffs—in the first two cases as custodians and in Surrey as a farmer.

In addition to the sixteen shrievalties where the sheriffs definitely became custodians there were four more whose sheriffs accounted for their profits. In Herefordshire and Worcestershire the seneschal of the royal household, William de Cantilupe, was not called a custodian but he accounted for his profits. In 1206 and 1207 he was called a custodian in Worcestershire but not in Herefordshire. In Wiltshire Earl William of Salisbury was not called a custodian in either 1205 or 1206, but he accounted for his profits. In 1207 the Wiltshire account has a strange heading—William, earl of Salisbury, John Bonet as custodian for him. Apparently the earl considered it beneath his dignity to be a custodian sheriff, but was willing to let his under-sheriff bear that designation. In Yorkshire Roger de Lacy, constable of Chester, was never called custodian, but in 1209 he admitted that he owed £200 a year from 1205 on as his profits.[63]

Leaving out London and Middlesex where the sheriffs were elected, Westmoreland that John had given as a fief to Robert de Vieuxpont, and the insignificant Rutland, there were twenty-seven royal shrievalties in England. In twenty of these John tried to apply his scheme. It is not difficult to explain why the remaining shrievalties were left alone. Cumberland and Northumberland were frontier shires under the command of tried soldiers, Roger de Lacy and Robert fitz Roger. Devonshire and Oxfordshire were in the hands of two royal favorites—William Brewer and Thomas Basset. Earl William Marshal had been replaced in Sussex by a custodian, and John probably felt it unwise to deprive him of Gloucestershire as well. Cornwall had offered a fine of 2,200 marks for the privilege of presenting several local men to the king and having him choose one as sheriff.[64] The result was the displacement of the little beloved William Brewer and the appointment of the Cornish lord, William de Botereaux. In the case of Essex and Hertfordshire Matthew Mantel had offered the king a fine of 100 marks and a palfrey and agreed to pay an in-

[63] Pipe roll 11 John, Public Record Office.
[64] *Pipe roll 6 John,* p. 40.

crement of 50 marks a year for a hereditary grant of the office of sheriff.[65] In short in five of the seven unaffected shrievalties John considered it wise not to disturb the incumbents with new ideas and in the other two he saw other ways of getting additional revenue.

At Michaelmas 1205 sixteen sheriffs accounted for the profits of their office. The custodians of Surrey never accounted for their profits and were replaced by a farmer sheriff. Reginald de Cornhill, who was sheriff of Kent until his death in 1210, was called a custodian in 1205 but never accounted for his profits. Nottingham and Derby and Yorkshire were special cases—their so-called profits during these years were in reality increments. Apparently John applied pressure on Robert de Vieuxpont and Roger de Lacy to answer for their profits and they offered him a fixed sum per year—£100 and £200 respectively.[66] If the profits reported by later sheriffs of Yorkshire are safe criteria, Roger de Lacy offered only a small part of his actual profits. The total sum yielded by the profits in 1205 was well over £1,500 or roughly a third of the net value of the county farms. By Michaelmas 1206 two shrievalties had disappeared from the list of those accounting for profits. The sheriff of Norfolk and Suffolk simply did not account for them. Lincolnshire dropped out because it had acquired a farmer sheriff. In December 1205 Thomas de Moulton offered 500 marks fine and a new increment of 100 marks a year to have the shire for seven years.[67] The total profits in 1206 were about £200 lower than in 1205. At Michaelmas 1207 four more sheriffs in addition to the sheriff of Norfolk and Suffolk failed to account for their profits, and the total sank below £900.

The exchequer year of 1207-1208 saw the liquidation of a large part of the experiment. Cambridgeshire and Huntingdonshire returned to a farmer sheriff—Fulk fitz Theobold offered a fine of 120 marks and 3 palfreys and 100 marks increment for the shires. Four shires were given at farm to the ever anxious William Brewer. John's mercenary captain, Gerard de Athies, became

---

[65] *Ibid.*, p. 32.
[66] *Rot. claus.*, I, 104; Pipe roll 11 John, Public Record Office.
[67] *Pipe roll 8 John*, p. 103; *Rot. pat.*, p. 57.

farmer sheriff of Herefordshire. In Worcestershire William de Cantilupe simply stopped bothering about his profits. Of the twenty shrievalties in which John had tried to collect the profits, all but nine were once more in the hands of farmer sheriffs. As hunting for the accounts of profits through the unpublished pipe rolls is an unprofitable business, I cannot say precisely how these nine fared during the rest of the reign. I can simply state that all of them were in the hands of custodians who accounted for their profits in at least some of the later years of the reign. In short John's experiment was continued in an attenuated form.

John did not take the collapse of his idea with good grace. Three sheriffs who simply stopped accounting for their profits paid large sums for "the king's benevolence." John de Cornard, sheriff of Norfolk and Suffolk, paid 1,200 marks, Walter de Clifford, sheriff of Herefordshire, 1,000 marks, and William de Montaigu, sheriff of Dorset and Somerset, £800.[68] In addition two sheriffs whose profits as accounted for by them shrank rather astonishingly between 1205 and 1207 offered similar fines. Roger fitz Ade of Hampshire offered 1,000 marks and Hugh de Chacombe of Warwickshire and Leicestershire 800 marks.[69] King John made far more money out of these fines than he would have out of the profits of the shires.

While it seems unlikely that an attempt to abolish farmer sheriffs could have been permanently effective without a complete reorganization of the English financial administration, John's limited experiment had been quite successful during its first year. Why then was it abandoned so rapidly? Apparently the answer lies in the unwillingness of barons, important knights, and high ranking royal officials to accept appointments as custodian sheriffs. Some of this feeling was undoubtedly the result of disinclination to hold profitless offices, but probably far more important was a general dislike of innovation and a belief that to act as a mere custodian was beneath their dignity. Thus the men of the class from which the English kings had always drawn their sheriffs

[68] *Pipe roll 9 John,* p. 63; *Pipe roll 10 John,* p. 191; Pipe roll 11 John, Public Record Office.
[69] *Pipe roll 9 John,* pp. 137, 149.

were in general unavailable for appointment as custodian sheriffs. Only one group seems to have entered into John's plan with any real desire to cooperate—men who were making their way in the world as professional administrators. Men of this type were the custodian sheriffs in the counties where the experiment was most successful and was continued longest—they held six of the nine shrievalties where profits were accounted for 1207. Robert de Braybrook was in 1199 the seneschal of William de Albini and had been his under-sheriff in Bedfordshire and Buckinghamshire.[70] He became under-sheriff again when Geoffrey fitz Peter succeeded William de Albini in 1200 and in 1205 became custodian sheriff. He continued in office until his death in 1211. In 1208 he was appointed custodian sheriff of Northamptonshire as well. John de Wickenholt had been under-sheriff of Berkshire for Hubert de Burgh. He became custodian sheriff in 1205 and continued in office until the end of the reign. Thomas de Eardington started his career in 1198 as Geoffrey fitz Peter's under-sheriff in Staffordshire. In 1205 he became custodian sheriff of both Staffordshire and Shropshire—an office he held until 1216. John de Cornard was in 1200 the seneschal of Earl Richard de Clare.[71] In 1204 he became sheriff of Norfolk and Suffolk. After the commission John had appointed in 1205 found that it could not manage the shires, John de Cornard became custodian sheriff. Although he only accounted for profits once and was obliged to offer a heavy fine for the king's benevolence, he held office until late in 1209. Here then was a small group of men who owed their position in society to their office as sheriff and hence could not decline to cooperate in the king's plans. Yet they had sufficient ability and prestige to run their shires effectively. But such men were rare. As a rule the man strong enough to control a shire did not need the office badly enough to accept it as a custodian sheriff.

When King John embarked on his experiment in the autumn of 1204, he was on comparatively good terms with his barons. England was peaceful and orderly and it seemed safe to risk a few

[70] *Memoranda roll 1 John*, p. 53; *Pipe roll 10 Richard I*, p. 8.
[71] *Ibid.*, pp. 22, 55.

shires in weak hands. But by the winter and spring of 1207-1208 the storm clouds were gathering rapidly. William Marshal, lord of Leinster, and Meiler fitz Henry, justiciar of Ireland, were at open war in that dominion of the crown. William de Briouse had quarreled with Meiler and was on steadily increasingly bad terms with the king. The Lacy lords of Meath and Ulster had shown clearly their intention of supporting the earl of Pembroke and William de Briouse. In short two of John's most intimate friends, between them masters of the south Marches of Wales and of much of Ireland, were becoming his foes. Both these great barons had extensive lands in south-west England. Then in addition to this baronial threat the king's quarrel with the papacy was reaching the acute stage. John had refused to accept Stephen Langton as archbishop of Canterbury and had expelled the monks of Christ Church from the realm. The interdict was clearly not far off. Thus in that winter and spring John clearly needed strong and completely loyal sheriffs—especially in the shires threatened by a Marshal-Briouse alliance. William Brewer, who was already sheriff of Devonshire, received Dorsetshire and Somersetshire, Hampshire, Sussex, and Wiltshire—the counties where the Briouse and Marshal lands lay. The mercenary captain, Gerard de Athies, was given the vital border counties facing the south Marches—Gloucestershire and Herefordshire. In addition Hubert de Burgh, ransomed and restored to favor, became sheriff of Lincolnshire, and a newly risen royal servant, John fitz Hugh, received Surrey. In short it seems clear that King John's reasons for so largely abandoning his experiment in custodian sheriffs were basically political. In the winter and spring of 1207-1208 he needed men as sheriffs who would not accept office as custodians. In a few shires where things looked peaceful and the custodian sheriffs seemed effective, the new system was continued.

In addition to demanding increments and appointing custodian sheriffs who accounted for their profits there was another method by which the king could increase the regular revenues of the crown. He could remove a borough or manor from the sheriff's custody and rent it to someone else at a higher rate. At times the new farmer seems to have been simply an optimist who hoped that the king had set the rent low enough to yield him a profit.[72] But more often the burghers or the men of the manor became a collective farmer. In February 1201 John rented ten Yorkshire and Northumberland towns and manors to their inhabitants at an average gain of 50 per cent in revenue.[73] By the end of his reign many royal boroughs were farmed by their citizens at a considerable profit to the royal treasury.[74] It is easy to understand why the men of the boroughs and manors of the royal demesne were willing to pay a higher rent direct to the exchequer—they got rid of the control of the sheriff. The king collected a fine for making the arrangement and enjoyed the increment on the farm as well.

At Michaelmas 1205 the increments on the county farms and the profits accounted for by the custodian sheriffs came to nearly £2,500.[75] It seems likely that the boroughs and manors removed from the sheriffs' custody yielded some £1,000 above the value assigned them in the farms. If this estimate is correct, Richard and John had increased the regular revenues of the crown by £3,500. I am inclined to believe that this general level of additional revenue was maintained until the beginning of the baronial revolt. While many counties were returned to farmer sheriffs, new increments made up for much of the loss in profits. The profits accounted for by the remaining custodian-sheriffs increased in several cases as time went on. Thus there was an enormous increase in the profits of Yorkshire after the removal of Roger de Lacy. Roger had settled with the king for a fixed £200 a year—his successor accounted for profits of £700 in his first year and £587 in his second.[76] In short while John's attempt to increase his regular revenues cannot be called an unqualified success, it was by no means a complete failure.

[72] As examples see the cases of Cheltenham in Gloucestershire and Rowde in Wiltshire. *Pipe roll 9 John*, pp. 202, 210.

[73] *Rot. chart.*, pp. 85-87.

[74] Adolphus Ballard, *British borough charters 1042-1216* (Cambridge, 1913), pp. 220-231.

[75] My actual totals are £1,539 for profits and £865 for increments or a total of £2,404.

[76] Pipe rolls 11, 12, 13 John, Public Record Office.

While £3,500 was an important sum when viewed as a percentage of the regular revenues of the crown, it was small in comparison to the cost of the unsuccessful defense of John's continental possessions and the probable cost of a serious attempt to recover them. If the king's war chest was to be kept full, special levies would have to supply the bulk of the funds. When John came to the throne, there were three types of special levies sanctioned by English political tradition—the hidage or carucage, the tallage, and the scutage. The hidages and carucages levied by Richard and John were the descendants of the ancient danegeld that had been abandoned early in the reign of Henry II. They differed from the older tax in only one respect. The danegeld had been based on a traditional assessment reaching far back into the Anglo-Saxon period. By the twelfth century it had little relation to actual plow teams or area of cultivated land. The new hidages and carucages were intended to be based on an actual count of teams. Tallage was the basic levy of the seignorial system. Every lord had the right to exact tallage from the inhabitants of his demesne. In the case of the English king this meant the inhabitants of the royal boroughs, of his demesne manors, of the demesne manors of escheated baronies, and of the demesne of fiefs in the custody of the crown. It was a tax on those direct tenants of the crown who did not hold by military service or by free alms. Scutage was a levy on those who held by military service and was assessed on the basis of knights' fees. Sometimes it was a true tax—at others an alternative to service in the host. The king, like other feudal lords, was entitled to demand aid from his vassals on certain occasions such as the knighting of his eldest son and the marriage of his eldest daughter. In such cases scutage was a general tax levied on knights' fees. These levies were by their very nature comparatively rare. Far more common was the use of scutage as a means of avoiding military service. King Henry II had adopted the custom of excusing vassals from service in the host in return for a fixed payment on every knight's fee for which they owed him service. Richard and John had continued this practice with ingenious improvements. As Professor Mitchell has treated the taxation of John's reign in great detail, my discussion of these levies will be very brief and general.[77]

In seven of the sixteen years of his reign John levied general tallages. While it seems that no one of these embraced all the counties of England, the most limited covered eleven shires. As a rule the tallage was assessed by the itinerant justices. Apparently a borough or manor was given an opportunity to offer a lump sum. If the offer was high enough, it was accepted, and the inhabitants could divide the tax among themselves, collect it, and give it to the sheriff. If a satisfactory sum was not offered, the justices assessed the tax themselves on individuals. The largest amount yielded by one of these tallages was £8,276 in 1210 and the smallest £1,500 in 1203.[78] The total yield of all seven was £25,518 or an average of £3,645. Thus a single tallage was roughly equivalent to the amount by which John had increased his regular revenues. In addition to these regular royal tallages levied fairly generally John raised large sums by special tallages on baronies that were in his custody. Every baron had the right to tallage his demesne. When a barony was in the custody of the crown, the king's agents who took the place of the baron usually tallaged with great enthusiasm. Thus when the lands of Roger de Lacy were in the king's hands in 1212 the demesne manors yielded £346 in ordinary revenue and £375 in tallage. In 1209 the manors of the bishopric of Durham produced £1,260 in ordinary revenue and £1,244 in tallage.[79]

Henry II had levied eight scutages—one at two marks or £1 6s. 8d. per knight's fee, three at £1 and four at one mark or 13s. 4d. Richard collected two at £1 per fee and one at ten shillings.[80] John levied eleven scutages—in 1206 and 1209 at £1—in 1199, 1201, 1202, 1203, 1205 and 1211 at two marks, in 1204 at 2½ marks, and in 1210 and 1214 at £2.[81] Thus by the end of his

[77] Sydney Knox Mitchell, *Studies in taxation under John and Henry III* (New Haven, 1914).
[78] *Ibid.*, pp. 31-32, 68, 76-77, 82, 98, 116-118; Ramsay, *Revenues of the kings of England*, I, 261.
[79] Pipe rolls 11 and 14 John, Public Record Office.
[80] Ramsay, *Revenues of the kings of England*, I, 195, 227.
[81] *Ibid.*, p. 261.

reign John had doubled the highest rate exacted by his brother. The £2 per fee demanded by John bore the same relation to the one mark per fee of most of Henry II's scutages as the two shillings per day that John paid his knights bore to the eight pence per day paid by Henry II. But if one assumes that the English barons owed forty days' service to the crown, it required a two mark scutage rate under Henry II and a £4 rate under John to pay substitutes for the knights buying exemption. Why then, one may well ask, did John not raise the rate still higher? One reason, of course, was the force of tradition—any raise in the rate met with protests. But a more important reason was probably the enormous variation in the value of knights' fees. Those who held the poorer fees could not pay a higher rate, and even the higher rate would not go far toward tapping the resources of those who held the richer fees. The king wanted to make his vassals support his military operations according to their ability to pay.

The same problem had faced King Richard and he had invented an ingenious device for solving it. The king's tenants-in-chief owed him service if he chose to demand it. To be allowed to buy exemption by paying scutage was a favor granted by the crown, not a right of the tenant. Moreover most barons made an actual profit out of paying scutage. They could collect from their vassals at the same rate, and they usually had more knights enfeoffed than they owed the crown. Thus a baron who owed the king the service of fifty knights but who had enfeoffed sixty made £20 profit on a £2 scutage and paid nothing himself. Richard adopted the practice of demanding a fine for the privilege of not serving in the host. The baron who paid such a fine was allowed to reimburse himself in part by collecting scutage from his vassals. John continued his brother's practice. When he summoned his host, some of his vassals were allowed to buy exemption by simply paying scutage, but others were obliged to offer fines that exceeded the scutage.[82] Thus in 1201 John levied £2,468 in ordinary scutage and £3,026 in fines. While the regular scutage was at two marks per fee, those who fined paid at a rate of three or four marks. As the

---

[82] For a full discussion see Mitchell, *Studies in taxation*.

reign went on the fines grew heavier.[83] In 1204 they ran from four to seven marks per fee and in 1210 they averaged ten marks.[84] Thus our baron who owed fifty knights would pay a fine of 500 marks or £333. He could collect £120 from his sixty knights' fees at £2 each, but the rest came out of his own pocket.[85]

If one assumes that all the sums charged on the rolls would be paid eventually, John raised £22,227 in scutage and £27,312 in fines from his eleven levies or an average of £2,020 in scutage and £2,483 in fines.[86] The grand total came to £49,539. Unfortunately it brought its full share of ill-will. While ordinary scutage was not a heavy financial burden on the great barons, collecting it from their vassals must have been a costly nuisance. The fines weighed heavily on the barons themselves. Moreover the scutage alone must have been a serious drain on many poor knights' fees. Then in order to collect scutage eleven times John had to squeeze the theoretical justification for such levies rather thin. From 1199 through 1203 he was conducting campaigns on the continent and the levies were probably justified. But the campaigns for which the scutages of 1204 and 1205 were collected never took place. While the host was summoned and scutage and fines assessed, no large-scale expedition was made. The last five scutages of the reign were connected with genuine military operations and hence were justified. But when one considers that Henry II took eight scutages in thirty-four years, Richard three in ten years, and John eleven in sixteen years, it is easy to see why the barons began to object to the levy. The king had developed scutage into an important source of revenue, but it had been done at a high political cost.

John levied only one carucage and very little is known about it. Early in 1200 he promised King Philip Augustus a relief of 20,000 marks for the fiefs which he held of the French crown and the

---

[83] *Ibid.*, pp. 36, 37-40.

[84] *Ibid.*, pp. 66, 99.

[85] For a general discussion of the military service due the crown see Painter, *Feudal baronies*, pp. 20-44.

[86] These figures are taken from Mitchell. Ramsay does not distinguish between scutage and fines and gives only the total actually collected the year the levy was made.

carucage was intended to raise money for this purpose.[87] The tax was referred to as "pennies assessed on ploughs for the king's aid," "pennies assessed on ploughs by the common assize of England," and the "aid from ploughs."[88] It was assessed and collected by special agents called "receivers of the carucage."[89] As these receivers did not render an account at the exchequer, there are only incidental references to the levy on the pipe rolls. The sheriff of Berkshire paid the tax on eleven ploughs on the royal demesne and claimed credit for it.[90] The custodians of the honor of Gloucester also claimed credit for the tax paid on its demesne ploughs.[91] Several prelates offered fines for exemption from the tax.[92] Some prelates apparently objected to paying the levy. John's half-brother, Geoffrey, archbishop of York, had his lands seized by the sheriff of Yorkshire, and refusal to allow the collection of carucage in his lands was at least one of the causes for the seizure.[93] But as John and his brother were always quarreling about something, it is hard to feel certain that opposition to the tax was the chief issue. Then a bitter and protracted feud between the king and the Cistercian order arose from John's financial exactions.[94] While the collection of carucage may have been the basis of this dispute, John was accustomed to demanding money from the Cistercians whenever his treasury looked empty and he may well have been seeking additional gifts at this time.

As there is no account of the carucage of 1200 on the pipe roll, we have no evidence as to how much money it yielded. In 1220 a carucage at the rate of two shillings brought in £5,483.[95] If John's tax of three shillings was assessed on the same basis, it should have yielded £7,524. While this was about twice the amount of the average tallage and 67 per cent more than the average scutage, it must have been far more difficult to assess and collect than the other levies. The fact that John did not again levy a carucage suggests that he did not consider it worth the trouble.

[87] Mitchell, *Studies in taxation*, pp. 32-34.
[88] *Pipe roll 2 John*, pp. 128, 185, 239.
[89] *Pipe roll 3 John*, p. 222.
[90] *Pipe roll 2 John*, p. 185.
[91] *Ibid.*, p. 128.
[92] *Ibid.*, pp. 47, 239.
[93] Hovedon, IV, 139-140.
[94] Coggeshall, p. 102.
[95] Mitchell, *Studies in taxation*, pp. 129-136.

While carucage, tallage, and scutage were the traditional special levies of the English monarchy, Henry II and Richard had experimented with taxes on income and movable property. The Saladin tithe of 1188 that was intended to raise money for the crusade called for the payment by everyone of one-tenth of his revenue and movables.[96] Then in 1193 Queen Eleanor and the commission of justices ruling England during Richard's absence levied a tax of one quarter of all revenues and movables to supply money for the king's ransom.[97] If effectively assessed and collected this would be an extremely heavy tax yielding an enormous sum. The one-thirteenth collected by John in 1207 brought in £57,421 and at that rate a tax of one-quarter should yield some £160,000. Actually the tax of one-quarter seems to have yielded somewhere between £50,000 and £60,000. As other levies were made during that same year, it clearly did not provide the full sum needed—£66,666. But the other taxes yielded no great amount and the bulk of the ransom must have come from the tax on revenues and movables. If it actually brought in £50,000, one can easily understand John's interest in such taxes.

According to Wendover when John returned to England in December 1203, he accused his earls and barons of deserting him and demanded from them one-seventh of their movable property. A later sentence indicates that ecclesiastics were also taxed.[98] But Wendover's account is too vague to be of much use in determining just what the tax consisted of. Moreover he is clearly wrong as to the time of the levy. As Mr. Mitchell has pointed out, the tax was being collected in the summer of 1203.[99] Beyond the statements in the chronicles we have only three references to this tax. Two of them suggest that Wendover may have been right in speaking of it as a levy on the movables of the barons.[100] Yet John ordered Geoffrey fitz Peter to allow the count of Aumale to have

---

[96] *Ibid.*, pp. 5-7; William Stubbs, *Select charters and other illustrations of English constitutional history* (Oxford, 1895), p. 160.
[97] Hovedon, III, 210.
[98] Wendover, I, 318.
[99] Mitchell, *Studies in taxation,* p. 62.
[100] *Rot. liberate,* p. 47; *Pipe roll 6 John,* p. 256.

the "seventh pence of his lands."[101] This seems to indicate a general levy. The problem cannot be solved on the basis of the evidence available. We do not know whether it was, like the earlier levies, a tax on both revenues and movables or on movables alone. Nor do we know whether it bore only on the personal property of barons and prelates or whether like its predecessors it was a general levy. And we have no idea how much it yielded. Considering our lack of information about the nature of the tax, Ramsay's estimate of its yield based on the return from the thirteenth of 1207 seems completely unjustified.[102] Yet the fact that John tried this type of tax again seems to indicate that the results were not too disappointing.

In the summer of 1206 John led an army to Poitou and conducted a campaign against his former vassals who had done homage to King Philip. He succeeded in getting a firm hold on Poitou and securing it for two years by a truce with the French king. But beyond the borders of Poitou his only success was a brief occupation of Angers. This expedition probably used up a good proportion of John's war-chest and showed him clearly how great an effort would be needed to recover Normandy, Maine, and Anjou. He returned to England determined to raise money for another and far larger venture when his truce with Philip expired. On January 8, 1207, the prelates and barons of the realm met in council at London. John asked the prelates to grant him as an aid a percentage of the revenue of every beneficed ecclesiastic in England. When the prelates hesitated to accede to this request, the council was adjourned. It met again in Oxford on February 2. The prelates then informed the king that they could not allow the clergy to pay a tax that had never before been demanded even from laymen.[103] The Saladin tithe and the tax for Richard's ransom had been forgotten. The statement of the clergy seems to indicate that the seventh of 1203 had taxed only movable property. John let the matter drop for the time being as far as the clergy

---

[101] *Rot. liberate*, p. 43.
[102] Ramsay, *Revenues of the kings of England*, I, 238.
[103] *Annals of Waverley* (ed. H. R. Luard in *Annales monastici*, II, Rolls Series), p. 258.

were concerned. Later in the year he used the familiar device of asking them for a gift.[104]

The lay barons were apparently unable to make an effective opposition to the king's demand, and on February 17 writs were issued providing for the collection of the tax.[105] John announced that the levy had been authorized by "the common counsel and assent of our council at Oxford for the defense of our realm and the recovery of our rights." Thus the king seemed to recognize that this was a special tax that he could not levy without the consent of his vassals. As a seigneur he could tallage his demesne and as a feudal lord he could collect scutage or fines from those who wanted to avoid the military service they owed. Perhaps he considered that the ancient tradition of the danegeld gave him the right to levy a carucage. But this tax was beyond the range of feudal and seignorial rights and of English political tradition. It required the assent of his feudal court.

Every layman in England was to pay twelve pence for every mark of annual revenue he enjoyed and twelve pence for every mark's worth of chattels he possessed on February 9, the day the council came to an end. Although the tax was generally called a thirteenth even in official documents coming from the royal chancery, it was actually not quite so heavy—a shilling out of every thirteen shillings and four pence. Groups of justices were to be sent into all the shires. The seneschal or other agent of each baron was to appear before these justices to swear to the value of his lord's and his own income and chattels. Every other layman was to appear to swear to his own income and movables. The justices were to keep a careful record of the assessments by parishes and by hundreds. At the end of every two weeks a copy was to be made of the justices' roll and turned over to the sheriff who was to proceed to collect the tax. Any one found guilty of avoiding "our convenience" by fraudulently removing chattels to some other place or concealing them in any way would have his chattels seized and be committed to prison at the king's pleasure. The same

---

[104] *Rot. pat.*, pp. 71-72; *Annals of Margam*, p. 28.
[105] *Rot. pat.*, p. 72; Gervase of Canterbury, II, lviii-lix.

penalty would be visited on those who underestimated their income or movables.

There was both covert and open opposition to the tax. On May 27 Hugh de Neville was ordered to seize Richmond castle because its hereditary constable, Ruald fitz Alan, had refused to swear to the value of his income and chattels. Ruald had to offer a fine of 200 marks and four palfreys to recover the castle.[106] William fitz Martin, a Devonshire baron, paid twenty marks to free his bailiff who was arrested for underestimating William's property by twenty shillings.[107] Another baron, Philip de Valognes, was forgiven a penalty for an unspecified offense in connection with the tax.[108] Several lesser men were clapped into prison and had to pay fines for their release.[109]

As the sanctity of monasteries made them comparatively safe from violence, they were favorite places for the deposit of money and valuables. The fact that ecclesiastical revenues and chattels were exempt from the tax made the monasteries excellent places of concealment for property subject to the thirteenth. On April 16 a royal writ directed the abbots, priors, and religious of Lincolnshire to turn over to the justices assessing the tax and the sheriff of the county all money deposited or concealed in their houses.[110] Since the Cistercians had no lay tenants, their lands were entirely free from the tax collectors. As a result Cistercian monasteries were ideal places of concealment. Chattels belonging to the countess of Aumale were seized at the Cistercian abbey of Vaudey.[111] Money belonging to her seneschal, Fulk de Oiry, was taken from Swineshead, another abbey of that order. Just to be on the safe side the king's officers seized the money the monks of Swineshead had been saving for a building fund. The chattels and the money were returned, but Fulk paid twenty marks as a fine.[112] The Cistercian abbey of Furness was also suspected of concealing laymen's chat-

[106] *Rot. pat.*, pp. 72-73; *Rot. oblatis*, p. 372.
[107] *Ibid.*, p. 374.
[108] *Rot. claus.*, I, 85.
[109] *Rot. pat.*, p. 73; *Rot. oblatis*, p. 430; *Pipe roll 9 John*, p. 45.
[110] *Rot. pat.*, p. 71; *Annals of Waverley*, pp. 258-259.
[111] *Rot. claus.*, I, 84.
[112] *Ibid.*, p. 85; *Rot. oblatis*, p. 393; *Pipe roll 9 John*, p. 29.

tels and it did not escape so easily. Two of its estates were seized and the chattels on them sold. The sheriff of Lancashire was ordered to credit the money received for the chattels against the abbey's debts to the crown and to keep any balance for the king's use.

Some at least of the prelates were not pleased at the idea of having the king's justices roaming over their lands assessing their tenants. The bishop of Bath offered 700 marks to cover the *dona* or gifts expected from him and from his churches of Bath and Welles and to obtain exemption from the tax for his tenants.[113] The abbot of Abingdon offered 600 marks to free his tenants from the tax and presumably this sum included his own gift.[114] The prior and monks of Christ Church, Canterbury, gave 1,000 marks "for the thirteenth" and it seems likely that this too represented their own gift and a fine to exempt their tenants.[115] The *Annals of Dunstaple* state that "the king had 100 marks from Dunstaple in addition to a bribe to the sheriff and a fine of eleven marks for our demesnes."[116] While this is rather vague, it apparently means that Dunstaple gave 100 marks to acquit its tenants and eleven as its own gift. The royal writ granting exemption for the tenants of the abbot of Abingdon shows that this prelate planned to raise at least part of the money for his fine by collecting the thirteenth himself from his tenants and it is probable that the other prelates who offered fines had the same intention. Their object was not to spare their tenants but simply to exclude the royal justices from their lands. The haughty and irascible archbishop of York followed his usual uncompromising course. He denied the king's right to tax the tenants of the lands held by the church and excommunicated the justices who entered his estates. John's natural answer was to seize the barony into his own hands and collect the tax with a heavy hand. Geoffrey and his suffragan, Philip, bishop of Durham, made a personal plea to the king, but John merely laughed

---

[113] *Rot. claus.*, I, 79; *Pipe roll 9 John*, p. 63; *Rot. oblatis*, p. 413.
[114] *Rot. claus.*, I, 84.
[115] *Rot. oblatis*, p. 413.
[116] *Annals of Dunstaple* (ed. H. R. Luard in *Annales monastici*, III, Rolls series), p. 29.

at them.[117] Geoffrey promptly left England, but Philip of Durham offered the king the enormous amount of £1,000 for his "benevolence" and the privilege of collecting the tax from his own tenants.[118]

Little is known about how the machinery set up for the assessment and collection of the thirteenth worked in practice. In Warwickshire and Leicestershire the first group of justices sent to assess the tax got into difficulties and on May 26 Robert de Ropsley and a royal clerk were despatched to straighten things out.[119] On July 13 Robert replaced Hugh de Chacombe as sheriff and Hugh offered a fine of 800 marks for the king's benevolence, but Hugh's fall from favor may have been the result of his poor record in accounting for his profits rather than his inefficiency in collecting the thirteenth.[120] We have already seen that there was trouble in Lincolnshire at least over chattels concealed in monasteries. A complete list of the assessing justices has been preserved for only one shire—Lincolnshire. The group consisted of fourteen men headed by Robert de Percy, a favorite servant of John, Simon de Kyme, a prominent Lincolnshire baron, and William de Cornhill, one of John's most trusted clerks.[121] It is interesting to see that Fulk de Oiry who was at least suspected of concealing his chattels and who paid a fine for it was one of the assessing justices.

An entry on the oblate roll states that the royal treasury had actually received £57,421 from the proceeds of the thirteenth and the gifts made by the prelates. Another £2,615 was still owed and two sheriffs had not yet rendered their accounts to the special exchequer set up to handle the tax.[122] Thus the total yield of the tax was over £60,000—a sum over twice as large as John's total income in any one of the first four years of his reign.[123] From the king's point of view this must have been the ideal tax. Those who lived from the produce of agriculture paid on their income, stock,

[117] Gervase of Canterbury, II, lix.
[118] Mitchell, *Studies in taxation*, p. 89, note 21.
[119] *Rot. pat.*, p. 72.
[120] *Ibid.*, p. 74; *Pipe roll 9 John*, p. 137.
[121] Gervase of Canterbury, II, lix.
[122] *Rot. oblatis*, p. 459; *Rot. claus.*, I, 86; *Pipe roll 9 John*, p. 63.
[123] Ramsay, *Revenues of the kings of England*, I, 261.

and stored grain. The merchant paid on his capital whether in cash or inventory. Thus the actual wealth of the country was tapped directly. But the tax was unpopular both because it was heavy and because it was unusual. It required complicated machinery to assess and collect it. Never again during John's reign was the condition of England to be stable enough for him to try another income and property tax. Nevertheless the memory of its success remained, and it became the model for later royal taxation. Moreover John's apparent recognition of the fact that he needed to obtain his vassals' consent before levying a special tax formed an important constitutional precedent.

The most novel of John's financial innovations were his experiments in levying import and export duties on a national scale. As customs revenues were soon to form an extremely important part of the income of the English crown, these early experiments are both interesting and significant. While foreign trade had not been entirely free under John's predecessors, the dues collected from it were local tolls of various kinds and the revenues went to local authorities.[124] Obviously some of this revenue found its way into the royal treasury through the farms paid by the king's ports, but the process was very indirect. It was extremely difficult to keep the farms of the ports adjusted to the volume of trade and the town's income from it. Not only was the total amount of trade expanding, but it was shifting from port to port. Dunwich in Suffolk was losing business and was in serious financial difficulty. John was obliged to reduce its farm.[125] On the other hand during his reign the farm of Newcastle-on-Tyne was advanced from £50 to £100.[126] But this was obviously an inefficient means of tapping the profits of England's growing foreign trade. Moreover a number of the richest ports including the second in respect to volume of foreign trade belonged to the king's vassals, and he obtained no revenue from their dues.[127] The only tax on trade that could

---

[124] See for instance the list of dues belonging to St. Augustine of Canterbury in certain ports in Dugdale, *Monasticon*, I, 142-143.
[125] *Rot. chart.*, p. 159.
[126] *Ibid.*, pp. 86, 190.
[127] Notably Boston and Lynn. *Pipe roll 6 John*, p. 218.

be called national was the king's *prise* on imported wine. While definite figures are unobtainable, it seems clear that this did not even supply the bibulous needs of the royal court and the king's garrisons.

In the summer of 1202 John established customs duties amounting to one-fifteenth of goods imported or exported.[128] Two years later detailed regulations were drawn up for its collection.[129] General responsibility for collecting the duties rested on three men—Reginald de Cornhill, William de Furnell, and William de Wrotham. It would be but a slight exaggeration to call Reginald de Cornhill John's business manager. Since the early twelfth century the Cornhills had been the chief merchant family of London. Under Richard and John they obtained a status that was practically baronial. Reginald was sheriff of Kent until his death in 1210. For considerable periods he was chamberlain of London—an office that made him the crown's chief purchasing agent. He was usually deeply involved in the operations of the king's mints and exchanges.[130] William de Wrotham was a man of even more varied activities. He held the high ecclesiastical dignity of archdeacon of Taunton, was hereditary royal forester of Dorsetshire and Somersetshire, and usually had the care of the tin mines of Cornwall and Devon. He also had his finger in the affairs of the royal mint. In addition he was John's First Lord of the Admiralty. He was ordinarily responsible for the building and upkeep of the king's ships and the hiring, paying, and disciplining of the crews.[131] Subject to the general authority of the king and the justiciar, these three "chief custodians" had complete control of the collection of the fifteenth.

The chief custodians were provided with deputies in every port. The men of each port were to select six or seven of the "wisest, most politically important, and richest" of their fellow citizens to act as local collectors in conjunction with a knight and a clerk who

[128] *Ibid.*
[129] *Rot. pat.*, pp. 42-43.
[130] *Rot. claus.*, I, 18, 27, 55, 88, 109; *Rot. pat.*, p. 54; *Pipe roll 7 John*, p. 10. *Rot. oblatis*, p. 297.
[131] *Rot. pat.*, pp. 54, 68, 86; *Pipe roll 1 John*, pp. 242-243; *Pipe roll 7 John*, pp. 10, 22, 27; *Pipe roll 10 John*, pp. 170-171.

were presumably the appointees of the chief custodians. No ship was to load or unload except under the supervision of these "bailiffs of the fifteenth." The collectors were to keep a careful record of the names of merchants and the sums paid by them. The money was to be kept in a chest with three or four separate locks. The local collectors could arrest those who tried to avoid the tax, but they could not accept fines for such offenses. This right was reserved to the chief custodians. Apparently John did not consider it safe to give the local collectors full power to assess and collect the duties on the most important of English exports—the large amounts of wool grown by the abbeys. No merchant was to take wool from an abbey until he obtained letters from the chief custodians stating the amount and the value. The local collectors levied the tax on the basis of these letters. In addition to collecting the customs duties the bailiffs of the fifteenth were expected to enforce a royal embargo on the export of arms and food stuffs. Arms could be taken from the realm only by those going abroad on the king's service and the export of food required a license from the justiciar.

While we can form a fairly clear picture of how the fifteenth was assessed and collected, its exact incidence is extremely hard to determine. John's original intention seems to have been to levy it on merchants from the lands of his enemy, Philip Augustus.[132] Wool was the chief English export, and Flanders which was the most important market for it was a fief of the French crown. Flemish merchants seeking wool and importing merchandise to pay for it were probably the largest group of foreign traders in England. Hence even this limited levy would tap a fair part of England's foreign trade. But it is clear that by 1204 the duties were being collected from all foreign merchants.[133] It is, however, impossible to be certain whether or not English merchants had to pay the duties. The only evidence that they did is the fact that the citizens of London offered a fine to be exempt from it.[134] I am inclined to believe that it became in 1204 a general levy on imports

[132] *Rot. pat.*, pp. 14, 42-43.
[133] *Ibid.*, pp. 39, 43, 44; *Rot. claus.*, I, 3, 7.
[134] *Rot. oblatis*, p. 341.

and exports. The almost complete lack of reference to English merchants in connection with the tax is probably explainable by the fact that most of the kingdom's external trade was carried on by foreigners.

An account has been preserved of the receipts from the fifteenth for the period extending from July 20, 1202, to November 30, 1204. The grand total was £4,958.[135] Although no further accounts seem to have survived, the duties were still in force in 1206.[136] On July 13, 1207, the bailiffs were summoned to appear before William de Wrotham to render their final accounts for the fifteenth.[137] One might well ask why John abandoned this fruitful source of revenue—some £2,500 a year was a decided addition to his exchequer. The answer apparently lies in the original purpose of the levy. In October 1206 John made a truce for two years with King Philip and one of its provisions was that there should be free trade between the two realms.[138] This was interpreted as banning duties like the fifteenth.

John seems to have conducted another more limited experiment in levying customs, but unfortunately very little is known about it. At Michaelmas 1210 the coasts of England were divided into districts and placed in charge of custodians. They collected duties on woad, a product used in dyeing wool, and on grain. A partial account of receipts for the period from Michaelmas 1210 to Mid-Lent 1211 appears on the pipe roll, and in a separate entry John fitz Hugh accounted for the duties on woad for a year and a half.[139] It is possible that when the pipe rolls for the later years of John's reign are published, some more information on these duties may come to light.

In addition to the regular revenues, the income from fines and penalties, and the receipts from various kinds of taxes, the financial resources of the English crown included several monopolies from which it drew profits. The most important of these was the Jews. The Jews were completely at the king's mercy. They were in England because he permitted them to be, and their safety de-

---
[135] *Pipe roll 6 John,* p. 218.
[136] *Rot. oblatis,* p. 341. [138] Rymer, *Foedera,* I, 95.
[137] *Rot. pat.,* p. 74. [139] Pipe roll 13 John, Public Record Office.

pended on his protection. The only occupation they were allowed to follow was money-lending, and they carried that on essentially for the king's profit. Whenever the crown was in need of funds the Jews were tallaged, asked for a loan, or persuaded to offer a large fine—it made little difference which method was used. Although the royal charters to the Jews promised free inheritance of property, in practice heirs had to buy their inheritance at any price the king asked. He usually took a third as his share and left the rest to the heirs as working capital.[140] A Jew had practically no chance of collecting a debt from a Christian without the king's aid, and he had to pay for that assistance. While the fee for this service varied, it was usually two shillings on the pound or 10 per cent.[141] It seems probable that John meant to establish this as a standard fee, but his greed often led him to demand more. When the king needed the friendship of a baron, he often forgave him his debts to the Jews.[142] On several occasions John freed men from their debts to the Jews in return for armed service in his host.[143] In short the crown regarded the property of the Jews as its own and simply allowed them to use it so that it might increase. If a Jew was suspected of concealing his resources, no torture was considered too savage to induce him to divulge the hiding place of his funds.

The machinery for exploiting the Jews of England had been developing gradually during Richard's reign. Its inauguration was the result of a series of anti-Semitic riots that occurred as the king's crusading companions were leaving England. While religious enthusiasm may have inspired the rioters, they were careful to destroy as many as possible of the documents that recorded the debts owed to the Jews. As the king regarded the Jews' money as his own, he was determined to prevent the destruction of their notes. In 1194 after his return to England Richard issued a decree setting up an organization to safeguard his interests. All the

[140] *Rot. oblatis*, pp. 391, 420.
[141] *Ibid.*, pp. 201, 205, 210, 231, 236, 246, 248, 297; *Pipe roll 2 John*, pp. 207, 234.
[142] *Rot. pat.*, pp. 16, 30, 82, 85; *Rot. liberate*, pp. 38, 48; *Rot. claus.*, I, 30; *Cartae antiquae rolls*, no. 308.
[143] *Rot. liberate*, pp. 42, 44.

property of the Jews, notes, pledges, lands, houses, revenues, and chattels were to be listed. There were to be six or seven places in England where the Jews could make loans. In each place two Christians, two Jews, and two scribes were to supervise the making of loans under the direction of a clerk appointed by the king's custodians of the Jews, William de Sainte-Mère-Eglise and William de Chemillé. One copy of the note promising payment of the loan was given to the Jew who loaned the money and another was to be kept in a chest with three locks. The two Christians had the key to one lock, the two Jews to the other, and the clerk of the custodians had the key to the third. The clerk was to keep a roll containing copies of all notes. All payments made to the Jews by their debtors were to be made before these groups and rolls were to be kept of such payments.[144] This system made certain that in the future nothing could be gained by killing your Jewish creditor and burning his records. The royal government always had another copy of the note and knew the exact unpaid balance. Moreover the king's officials could form a pretty accurate estimate of the individual and combined resources of the Jews.

Shortly before Richard's accession the death of Aaron of Lincoln who had conducted his money-lending business on a vast scale brought into the hands of the crown a large number of notes, and the royal government proceeded to collect them. It was a long, slow process. By the latter years of Richard's reign the remnants of the obligations to Aaron had combined with notes due to other Jews to make a formidable total. Apparently the collection of these debts was until 1198 in the hands of William de Sainte-Mère-Eglise and a Jew called Jacob of London who bore the title of priest of all the Jews of England.[145] Jacob's office seems to have gone back to the reign of Henry II. In February 1198 Richard set up a more complicated central organization. Two royal justices, Simon de Pattishall and Henry de Wickenton, and a Poitevin Jew called Benedict de Talmont were appointed custodians of the Jews.[146] Joseph Aaron, apparently a converted Jew who even-

---

[144] Hovedon, III, 266-267.
[145] Richardson, Introduction to *Memoranda roll 1 John*, pp. xc-xcii, 72.
[146] *Pipe roll 10 Richard I*, pp. 125, 165, 210.

tually died a canon of Shrewsbury, was listed with them at times.[147] As the two royal justices were busy officials, it seems likely that Benedict did most of the work.[148] Certainly he presented the only account preserved of their collections.

Shortly after John came to the throne he confirmed Jacob of London in his office as priest of the Jews, but he does not seem to have restored to him his duties as debt collector.[149] Then in April 1200 the king appointed a new group of custodians or justices of the Jews—William de Albini, William de Warren, Thomas de Neville, and Geoffrey de Norwich.[150] William de Albini was an important baron known for his military prowess. After the charter of appointment he is never mentioned again as a justice of the Jews. William de Warren, lord of Wormegay, was also a baron, but he continued to serve at least nominally until his death in 1209.[151] Thomas de Neville continued as a justice of the Jews throughout John's reign. In 1205 he was given a manor in Essex and in 1212 he became archdeacon of Shropshire.[152] Geoffrey de Norwich became involved in the conspiracy of Robert fitz Walter in 1212 and died in a royal prison.[153] These three men had charge of the king's copies of notes recording debts to Jews, kept track of payments made, and generally supervised the king's interests. They were sometimes spoken of as the "exchequer of the Jews." Their designation as justices of the Jews suggests that part of their work was to settle disputes arising from the money-lending operations. The king's writs dealing with debts owed to the Jews were addressed to them. While some of the debts of the Jews were collected by the regular exchequer and appear on the pipe rolls, it seems probable that many more were collected by the justices.

As the Jews were a valuable source of revenue, John was determined to protect them against everyone except himself. On April

[147] *Ibid.*, p. 210; *Memoranda roll 1 John*, p. 72; *Rot. claus.*, I, 116.
[148] *Memoranda roll 1 John*, p. 69.
[149] *Rot. chart.*, pp. 6-7.
[150] *Ibid.*, p. 61.
[151] *Rot. oblatis*, p. 425.
[152] *Rot. claus.*, I, 19, 220, 223; *Rot. chart.*, pp. 141, 187.
[153] See below, pp. 270-272.

10, 1201, he issued a formal charter for the Jews of England and Normandy.[154] The Jews of England offered a fine of 4,000 marks for this grant.[155] The wording of the document suggests that it was essentially a renewal of a charter of King Henry I. The Jews were to live "freely and honorably" in John's lands and to hold their property. They were to have all the privileges they possessed in the reign of Henry I. If a Jew accused a Christian or a Christian a Jew of a criminal offense, the accuser was expected to produce two witnesses—one Christian and one Jew. If a Jew was accused and no witnesses were produced, he could free himself by an oath "on his book." When a Christian accused a Jew, the Jew was to be judged by his peers—that is by other Jews. No Jew was to be involved in a civil plea except before the king or "those who guard our towers in which the bailiffs of the Jews stay." This seems to mean that such cases would be heard by the constables of royal castles rather than the bailiffs themselves. Actually in John's reign this function was clearly performed by the justices of the Jews or by the ordinary royal justices. On the economic side the charter promised that a Jew's heir would inherit his money and his notes. The Jews could buy and receive anything except sacred objects. A Jew could sell anything pledged to him for a loan after he had held it a year and a day—presumably after the note was due. Jews could travel with their property wherever they pleased. They were to be quit of all tolls in England and Normandy. In short John made sure that his subjects would not exploit his Jews. Another charter issued the same day allowed the Jews to settle by their own law in their own courts all quarrels among themselves that did not involve pleas of the crown.

In the summer of 1203 John apparently received complaints that his Jews were being molested in London. The result was a strong letter of reproof addressed to the mayor and barons of the city. The king reminded them that the Jews were in his special protection. Attacks upon them were a violation of the peace of the realm. "If we give our peace to a dog, it ought to be preserved inviolate." The mayor and barons of London were to defend the Jews and prevent foolish men from harming them.[156]

[154] *Rot. chart.*, p. 93.   [155] *Rot. oblatis*, p. 133.   [156] *Rot. pat.*, p. 33.

Except for scattered notices of fines offered by Jews and fees paid by them to collect the debts owed them there is little information about John's financial relations with his Jews. The chroniclers state that in 1210 he levied a tallage on them of 66,000 marks, but this looks like one of the round figures so well liked by mediæval writers and may mean simply a very large sum.[157] In 1211 John fitz Hugh accounted for £430 collected by him of a tallage placed on the Jews at Bristol on November 1, 1210. The roll carries the tallage paid by some Jews, amounts raised by selling the chattels of others, and several fines offered presumably in lieu of tallage.[158] On July 26, 1213, the constable of Bristol was ordered to hold in prison all Jews who had not paid their tallage, and the sheriffs were ordered to send all such culprits to Bristol.[159] There are references to tortures inflicted on the imprisoned Jews.[160] In 1215 Thomas de Neville, the last survivor of John's justices of the Jews, was directed to accept pledges for future payment from poor Jews who had fled England because they could not pay the tallage.[161] It is far from clear whether all these references refer to a single tallage or several. On the whole it seems probable that an extremely heavy tallage was levied in 1210 and that a long period was covered by the attempts to collect it. While this tallage is the only one for which there is solid evidence, it is clear that John was engaged in wringing money from the Jews in 1204-1205, and there may well have been a tallage at that time.[162]

Another monopoly from which John drew revenue was the exchange and minting of money. This was not an absolute royal monopoly. A small number of great ecclesiastics had their own mints and exchanges. The mint and exchange at Durham belonged to the bishop of Durham and the abbot of St. Edmunds had these facilities in his town.[163] The archbishop of Canterbury had a mint

---

[157] Wendover, II, 54-55; *Annals of Waverley*, p. 264; *Annals of Margam*, p. 29.
[158] Pipe roll 13 John, Public Record Office.
[159] *Rot. pat.*, p. 102; *Rot. claus.*, I, 139.
[160] Wendover, II, 54-55. In 1226-1228 several houses in Lincoln were escheats because of Jews slain at Bristol. *Book of fees*, I, 365.
[161] *Rot. claus.*, I, 186.
[162] *Ibid.*, pp. 20, 25; *Rot. pat.*, p. 38.
[163] *Pipe roll 8 Richard I*, p. 261; *Rot. chart.*, p. 156.

and an exchange in Canterbury, but the crown had its own there as well.[164] In Chichester the king had two dies for making money and the bishop one.[165] But with these few exceptions the privilege of exchanging and making money was reserved to the crown. The profits from this monopoly seem to have fluctuated greatly from year to year, and it is difficult to estimate them with any confidence. As the chief business of the exchanges was to handle the wide variety of coins brought to England by foreign merchants, their income would vary with the amount of foreign trade. The accepted fee for exchanging money was apparently six pence in the pound.[166] As the moneyers struck 240 twenty-two and a half grain pennies out of a pound of silver, there should have been a 6 per cent profit in minting coins.[167] When John came to the throne he owed Hugh Oissel, an enterprising Flemish merchant who had settled in England, 1,700 marks and gave him the profits of the exchange for two years to discharge the obligation.[168] But Hugh may have been simply writing off part of a dubious debt. During the year 1201-1202 he ran the exchanges and mints of England as custodian and accounted for profits of £166.[169] Reginald de Cornhill who succeeded him accounted for £378 for twenty-one months.[170] John's reform of the coinage that we shall discuss in the next paragraph raised the profits greatly. In 1205-1206 the mint and exchange of London alone brought in £710 and in 1211 John fitz Hugh accounted for their profits for a year and a half at £1,132.[171]

There is a fair amount of evidence to indicate that the English currency was in a bad state when John came to the throne.[172] There had not been a new coinage since the time of Henry II, and Englishmen were enthusiastic clippers of the king's silver pennies.

---

[164] *Ibid.*, p. 24.
[165] *Rot. claus.*, I, p. 32.
[166] *Rot. pat.*, p. 54.
[167] A. E. Feavearyear, *The pound sterling* (Oxford, 1931), pp. 7, 350.
[168] *Rot. chart.*, p. 12.
[169] *Pipe roll 4 John*, p. 289.
[170] *Pipe roll 7 John*, p. 10.
[171] *Ibid.* Pipe roll 13 John, Public Record Office.
[172] Coggeshall, p. 151; *Annals of Waverley*, p. 256; *Rot. claus.*, I, 3, 28.

As Mr. Sidney Smith has suggested, this situation undoubtedly complicated foreign trade, but I suspect that was not what really troubled King John.[173] While some of the royal revenue was payable by weight, a much larger part was payable in standard currency. Thus John lost through the lightness of the pennies. The fact that reform of the coinage took place at the same time as the experiments with custodian sheriffs seems to indicate that it was essentially part of the general effort to improve the royal revenue. Moreover the very process of reform swelled the profits of the exchange.

On November 9, 1204, King John took the first step toward currency reform. The sheriffs of England were directed to proclaim at markets, fairs, and religious celebrations that no one should possess clipped money after January 13, 1205. If clipped pennies were found in the possession of a burgher, they should be pierced and seized for the king's benefit. The burgher should be arrested and released in the care of pledges and his chattels should be seized. A Jew should be thrown in prison and his goods seized. But if the clipped money was found in the possession of a country gentleman or peasant, it should be pierced and returned to him. The countryman who was presumably unused to handling money escaped more easily than those who lived by commerce and moneylending. Four good men were to be appointed in every borough, castle, and market town to enforce these regulations.[174]

Then on January 26, 1205, John issued his "assize of money." Old money, that is pennies of previous coinages, were to continue to be acceptable if they were not underweight by more than one-eighth. If anyone was in doubt as to whether or not his coins came up to this standard, he could obtain from the mint a penny-weight that represented the minimum acceptable. With this he could test his coins. Pennies that were more than an eighth underweight were to be pierced. The new money was to be made with a rim and no part of the coin was to protrude beyond the rim. This device was obviously intended to discourage clipping. Moreover if anyone was found with clipped pennies of the new coinage,

[173] Sidney Smith, Introduction to *Pipe roll 7 John,* pp. xxvii-xxxii.
[174] *Rot. pat.,* pp. 47-48.

he was to be arrested as a thief. A later sentence made this more specific—the culprit was to have all his chattels seized and he was to be thrown in prison at the king's mercy. Thus clipping was made more difficult and the penalties for it increased. Finally the assize reserved for the royal exchanges and the exchange of the archbishop of Canterbury the right to issue new pennies in exchange for the old. The fee for this service was set at six pence for each pound.[175] As Hubert Walter died some six months later and his exchange and mint came into the king's hands, John got all the profits from his new coinage.[176]

The enforcement of the assize of money was placed in the hands of two of the men who had supervised the collection of the fifteenth —William de Wrotham and Reginald de Cornhill.[177] They personally ran and accounted for the exchanges and mints at London and Canterbury including those of the archbishop at the latter place.[178] The bishop of Chichester was given the farm of the two royal dies in his town.[179] The seneschal of the household, Peter de Stoke, offered sixty marks for the mint and exchange of Northampton for one year.[180] Reginald de Cornhill acting without his fellow custodian apparently as a private venture gave a fine of sixty marks to have the mint and exchange of Oxford for a year.[181] Two men offered 400 marks for those at York while 240 marks and a dolia of wine were given for the mint and exchange at Winchester.[182] Apparently the opportunity for profit in connection with exchanging new money for old made men anxious to buy the farm of the king's mints and exchanges. Except for London and Canterbury all of them were let at farm in 1205.[183] But as mints could be and were closed and reopened easily, it is difficult to be certain how many were in operation at any one time. Eight mints are

---

[175] *Ibid.*, p. 54.
[176] *Pipe roll 7 John*, p. 10.
[177] *Rot. pat.*, p. 54.
[178] *Pipe roll 7 John*, p. 10.
[179] *Ibid.*, p. 110; *Rot. oblatis*, p. 303.
[180] *Pipe roll 7 John*, p. 262; *Rot. oblatis*, p. 294.
[181] *Pipe roll 7 John*, p. 117; *Rot. oblatis*, p. 297.
[182] *Pipe roll 7 John*, pp. 59, 129; *Rot. oblatis*, pp. 299, 303.
[183] *Pipe roll 7 John*, p. 10.

mentioned on the pipe roll of 1205—Canterbury, Chichester, London, Northampton, Oxford, St. Edmunds, Winchester and York.[184] Lincoln should probably be added though the word in the roll is London.[185] A royal writ of October 7, 1207, summoning all moneyers to London mentions seven more—Carlisle, Durham, Exeter, Norwich, Ipswich, Lynn and Rochester.[186] There is reason for thinking that the mint at St. Edmunds was opened or reopened in 1205.[187] Those at Ipswich, Lynn, and Rochester do not seem to have been in operation under Richard. But all one can say positively is that there were apparently sixteen mints and exchanges in 1207.

One of the most interesting political events of the early years of John's reign and one that had important financial implications for the kings of both France and England was the separation of England from Normandy. This separation deprived Normandy of a large proportion of its major barons. Outside of the great border lords of southern Normandy, the counts of Perche, Alençon, and Seez and Gilbert de Laigle, the only Norman barons of the first rank who stayed in the duchy were the count of Eu and the chamberlain of Tancarville. The ease with which Philip Augustus and his successors held the duchy was in all probability largely the result of the lack of really powerful lords with whom the English kings could intrigue. After 1204 the greatest lords of Normandy were secondary barons like Ralph Taxon and Fulk Painel. Philip Augustus had a magnificent opportunity and made full use of it. William Marshal and Earl Robert of Leicester made arrangements by which they could stay in England and still keep their Norman lands.[188] Robert Marmion left his eldest son in Normandy.[189] But in general the lands of the great barons who chose to stay in England fell into the hands of King Philip. And the king showed no great generosity in granting them to his followers. A few Normans were bought with modest fiefs—Warin

[184] *Ibid.*, pp. 10, 59, 110, 117, 129, 236, 262.
[185] *Ibid.*, p. 11.
[186] *Rot. pat.*, p. 76.
[187] *Pipe roll 7 John*, p. 236.
[188] Painter, *William Marshal*, pp. 138-139.
[189] Pipe roll 1 Henry III, Public Record Office.

de Glapion, John's last seneschal and Philip's first, John de Rouvrai, and Richard de Argences.[190] Count Reginald of Boulogne received the county of Aumale and a fair part of the Mortimer lands.[191] On the whole, however, the forfeited fiefs seem to have slipped gently into King Philip's demesne.[192]

King John was in a more complicated position than his rival. As far as Philip was concerned the separation of England and Normandy was permanent. There was no reason for him to regard his disposal of the lands of the English barons as temporary and he had no strong reason for desiring to court their favor. His arrangement with William Marshal seems to have been entirely the result of personal friendship. But John did not regard the separation as permanent. He was full of plans to recover the duchy, and the good-will of the Norman lords was very important to him. All grants made by John from the possessions of his vassals who remained in Normandy were probably regarded as valid only until the recovery of the duchy and in many of them this condition was expressly stated.[193] And the English king was always ready to be generous to lords like Reginald of Boulogne and Thomas de St. Valéry who showed an inclination to carry on intrigues with him. The latter seems to have managed in one way or another to keep his English barony in the hands of himself or his brother Henry during most of John's reign.[194] Then many English lords produced reasons why they should have lands abandoned by the Normans. Ranulf of Chester received Richmondshire either because of his former wife or as compensation for his Norman fiefs. The Earl Warren received the custody of Gilbert de Laigle's barony of Pevensea because his sister was Gilbert's wife.[195] He was given Grantham and Stamford as compensation for his losses.[196] These two towns had belonged to the Humets. The rest of the Humet

---

[190] *Recueil des actes de Philippe Auguste* (ed. Delaborde, Petit-Dutaillis, et Monicat), II, nos. 793, 797, 903.
[191] *Ibid.* no. 862.
[192] *Ibid.*, no. 901.
[193] *Rot. pat.*, pp. 92, 128.
[194] *Ibid.*, pp. 108, 128-129; *Rot. claus.*, I, 43, 82, 161, 232.
[195] *Rot. oblatis*, p. 401-402.
[196] *Rot. pat.*, p. 92.

lands were absorbed by Richard de Canville who was a relative of the Humets.[197] Geoffrey de Mandeville had before the loss of Normandy sued Henry de Tilly for the barony of Merswood. When Henry stayed in Normandy, his barony went to Geoffrey's son Robert while his lesser fiefs were kept by his younger brother William fitz John.[198] Hugh Painel of West Rasen in Lincolnshire received his cousin Fulk's manor of Drax in compensation for his Norman lands.[199] In short many of the fiefs lost by the Normans were taken over by English claimants.

There is, unfortunately, no way of discovering the total value of the English lands of those who remained in Normandy. Late in 1204 or early in 1205 John ordered his justices to list these lands with an estimate of their value.[200] A roll carrying this information has survived, but it is clearly not complete.[201] The values given on it come to a total of £1,512. As the honor of Richmond alone was worth almost that much, the sum of all the forfeited estates must have come to something like £4,000. If John had kept these in his own hands, it would have made a decided increase in the royal revenue. Actually little remained in the king's hands. The estates that did not go to English lords who had some claim to them were given to men whose services the king wanted to reward or whose loyalty he hoped to buy. The lands of the Normans were dissipated, and John lost an excellent opportunity to enlarge his demesne.

---

[197] *Rot. claus.*, I, 1.
[198] *Ibid.*, p. 51; *Rot. pat.*, p. 61; *Rotuli Normanniae*, I, 8; *Pipe roll John*, p. 32.
[199] *Rot. claus.*, I, 108.
[200] I can find only one reference to these justices. *Rot. claus.*, I, 19.
[201] *Rotuli Normanniae*, I, 122-143.

Chapter V

KING JOHN AND THE CHURCH

THE spectacular nature of John's quarrel with Innocent III over the election of Stephen Langton to the see of Canterbury and the mixture of cunning and ferocity with which he conducted it has tempted men to forget that it was but one episode in a long, bitter struggle. Between the sixth and the eleventh centuries the bishops and abbots of Western Europe had built up immense landed estates and extensive political privileges. When strong feudal states began to appear, their rulers were determined that the property held by the church should contribute to their resources. Moreover the feudal princes were jealous of the political privileges of the church. At times they sought to limit them as in Henry II's Constitutions of Clarendon, but more often they simply tried to neutralize them by controlling the appointment of the prelates who wielded these powers. Control of the church was an extremely vital element in the power of a feudal prince. The feudalized church had great military resources, and a wise selection of prelates could keep these resources available to the prince. Then any government above the most primitive needs the service of some literate officials, and literacy was practically a clerical monopoly.

As long as bishops and abbots stood in comparative isolation, their control by the prince was not very difficult. But in the eleventh century a reformed papacy renewed the attempt to make the church into a centralized organization with common laws, practices, and beliefs. The result was a long struggle between the popes and the feudal princes—in particular the feudal monarchs of England, France, and Germany. For the most part this contest was a matter of relatively obscure skirmishes, but occasionally a disagreement between an able and determined pope and an able and ambitious monarch would lead to a major battle like the quarrel between Gregory VII and the Emperor Henry IV. Behind these skirmishes and battles both parties steadily built up their strength. Through the system of judges delegate the popes acquired effective control of the administration of canon law. Their legates tightened the bonds of church discipline. The papal treasury began to devise the means by which the church was to contribute to the support of the steadily growing papal administration. At the same time, at least in France and England, the feudal monarchs were developing their power and forging effective agencies of government.

With the possible exception of Stephen, the Norman and Angevin kings of England had consistently resisted the development of papal power within their domains. They kept close control of the election of bishops and abbots. In general they would not permit the presence in England of a foreign legate, but insisted that the legatine commission be given to an English prelate. They had obliged the church fiefs to perform their full feudal obligations. Henry II had gone farther—in his Constitutions of Clarendon he tried to reduce the privileges enjoyed by the church. Later in his reign he had scandalously abused his right of custody by leaving sees vacant for years while he enjoyed their revenues. Richard quarreled with his prelates over the knight service owed him and exacted huge sums from the church for his ransom. Thus when John came to the throne, the general tone of the policy of the English crown toward the papacy and the church was well set by tradition. An English king could be expected to use episcopal appointments as rewards for his servants, to draw money and men from the lands of the church, to insist to the full on all his rights and to resist fiercely any extension of the papal authority.

There was nothing in John's character to suggest that his policy would be less vigorous than that of his predecessors. He was certainly no model of piety. While one may discount the statement of the biographer of St. Hugh of Lincoln that John never took the sacrament after he reached maturity, it clearly indicates what people thought of his religious practices. Moreover there seems no reason for rejecting the same author's account of John's frivolous behavior at the Easter mass conducted by St. Hugh.[1] In general his religious activities seem to have been confined to some of the more superficial forms. He occasionally visited shrines.[2]

---

[1] *Magna vita sancti Hugonis*, pp. 291-293.
[2] Jocelin de Brakelond, p. 86.

King John and the Church

When he ate meat on Friday, he did penance by feeding some poor people.[3] Frequently during his travels about his realm he gave small sums in alms to the members of obscure monastic houses—usually to houses of nuns.[4] The frequency of these gifts would seem to rule out the scandalous explanation for them that John's reputation suggests. He founded one monastery, the Cistercian abbey of Beaulieu in Hampshire, but it was the result of a semi-political bargain, and he did it as cheaply as he could.[5] In short outside of the giving of comparatively small sums in alms, one can find no evidence of any acts of piety on John's part. At the best his attitude toward the church and its clergy was coldly practical—at the worst it was almost insanely ferocious.

When John ascended the English throne, the general political situation in Europe made Pope Innocent III inclined to favor him in every possible way. Innocent was a firm supporter of the claims of Otto of Brunswick to the Imperial throne against those of Philip of Hohenstaufen, duke of Swabia. Philip Augustus of France, who was in the bad graces of the papacy because of his efforts to set aside his queen, Ingelborg of Denmark, had formed an alliance with Duke Philip. Otto was John's nephew and had been a prime favorite of King Richard who had bequeathed him a large part of his money and jewels. While John's political support would be useful to Otto as a partial balance to the enmity of King Philip, the prompt payment of Richard's legacy was even more important to the impecunious prince and his papal ally. The earliest letters of Innocent to John that have been preserved are exhortations to hasten full payment to Otto.[6]

Unfortunately it is impossible to determine the extent of John's obligations to his nephew. Richard's will has not been preserved, and we have to rely on Hovedon's account of it. He seems to state that Richard bequeathed Otto all his jewels and three quarters of his treasure.[7] The same chronicler reports that in 1200 Otto

---

[3] "Rotulus misae 14 John," pp. 231-238, 242-243; *Rot. liberate*, pp. 110, 11, 117, 120, 136.
[4] "Rotulus misae 14 John," pp. 233-235, 237, 240, 242; *Rot. liberate*, pp. 2, 84.
[5] Coggeshall, pp. 102-110; Migne, *Patrologia*, ccxiv, 972-973.
[6] *Ibid.*, columns 1023, 1050-1051.
[7] Hovedon, IV, 83.

claimed the jewels and half the treasure.[8] Even if we knew the precise terms of Richard's will, there would be no way to discover the value of his jewels and the amount of money in his treasury. From what is known of Richard's financial habits one would not expect him to have any very large cash reserve. Hovedon states that in addition to the money and jewels Otto claimed to be earl of Yorkshire and count of Poitou.[9] It is clear that the claim to Yorkshire, if Otto really made it, was groundless.[10] But King Richard had formally invested his nephew with the county of Poitou, and Otto had borne the title for several years and issued charters under it.[11] On the other hand there is evidence that Richard considered that Otto had given up Poitou when he became king of the Romans.[12]

During the first year of his reign John spent very considerable sums for Otto's benefit. Hugh Oissel was given the exchange of England as payment of 1,700 marks owed him by John. Of this sum 1,000 marks represented money owed Hugh by Otto.[13] Then the king agreed to pay 2,125 marks that were expended by the bishops of Angers and Bangor and Stephen Ridel who were in Rome on Otto's behalf.[14] An unknown amount of treasure was despatched to Otto from England and several payments recorded on the pipe roll appear to have been made to creditors of Otto.[15] While the emperor-elect and the pope were still unsatisfied, and John never seems to have claimed that he had paid the legacy in full, I suspect that Otto got a very considerable portion of what he was entitled to. Moreover John continued to pay debts incurred by Otto and in 1202 he asked the English clergy to contribute money to aid him.[16] But the English king was not willing to in-

[8] *Ibid.*, p. 116.
[9] *Ibid.*
[10] *Ibid.*, III, 86.
[11] *Ibid.*, IV, 7. *Layettes du trésor des chartes*, I, 192.
[12] During 1197 Otto attested charters of Richard as count of Poitou. Landon, *Itinerary*, pp. 118, 123. He was crowned king of the Romans on July 12, 1198. On August 1198 he attested a charter as *Otone filio ducio Saxonie. Cartae antiquae rolls*, no. 315.
[13] *Rot. chart.*, pp. 11-12.
[14] *Ibid.*, p. 31.
[15] *Pipe roll 1 John*, pp. 59, 129, 243.
[16] *Rot. liberate*, p. 46; Rymer, *Foedera*, I, 87.

convenience himself too much for his nephew's cause. In concluding his treaty with Philip Augustus in 1200 he solemnly promised not to give aid to Otto.

In the first two years of his reign John was faced with the need to make decisions in the most important realm of ecclesiastical policy—the selection of bishops. The see of Hereford was vacant at his accession and St. Hugh of Lincoln and John of Norwich died before the end of the year 1200. Hereford was used to pay part of his debt to William de Briouse—it went to his son Giles. Little is known of the personal characteristics of Giles de Briouse, but there is no reason for thinking that he was not simply a wild marcher lord covered with clerical vestments. The see of Norwich was given to the bearer of the royal seal, John de Grey. John was a man of purely secular interests—a competent captain and efficient civil servant. There was no man in England whom King John trusted so completely and so consistently as he did John de Grey. Yet John seems to have made a reasonably acceptable bishop and to have been well liked by the clergy of his diocese.[17] In the case of Lincoln the king was not so successful in imposing his will. Early in 1201 he visited the chapter and sought to persuade them to elect as St. Hugh's successor Roger, bishop of St. Andrews in Scotland, brother of Earl Robert of Leicester.[18] This was clearly part of his campaign to win the firm support of Earl Robert against his baronial foes. In a military sense the see of Lincoln with its hundred odd knights' fees and three demesne castles was the most important in England. Little is known about the details of the affair, but the canons resisted the king, insisted on their freedom to elect, and chose one of their number, William de Blois, who was finally accepted by John. If one may judge by his later behavior, the king must have decided that he would never again let a chapter get the best of him.

Towards the end of the first year of his reign John became engaged in a quarrel with the Cistercian order. When in the spring

[17] *The first register of Norwich cathedral priory* (ed. H. W. Saunders, Norfolk record society), p. 89.
[18] Hovedon, IV, 156; *Magna vita sancti Hugonis*, pp. 234-235. Migne, *Patrologia*, ccxiv, 1175-1178.

of 1200 the king levied a carucage to pay the relief he had promised King Philip, the Cistercians stated that they could neither pay the tax nor a fine for exemption without special permission from the general chapter of their order. Only the pleas of the Cistercians' most powerful friend, Hubert Walter, prevented the king from issuing orders that would have practically outlawed the order. According to Coggeshall the archbishop offered the king a fine of 1,000 marks in behalf of the Cistercians for his favor, but apparently it was rejected. John left England full of anger. When he returned in the autumn, he ordered Hugh de Neville to direct the Cistercians to remove all their stock from the royal forests within two weeks of Michaelmas or have their animals taken for the king's use. Once more the abbots of the order appealed to the primate. He suggested that the abbots approach the king in person at Lincoln on November 20. The occasion turned out to be even more propitious than the archbishop had hoped. John journeyed to Lincoln to meet King William of Scotland, but shortly before the appointed day he heard that St. Hugh had died in London. The death of the most revered of English prelates seems to have softened John for the time being. He allowed Hubert to reconcile him with the Cistercian abbots. He even begged their forgiveness for any harm he had done them and promised to found a house of their order.[19] Thus the quarrel ended amicably, but it showed John's capacity for violent measures when he was aroused.

During these same early years of his reign John was at odds with two of his chief ecclesiastical dignitaries, but the issues involved had little to do with broad questions of policy. Before Richard's death John as lord of Ireland had expelled the archbishop of Dublin from his domains.[20] This quarrel he simply kept boiling merrily by refusing to make terms with the exiled prelate. The other feud was with his half-brother, Geoffrey Plantagenet, archbishop of York. Geoffrey was no easy man to get on with. He was arrogant and arbitrary with a high idea of his rights, liberties, and prerogatives and no inclination to compromise. He had quarreled heartily with Richard. He and his chapter were continu

---

[19] Coggeshall, pp. 102-110.
[20] Migne, *Patrologia,* ccxiv, 1175-1178.

ously at odds, and when times grew dull, he had conflicts with his vassals and townsmen.[21] When John came to the throne, the see of York was in the hands of the crown while Geoffrey conducted his litigation at Rome with his numerous foes. The new king immediately turned the archbishop's barony over to his agents.[22] Geoffrey returned to England early in 1200 and for the moment made peace with his chapter.[23] But he could not stay out of trouble long. When John asked him to go with him to meet Philip Augustus, he refused. He also refused to allow his lands to be assessed for the carucage, and his men offered violent resistance to the collectors.[24] Finally he lost a court case with his burghers of Beverley and excommunicated the sheriff of Yorkshire who tried to enforce the orders of the royal justices. John promptly seized his barony.[25] The two brothers made peace at Portsmouth in May 1201, and Geoffrey offered £1,000 for the king's benevolence.[26] John crossed to Normandy while Geoffrey returned with renewed energy to his quarrels with his chapter.[27]

As we have seen in an earlier chapter the spring of 1201 was a difficult time for King John. The barons of England showed no enthusiasm for crossing to the continent to aid him in suppressing the revolt of the Lusignans in Normandy and Poitou. Fulk fitz Warin and William Marsh were in open revolt. Apparently John decided that he needed the active support of the papacy. He confessed his sins to Hubert Walter and expressed his desire to give satisfaction to God and His church. Hubert suggested that he send 100 knights to the Holy Land for a year and found a Cistercian house.[28] The archbishop then informed Pope Innocent of John's burst of piety and apparently suggested at the same time that the barons were not behaving very well. On March 7, 1202, Innocent directed the archbishops of Rouen and Canterbury to use all

---

[21] *Ibid.*, columns 1029-1030; *Curia regis rolls,* I, 385.
[22] Hovedon, IV, 92.
[23] *Ibid.*, p. 126.
[24] *Ibid.*, pp. 139-140.
[25] *Ibid., Curia regis rolls,* I, 385.
[26] Hovedon, IV, 163; *Rot. oblatis,* p. 146.
[27] Hovedon, IV, 174
[28] Migne, *Patrologia,* ccxiv, 972-973.

their spiritual powers to force any rebels against John to return to their allegiance.[29] On the twenty-seventh of the same month he wrote a warm letter to the king welcoming him into the fold with the reminder of how greatly God loves a repentant sinner.[30] The pope was still hopeful of persuading John to aid Otto, and it seems likely that the only offense of the English king that he knew of at the time was the long-standing quarrel with the archbishop of Dublin. As Innocent was at the moment annoyed to the point of desperation over Geoffrey of York's everlasting quarrels with his clergy, it seems doubtful that he would have taken the king's difficulties with that turbulent prelate very seriously even if he had known of them.[31]

By the end of another year, however, Innocent's patience began to wear thin. On February 20, 1203, he despatched a long letter to John reciting his misdeeds. He had made a treaty with Philip Augustus that bound him not to aid Otto. He had publicly announced that he would not permit a papal legate to enter his lands. While the king had later changed his stand on this point, the pope was offended. Then John had interfered with the activities of the papal delegates hearing cases in England. He had expelled the bishop of Limoges from his diocese and had injured the bishop of Poitiers. At Lincoln in England and at Seez in Normandy he had interfered in episcopal elections. Finally he paid no attention to the pope's pleas to make peace with the archbishop of Dublin.[32] John was called upon to mend his ways.

The papal admonitions had little effect on King John. In 1206 Innocent was still trying to persuade him to pay the legacy to Otto.[33] Papal letters of the summer of 1203 sternly directed the king to make peace with the archbishop of Dublin.[34] These letters supported by the personal pleas of a legate moved the king to arrange a conference with the exiled prelate, but the meeting was fruitless and late in 1204 Innocent despatched even stronger letters. John was to make peace with the archbishop within two months or whatever diocese he might be in would be placed under

[29] *Ibid.*, column 984.
[30] *Ibid.*, columns 972-973.
[31] *Ibid.*, columns 1029-1030.
[32] *Ibid.*, columns 1175-1178.
[33] *Ibid.*, ccxvi, 1129-1130.
[34] *Ibid.*, ccxv, 61-62.

an interdict while he resided there. If this was ineffective, the interdict was to be placed on the whole province of Dublin.[35] John ignored these letters as cheerfully as he had the earlier ones. It was only a year later when a matter of far greater importance, the succession to the see of Canterbury, was at stake that John decided to obey the papal mandates about the archbishop of Dublin. On December 6, 1205, the king officially notified the justiciar of Ireland that he had made peace with the archbishop.[36]

In December 1204 Pope Innocent approached John on another subject—the dower of his sister-in-law Berengeria of Navarre.[37] A dowager whether royal or baronial often had difficulties when her husband was succeeded by someone other than her son. Berengeria was childless, had married Richard in far off Cyprus, and had been crowned there by the bishop of Evreux. She had never been formally crowned in England. Moreover Queen Eleanor still held her munificent dower in England as well as her broad continental lands. John may well have felt that his obligation to Berengeria was slight and that two dowers would be too great a burden on his resources. But in 1201 he had come to an agreement with Berengeria. She was to have the city of Bayeux, two Angevin castles, and 1,000 marks annual pension to be paid at the Norman exchequer in Caen.[38] Innocent's letter of 1204 suggests that this pension was never actually paid. Certainly John's interest in it would disappear when he lost Normandy and Anjou. The papal letter of 1204 had no effect nor did succeeding ones on the same subject. King Philip dowered Berengeria with certain rights that had belonged to the counts of Maine in Le Mans and its vicinity, and John was glad to leave his sister-in-law in his enemy's care. Philip's generosity was probably not entirely inspired by his sense of justice. Berengeria's sister was the countess of Champagne whose good-will was useful to the French king.

On September 11, 1204, the death of Godfrey de Lucy, bishop of Winchester, left vacant one of the richest and most powerful of the English episcopal baronies. The see of Winchester yielded its lord some £3,000 in annual revenue, had four castles, Wolvsey in

[35] *Ibid.*, columns 483-486.
[36] *Rot. pat.*, p. 56.
[37] Migne, *Patrologia*, ccxv, 475-477.
[38] Hovedon, IV, 164, 173.

Winchester itself, Downton, Taunton and Farnham and contained nearly a hundred knights' fees. It was thus one of the great baronies of the realm. John was determined to secure this rich prize for one of his intimates. He nominated Peter des Roches, precentor of Lincoln, whom we have already heard of as one of John's most trusted officials. The prior and monks as a whole seem to have been ready to accept the king's nominee, but the archdeacon of Winchester and some other members of the chapter held out for the election of Richard Poor, dean of Salisbury. There was doubt of the legitimacy of both candidates. John seems to have acted with savage vigor. Papal letters speak of supporters of the dean of Salisbury imprisoned in chains and driven into exile. The case was appealed to Rome and Peter des Roches departed to press his claim in person. Pope Innocent voided both elections and ordered the delegation of the monks that was in Rome to elect a bishop. They chose Peter des Roches, and he was duly confirmed by the pope who had received letters from the archbishop of Tours vouching for his legitimate birth. John had won the contest. Six months later Innocent was still trying to persuade him to forgive those who had supported Richard Poor.[39] The pope did what he could to comfort the loser—he gave him letters permitting his promotion despite his illegitimate birth.[40]

While the chief cause of Peter's victory in Rome was undoubtedly the pope's desire to be at peace with John, some credit probably belongs to his own skill as a diplomat. During his stay in Rome he seems to have won the confidence of Pope Innocent. When he departed for England, he bore papal letters protecting him from excommunication by anyone except the pope himself.[41] Moreover he was entrusted with a very delicate task for which he probably had little enthusiasm. The ancient tax known as *Romescot* or Peter's Pence was collected in every English diocese except Carlisle and Durham.[42] In theory every house paid a penny to the

---

[39] Migne, *Patrologia,* ccxv, 562-563, 671-673, 792-793.
[40] *Ibid.,* column 759.
[41] Migne, *Patrologia,* ccxv, 754-755
[42] William E. Lunt, *Papal revenues in the middle ages* (Records of civilization, no. xix, New York, 1934), II, 65.

parish priest who passed the receipts on through the hierarchy to the bishop. The archbishop of Canterbury or some prelate appointed in his place sent the contribution to Rome. But tradition had set the sums due from each diocese so that Peter's Pence yielded the pope £200 a year.[43] Innocent suspected, undoubtedly with justice, that most of the money collected got lost in its passage through the English ecclesiastical hierarchy.[44] Bishop Peter was appointed official receiver of the money and was directed to see that it was faithfully paid.[45] Perhaps Innocent hoped that Peter's high favor with John would enable him to carry out this highly unpopular commission. Peter himself was not burning with enthusiasm. He reached England in the spring of 1206, but it was not until May 1207 that he summoned a council at St. Albans to discuss the question of Peter's Pence.[46] He must have realized that the whole proceeding was only a pleasant formality. John sternly warned the assembled clergy not to alter the custom of the realm.[47]

While Peter des Roches was in Rome seeking the confirmation of his election as bishop of Winchester, King John plunged into his longest and bitterest quarrel with the church—the contest over the succession to the see of Canterbury. The fiercely intransigent attitude of the king in this dispute can only be understood in the light of his relations with Hubert Walter. Hubert's interests were almost entirely secular. When he took a firm stand on an ecclesiastical question, it was because his personal power and prestige were at stake. He bitterly and successfully opposed the elevation of Giraldus Cambrensis, archdeacon of Brecon, to the see of St. David's because Giraldus believed that the Welsh church with the bishop of St. David's at its head should be independent of Canterbury.[48] While he might intercede with the king to persuade him to pay for the wine taken from a French abbot or to make peace between him and the Cistercians, he never hindered John's policy

[43] *Ibid.* The sums given in this papal letter of 1273 add up to £200 1s. 8d. In 1214 Innocent stated that he received 300 marks a year. *Ibid.,* p. 64.
[44] In 1214 he estimated the leakage at 1,000 marks. *Ibid.*
[45] *Ibid.,* pp. 62-63.
[46] *Rot. claus.,* I, 71; *Rot. pat.,* p. 72.
[47] Lunt, *Papal revenues,* II, 63-64; *Rot. pat.,* p. 72.
[48] Giraldus Cambrensis, *Opera,* I, 95-96, 120-121, 289-296; III, 164-176.

toward the church in any matter of importance.[49] It was as a great official and secular baron that he aroused the king's jealousy and hatred.

During the last twelve years of his life Hubert Walter wielded more power than any other subject of the English crown. He started his career as a clerk of Henry II's justiciar, Ranulf de Glanvill.[50] In 1186 Henry II made him dean of York, and in 1189 King Richard elevated him to the see of Salisbury.[51] Having accompanied Richard on his crusade he returned to England in 1193 to become archbishop of Canterbury and justiciar.[52] In 1195 the pope added a legatine commission to this amazing combination of offices.[53] Even Hubert was aware that it was improper for the same man to head both the ecclesiastical and secular administrations and in 1196 he sought to resign the justiciarship, but Richard would not hear of it.[54] Not until 1198 when papal protests against the situation grew insistent did Richard accept his resignation.[55] As the new justiciar, Geoffrey fitz Peter, was a friend and colleague of Hubert, the archbishop retained an important position in the administration of the realm. This position was vastly strengthened when John made him chancellor. Thus in the early years of John's reign Hubert combined the dignity, prestige, wealth, and secular and spiritual power of the archbishop of Canterbury with the authority and influence of the chancellor. When one considers in addition his knowledge of the law and his extensive administrative experience, it is easy to see that he was bound to have a dominant influence over a young and inexperienced king.

Hubert Walter used his influence to increase his power and revenue and the resources of his see. He obtained possession of Rochester castle and the suzerainty over the earl of Clare's castle of Tunbridge. The manor of Saltwood with its ancient *motte* was returned to his barony.[56] He was also granted dies to make money and the exchange of Canterbury.[57] John confirmed to him and

---

[49] Coggeshall, pp. 102, 108-109; *Rot. liberate,* p. 47.
[50] Hovedon, II, 310.
[51] *Ibid.,* II, 310; III, 15.
[52] *Ibid.,* III, 213, 221, 226.
[53] *Ibid.,* pp. 290-293.
[54] *Ibid.,* IV, 12.
[55] *Ibid.,* p. 48.
[56] Gervase of Canterbury, II, 409, 411.
[57] *Rot. chart.,* p. 68.

his church all their extensive franchises.[58] Moreover from John's accession to his own death Hubert had the custody of the baronies of Cainhoe, Wahull, and Vaux and the important mesne fief of the Aubervilles—a total of some seventy knights' fees.[59] When William de Stutville died he was allowed to buy the custody of that extremely rich barony.[60] In June 1200 John issued a charter granting these fiefs freedom from suit at shire and hundred courts and from the payment of the sheriff's aid as long as they were in Hubert's hands.[61]

The mere fact that Hubert possessed such vast wealth and power was enough to make King John jealous of him, and the archbishop took no pains to assuage the king's feelings. He openly vied with John in pomp and magnificence of life and boasted that he was the richer of the two.[62] While Hubert's income certainly was not so large as the king's, he may well have had more to spend on personal extravagance. Then the archbishop had no hesitation in opposing John on questions of state policy. If the biographer of William Marshal is correct in stating that Hubert originally favored the succession of Arthur, that would, if the king knew of it, have aroused his permanent distrust of the primate.[63] Then Hubert had opposed John's tentative efforts to make peace with Philip Augustus and had interfered to nullify the efforts of a royal embassy sent to France for that purpose.[64] But he had also opposed John's expedition to Poitou in 1205 and was one of those whose advice finally persuaded the king to abandon it.[65] In short he saw no point in officially giving up Normandy by making peace, but he had no desire to spend English treasure in trying to reconquer John's continental fiefs. On the whole it is not difficult to understand why John rejoiced at Hubert's death and why he was de-

[58] *Ibid.*
[59] *Pipe roll 1 John*, pp. 105, 211; *Pipe roll 2 John*, p. 209; *Rot. claus.*, I, 42, 44; *Memoranda roll 1 John*, p. 64; *Rot. oblatis*, p. 307.
[60] *Rot. chart.*, p. 108.
[61] *Ibid.*, p. 68.
[62] *Histoire des ducs de Normandie*, pp. 105-107; Wendover, I, 311.
[63] *Histoire de Guillaume le Maréchal*, lines 11880-11882.
[64] Painter, *William Marshal*, pp. 137-139.
[65] Coggeshall, p. 152; Wendover, II, 9-10.

termined that the next primate should be a man in whom he had complete confidence and who owed his position to his favor.

Hubert Walter died at his manor of Tenham on July 13, 1205.[66] The close roll indicates that John was at Brill in Buckinghamshire on July 14 and at Canterbury on July 15. As the distance between these places was about a hundred miles, I suspect a mistake in the close roll, but the king was certainly in Canterbury by July 17.[67] He had no intention of endangering the success of his plans by unnecessary delay. When he arrived at Canterbury, John found the monks of the monastery of Christ Church, the cathedral chapter of Canterbury, already engaged in their ancient argument with the suffragans of the province. The monks claimed the right to elect one of their own number to the archepiscopal throne without outside interference. The bishops of the province maintained that they had the privilege of participating in the election. As the bishops were by and large his men, the king was inclined to favor their claim, but for the time being he postponed the question—everyone promised to do nothing before December.[68]

While the course of events between July and December is not entirely clear, its chief features can be ascertained.[69] Both monks and bishops decided, apparently without the king's knowledge, to send delegates to Rome to plead for their respective ideas as to the proper electoral procedure.[70] The bishops of London, Rochester, Exeter, Salisbury, Landaff, Coventry, Ely, Worcester, St. David's, and Chichester met at St. Paul's in London and composed a solemn letter to Innocent III. They claimed that from the most ancient times the bishops had participated with the monks in the election of the archbishop. The result was always announced by the dean of St. Paul's. They begged the pope not to change the

---

[66] In my account of the events leading to the election of Stephen Langton I have leaned heavily on Dom M. D. Knowles, " The Canterbury Election of 1205-6," *English historical review*, LIII (1938), 211-230. Gervase of Canterbury, *Actus pontificum*, II, 413.

[67] *Rot. claus.*, I, 42.

[68] Migne, *Patrologia*, ccxv, 834-835; Gervase of Canterbury, II, 98.

[69] For a detailed account see Knowles, " The Canterbury election of 1205-6," pp. 211-220.

[70] *Rot. pat.*, p. 56; Migne, *Patrologia*, ccxv, 740-742.

traditional custom. This letter was entrusted to Master Peter de Englosam who was despatched to Rome.[71] The monks, or at least a fair part of them, decided to be extremely clever. They chose Reginald, their sub-prior, to head their delegation. Then they went through the forms of an election and gave him letters certifying that he was the archbishop-elect and asking the pope to confirm his election.[72] Reginald's friends steadily insisted that this was a proper, canonical, unconditional election, but the other monks maintained that Reginald was obliged to swear that he would not use the letters unless when he reached Rome he found the pope considering the confirmation of someone nominated by John or the bishops. According to this version the monks had elected Reginald conditionally because they heard that the king had sent delegates to persuade Innocent to give the office to "a certain man"—presumably John de Grey, bishop of Norwich.[73] Neither of these versions sounds very probable. The monks knew perfectly well that they had no right to hold an election until they had secured the king's permission—the *congé d'elire*. They must have realized from the beginning that Reginald's election was a dubious trick. The second story is even more implausible. It is incredible that the monks believed there was any danger that Innocent III would confirm anyone as archbishop of Canterbury without assuring himself that the candidate had been elected by the monks. The bishops did not claim the right to elect the archbishop but simply the privilege of participating in the election. It seems clear to me that some of the monks hoped that if Reginald had letters certifying his election, he might persuade the pope to confirm him without further investigation. As we shall see, this trick almost worked.

On December 13, 1205, Pope Innocent despatched letters to the abbots of St. Albans and Reading and the dean of St. Paul's. The delegation of Canterbury monks had arrived in Rome and requested him to confirm the election of the sub-prior. But the agent

[71] *Ibid. Early charters of the cathedral church of St. Paul's, London* (ed. Marion Gibbs. Camden society, third series, LVIII), p. 140.
[72] Migne, *Patrologia,* ccxv, 740-742.
[73] *Ibid.,* columns 834-838.

of the bishops, Master Peter de Englosam, had insisted that their rights had been infringed in the election. Peter had lost his credentials on his journey. Fortunately Peter des Roches was still in Rome and was able to guarantee that he was the authorized delegate of the provincial bishops. Innocent directed the three English ecclesiastics to collect all available evidence concerning the dispute between the bishops and the chapter and despatch it to Rome.[74] Dom Knowles feels that the tenor of this letter indicates that the pope was ready to confirm Reginald's election as soon as the question of the bishops' rights was settled. Certainly there is no mention of the lack of the royal leave to elect. Either the monks deceived Innocent or he chose to ignore this well recognized requirement.

King John had postponed the discussion of the Canterbury succession to early December. On the first day of that month he journeyed from London to Canterbury, on the fourth he returned to London, and on the tenth he was back in Canterbury to finish the business.[75] Gervase of Canterbury states that the king's agents in Rome had informed him of Reginald's claim to be archbishop-elect, that he asked the monks if such an election had been made, and that they discreetly denied it.[76] When the king returned to London on December 4, he took with him a delegation of the monks. On December 6 the monks and the bishops of the province met in London and solemnly renounced their mutual appeals to Rome.[77] Then on December 10 the chapter formally elected John de Grey, bishop of Norwich, and the election received the royal assent. King John recounted these events in a letter addressed to the pope on December 11.[78] He appointed Honorius, archdeacon of Richmond, to carry the letter to the pope and to secure the confirmation of John de Grey. The bishops of the province of Canterbury were directed to write to the pope expressing their approval of John's election. Finally six monks of Christ Church were despatched to Rome under the conduct of Master Geoffrey de Der-

[74] *Ibid.*, columns 740-742.
[75] T. D. Hardy, *Itinerary of King John* in *Rot. pat.*
[76] Gervase of Canterbury, II, 99.   [77] *Rot. pat.*, p. 56.   [78] *Ibid.*

ham who as the chancellor of the diocese of Norwich was presumably a strong supporter of John de Grey.[79]

King John must have been fully aware that the affair had become a magnificent mess. From his point of view the election of Reginald was entirely illegal. He had neither given the monks leave to elect nor his assent to their choice. But he must have known that when papal confirmation was requested even for an invalid election, no valid election could be held until the pope had made his decision. Essentially the king was sending a carefully chosen body of monks to hold the election in Rome under the eye of his agents, Honorius and Geoffrey de Derham. The election of John de Grey at Canterbury was simply a formality to strengthen his bargaining position. Dom Knowles points out that there is evidence that the king used threats to obtain John's election by the chapter, but this can hardly have troubled the royal conscience. Use of pressure in support of the king's candidate was a regular feature of episcopal elections. Far more violent means had been used to persuade the chapter of Winchester to choose Peter des Roches.

John's plan almost worked. When Innocent had despatched his letters to the abbots of St. Albans and Reading and the dean of St. Paul's, he had entrusted them to Master Peter de Englosam and the monks who had accompanied the sub-prior. Only one monk had remained in Rome with Prior Reginald. But this monk vigorously opposed the confirmation of John de Grey. He claimed that the archbishop should be chosen from among the monks, that John's election had been held while a previous election was under papal consideration, and that the king had used pressure to secure John's election. No one can have taken the first argument very seriously and the third was little stronger, but the second was undoubtedly sound. Then the new delegation proceeded to point out that Reginald's election had been conditional and that the conditions had not been met—he had announced his election before there was any danger that the pope was about to confirm someone else.[80] Hence all was confusion once more, and Innocent decided

---

[79] *Ibid.*, p. 57. *First register of Norwich cathedral priory*, pp. 98-101.
[80] Migne, *Patrologia*, ccxv, 836-838.

on another postponement. In letters of March 30, 1206, he instructed the chapter of Canterbury to send a new delegation to Rome. The pope named ten monks who were to be sent and directed the chapter to choose six more. Presumably the ten named were supporters of the sub-prior, and Innocent's purpose was to prevent the packing of the delegation by royal influence. The bishop of Rochester and the abbot of St. Augustine of Canterbury were ordered to proceed to Canterbury to gather evidence concerning the questions at issue and to transmit their findings to the pope. The king and the bishops of the province were directed to send proctors to guard their interests. All these people were to be in Rome by the end of September.[81]

On May 26, 1206, King John despatched the proctors called for by the pope's letters. The chief of these was one of John's favorite prelates, Hugh, abbot of Beaulieu, the king's own Cistercian foundation. With him went Thomas de Eardington, sheriff of Shropshire and Staffordshire, and Amfrid de Dene, a Sussex knight who had once been Count Ralph de Lusignan's seneschal of the rape of Hastings. Presumably Thomas and Amfrid were chosen because of their imperviousness to ecclesiastical wiles. These delegates were supplied with the generous sum of 3,000 marks.[82] Whether justly or not John and his subjects were firmly convinced that ready cash was a great assistance in dealing with the papal court.[83]

If the various delegations actually arrived in Rome by the end of September, no one can charge the pope with acting hastily. His decision was announced in letters addressed to John on December 21. Innocent had first examined the dispute between the monks and the provincial bishops and had come to the conclusion that the right to elect the archbishop belonged solely to the monks. In March the pope had declared invalid the election of John de Grey. In December he also nullified the election of Reginald. He then directed the monks to hold a new election. But the two parties

[81] *Ibid.*, columns 834-840.
[82] *Rot. pat.*, p. 65.
[83] As a sample of contemporary opinion see *Histoire de Guillaume le Maréchal*, II, lines 11355-11372.

were still divided between John de Grey and Reginald. When he saw that no decision could be reached between these two, Innocent suggested a third candidate, Stephen Langton, cardinal priest of St. Chrysogonus. Langton was an Englishman and a canon of York. He had had a distinguished career as a professor of theology at the University of Paris and as a member of the papal court. The divided monks yielded to the pope's wish and unanimously elected Stephen as archbishop of Canterbury. Innocent then asked the royal proctors to give John's assent, but they refused to do so. Clearly they had been authorized to assent to no archbishop-elect except the bishop of Norwich. In his letters to the king Innocent pointed out that when an episcopal election was held in Rome, the royal assent was not necessary. He had been leaning over backward to respect John's rights and had assumed that the royal proctors had full power to assent to any election made. John was called upon to give his assent and to receive Stephen with open arms.[84]

It is difficult to believe that this papal missive was entirely candid. Innocent must have had a fairly good knowledge of John's character and policy. He must have realized how anxious the king was to have a man on whom he could rely as primate of all England. To believe that John would authorize his proctors to assent to any election would have been incredibly naïve. Moreover it is perfectly clear that Innocent could have persuaded the monks to elect John de Grey. Instead he threw his influence behind Stephen Langton. Now there can be no question that Langton was a far more worthy candidate for high ecclesiastical office than the worldly bishop of Norwich, and it seems probable that Innocent knew of no reason why he should be particularly objectionable to John. But it was politically impossible for the king of England to allow an outside authority to control the choice of the archbishop of Canterbury. Whatever its status in canon law, the royal assent was a practical necessity. As Dom Knowles states,

---

[84] Migne, *Patrologia*, ccxv, 1043-1047. The appendix to the preface of volume II of the rolls series edition of Gervase of Canterbury contains many letters dealing with this controversy. In general I shall cite this rather than Migne. Gervase of Canterbury, II, lxviii-lxxii.

Innocent had acted throughout the affair in perfect accord with the rules of canon law, but in doing so he raised an issue that constituted a vital threat to the political authority of the king of England. An archbishop of Canterbury had been chosen without John's consent.

We do not have John's reply to Innocent's letter except in a summary given by Wendover, but the chronicler's account of the king's remarks sounds reasonable.[85] John objected to Langton personally as a man almost unknown to him who had lived for a long time among his French enemies. As the election had been made without his assent, it was a violation of his rights. If necessary he would stand until death for the privileges of his crown. Moreover, he would not renounce the election of John de Grey as he believed it useful for him. Now it is fairly clear that "unknown" as used in this context should not be taken to mean "unheard of" but rather "unacquainted with." As Innocent was to point out in his reply John knew about Langton and had written a letter to him. The king would hardly tell the pope he had never heard of a man whom he had congratulated on his elevation to the cardinalate. But Langton had been out of England since about 1180 and John did not know him personally—he was not one of his familiars. Moreover Langton had received an appointment as canon of Notre Dame of Paris.[86] This could only have been given with the approval of John's bitter foe, Philip Augustus. Finally the king's argument about his rights was entirely sound from his point of view—he could not have an archbishop of Canterbury chosen without his approval.

These two letters show very clearly what the issue was in this bitter controversy. Innocent was taking the position that the election of the archbishop of Canterbury was a purely ecclesiastical affair and that the king's right to participate consisted at most in giving formal assent to the result. The election of Reginald had been made without seeking John's leave to elect and hence was a clear violation of English custom. John stressed this point in his

[85] Wendover, II, 40.
[86] F. M. Powicke, *Stephen Langton* (Oxford, 1928), pp. 10, 31.

letter certifying the election of John de Grey.[87] Yet in declaring Reginald's election invalid, Innocent did not mention this feature of it.[88] Now there is no question that the principle for which Innocent was fighting was important for the welfare of the church. But it is equally clear that no English king could accept it. The archbishop of Canterbury was far more than the primate of the English church—he had by tradition an important place in the secular government of the realm and he held a great barony with almost palatine franchises. No English king could allow this great office to be filled without his approval. Throughout his long controversy with Innocent John was to stick to this point tenaciously.

Innocent did not wait to learn the result of his letter of May 26—perhaps he realized how feeble his arguments were. On June 17, 1207, he consecrated Stephen Langton and gave him the pallium. On June 24 he announced his action to the bishops of the province.[89] The pope had thrown down the challenge—he had consecrated an archbishop of Canterbury without the assent and in opposition to the known wishes of the king of England. Any English king would have resisted. With John the resistance was almost certain to be both violent and stubborn.

When King John learned of Langton's consecration, he acted with his customary savage decision. As the chief objects of his anger, the new archbishop and the pope, were beyond his reach, he vented his rage on their instruments, the monks of Christ Church. Reginald de Cornhill, sheriff of Kent, and Fulk de Cantilupe, one of John's household knights, were sent to Canterbury with a force of men-at-arms. They were ordered to expel the monks from England.[90] All but thirteen aged monks who could not leave fled before the king's wrath. They crossed to Flanders and took refuge in the monastery of St. Bertin while John's agents took over their vast and flourishing estates.[91] About this same time the king seems to have seized the English benefices held by Italian ecclesiastics and forbidden papal delegates to hear cases in England.[92]

---

[87] *Rot. pat.*, p. 56.
[88] Migne, *Patrologia*, ccxv, 1043-1047.
[89] Gervase of Canterbury, II, lxxiv-lxxv.
[90] *Rot. pat.*, p. 74; Wendover, II, 39.
[91] Gervase of Canterbury, II, 100.
[92] *Rot. claus.*, I, 90; *Annals of Waverley*, p. 259.

Pope Innocent waited until August 27, 1207, to see whether or not John would show some sign of giving way. Then he addressed a long letter to the bishops of London, Ely, and Worcester. He loved John very much. When there had been revolts in his realm, he had aided him. But the king had shown himself ungrateful. He had violated the liberties of the church and had refused to accept the archbishop duly elected by the monks of Canterbury and consecrated by the pope. The bishops were directed to urge the king to receive Stephen Langton. If he refused, they were to lay an interdict upon all England and see that it was observed.[93] Innocent had chosen his three bishops carefully. William de Sainte-Mère-Eglise, bishop of London, Eustace, bishop of Ely, and Mauger, bishop of Worcester, were with the exception of Herbert Poor, bishop of Salisbury, and the very aged Gilbert de Glanvill, bishop of Rochester, the only suffragans of Canterbury on whom the pope could rely. The sees of Exeter and Lincoln were vacant. Bath, Chichester, Norwich, and Winchester were held by creatures of King John. While Giles of Hereford was soon to break with the king, it was to be for reasons entirely non-ecclesiastical. Little is known of Geoffrey de Muscamp, bishop of Chester, but he too was probably well advanced in years as he died a little more than a year later. Another letter of the same date directed the bishop of Rochester to excommunicate Fulk de Cantilupe, Reginald de Cornhill and all others who had laid violent hands on the property of the monks of Christ Church.[94]

By the autumn of 1207 Inocent had learned that John's obduracy was viewed with indifference if not with actual favor by the prelates and barons of his realm. On November 19 the pope despatched a number of letters designed to remedy this situation. The bishops of England and Wales were ordered to abandon their "tepid and remiss" attitude and to support Stephen's cause vigorously. The "magnates" of John's realm were informed that they should place their duty to the "king of Heaven" before their obligation to their "terrestrial king." They should decline to support John's impious policy and should urge him to yield. Fin-

---

[93] Gervase of Canterbury, II, lxxvi-lxxviii.
[94] *Ibid.*, pp. lxxxix-xc.

ally the bishops of London, Ely, and Worcester were ordered to permit no privileges, not even those of the Templars and Hospitallers, to interfere with the effectiveness of the interdict that they were to proclaim unless John gave way.[95]

Early in 1208 King John modified his position. On January 21 he informed the bishops of London, Ely, and Worcester that he was ready to obey the pope if his "rights, dignity, and liberties" were preserved. As a sign of his good intentions he removed Fulk de Cantilupe and Reginald de Cornhill as custodians of the archepiscopal barony and the monastery of Christ Church and replaced them with agents less deeply involved in his previous violent policy. Then on February 19 the king issued letters patent of safe-conduct for the archbishop's brother, Master Simon Langton, to come to England for a conference.[96] The meeting took place at Winchester on March 12. In a letter to the men of Kent John described the crucial point of the negotiations—"When we spoke to him about preserving our dignity, he said to us that he could do nothing for us in that respect unless we placed ourselves entirely at his mercy."[97] In short John demanded some guarantee that Simon lacked either the power or inclination to give and the conference ended in failure.

Shortly after his meeting with Simon Langton at Winchester King John despatched the abbot of Beaulieu to offer his terms to the pope. John would receive Stephen as archbishop, restore the money and property he had taken from the church, and allow the monks of Christ Church to return to their house. Stephen would give security for the loyalty of himself and his followers. The king would surrender the "regalia" of the archepiscopal see to the pope by the hands of the abbot of Beaulieu and the pope could have them given to Stephen. John would never willingly show friendship for Langton and had no intention of presenting him with the "regalia."[98] These were John's terms as outlined in Innocent's reply, but it is clear that the king set another condition that the pope saw fit not to mention. The abbot of Beaulieu was

---

[95] *Ibid.*, pp. lxxxv-lxxxix.
[96] *Rot. pat.*, pp. 78-79.
[97] *Ibid.*, p. 80.
[98] Gervase of Canterbury, II, xc-xci.

to obtain formal letters safeguarding John's "rights."[99] While there is no clear evidence as to just what the king had asked Simon Langton to promise and was now demanding from the pope, there seems to be a good basis for speculation as to the nature of John's desires. He was willing to accept Langton and to restore what he had taken from the church. He would overlook the violation of his royal privilege on this occasion. But he wanted to be assured that it would not establish a precedent. He insisted that Innocent should admit his right to participate in the election of English prelates by giving or withholding his assent. On May 27, 1208, Innocent wrote to the bishops of London, Ely and Worcester accepting John's terms as he outlined them and directing them to confer the "regalia" on Stephen Langton.[100] As we shall see later he also made a gesture toward satisfying John's demand for a guarantee of his rights.

Meanwhile in England the quarrel had reached an acute stage. Two days after his futile conference with Simon Langton John had returned the lands of the archbishop and the monks to the custody of Reginald de Cornhill.[101] Three days later, on March 17, he placed the sees of Bath and Exeter in the custody of heavy-handed mercenary captains.[102] By March 18 John knew when the interdict would be declared and had decided on his countermeasures. On that day he issued letters patent addressed to the clergy and laity of the see of Lincoln informing them that William de Cornhill, archdeacon of Huntingdon, and Gerard de Canville, sheriff of Lincolnshire, had been ordered to seize on the Monday after Easter the property of all clergy whether regular or secular who refused to perform the services of the church. While the only similar letter entered on the roll gives the same function in the see of Ely to Earl William of Salisbury, it seems clear that the same arrangements were made for all the sees of England.[103] An interdict forbade the clergy to perform their functions. But they held their property in consideration of performing religious services. Hence the answer to the interdict was to seize all ec-

[99] *Ibid.*, pp. c, cx.
[100] *Ibid.*, pp. xc-xci.
[101] *Rot. pat.*, p. 80.
[102] *Ibid.*
[103] *Ibid.*

clesiastical property. While the assumption that the clergy held their property solely because they said mass and administered the sacraments is debatable, there was clearly much to be said for John's argument. Confiscation for default of service was an idea that was easily grasped by the feudal world.[104]

Apparently John accompanied these orders with instructions that seemed at least to his more enthusiastic followers to put the clergy outside the protection of the law. On April 11 the king either changed his mind or made his original meaning clear. Anyone who harmed a clerk in violation of the king's peace would be hanged on the nearest oak tree.[105] He also began to mitigate his orders in regard to the property of ecclesiastics. The bishops of London, Ely, and Worcester had discreetly retired to the continent after publishing the interdict on March 24.[106] On April 5 the king's two favorite bishops, those of Winchester and Norwich, were given possession of their sees.[107] On April 10 the same courtesy was extended to the bishops of Bath and Salisbury.[108] A little later Giles de Briouse, bishop of Hereford, was given his lands, but the king kept his castles.[109] John feared Giles as a Briouse, not as a churchman. During this same month a host of clerks who had remained loyal to the king had their property returned to them.[110] The Cistercians, who claimed that their privileges exempted them from observing the interdict, received their property on April 4.[111]

While the interdict gave John an opportunity to vent his savage rage, it also allowed him to demonstrate his curiously wry sense of humor. He ordered his agents to seize the mistresses of the members of the clergy and to hold them until their lovers ransomed them. If we are to believe a sermon preached by the abbot

---

[104] On the general subject of the interdict see C. R. Cheney " King John and the papal interdict," *Bulletin of the John Rylands Library*, xxxi (1948).

[105] *Rot. claus.*, I, 111. This should be viewed in the light of John's letters patent of June 1213 in which he promises never again to outlaw clerks. *Rot. pat.*, p. 100.

[106] Gervase of Canterbury, II, 100-101.
[107] *Rot. claus.*, I, 108.
[108] *Ibid.*, p. 111.
[109] *Ibid.*, p. 113.
[110] *Ibid.*, p. 112.
[111] *Ibid.*, p. 108.

of Ford, this provided a considerable source of revenue as well as of entertainment to the king.[112] It was a perfectly magnificent idea. The clergy was harassed, money was extorted from them, and yet no ecclesiastical authority could gracefully protest.

The ecclesiastics who were given actual possession of their lands were a small minority. The property of the rest of the clergy was handled in three different ways. In every see there was a royal custodian who had charge of the property not entrusted to anyone else.[113] It was his duty to feed and clothe the clergy and retain the rest of their income for the king. Then various royal servants were given special custodies. The lands of the Knights Templar were entrusted to Geoffrey fitz Peter and the abbey of St. Edward to Hugh de Neville.[114] But most abbeys that depended directly on the crown were placed in the custody of their own abbots.[115] The Knights Hospitallers were also left in charge of their property. The canons of the vacant see of Exeter and the dean and chapter of Lincoln also had custody of their lands.[116] When a monastic house depended on a baron, it was usually placed in his care.[117] Finally a number of favored barons were given the custody of church property lying in their fiefs.[118] In theory all these people were custodians who would account to the crown for any income above what was needed to support the clergy, but it seems unlikely that the barons at least ever rendered any accounting. In all probability the ecclesiastical revenues in their lands served to quiet any tremors of conscience that might trouble them.

Simon Langton had gone to Rome after his interview with John in March—presumably to argue against the acceptance of the offer carried by the abbot of Beaulieu. When Innocent decided to accept John's terms, he sent both the abbot and Simon back with his letters.[119] On July 14 the king issued safe conducts for Simon, two monks of Canterbury, and the bishops of London, Ely, and

[112] Cheney, "King John and the papal interdict," p. 306.
[113] *Rot. claus.*, I, 107, 110; *Rot. pat.*, p. 80.
[114] *Rot. claus.*, I, 108, 110.   [117] *Ibid.*, pp. 107-110.
[115] *Ibid.*, pp. 108-113.   [118] *Ibid.*, pp. 109-113.
[116] *Ibid.*, pp. 108, 110, 112.   [119] Migne, *Patrologia*, ccxv, 1422-1423.

Worcester.[120] The purpose of the proposed meeting must have been to conduct final negotiations on the basis of the pope's letter of May 27. While there is no positive evidence that this conference was actually held, it seems likely that it was. On September 9 John issued a conduct for Stephen himself.[121] But apparently the report of his emissaries did not satisfy the archbishop, and he did not use the conduct. In all probability John purposely delayed a conclusion. He was enjoying a large part of the revenues of the English church and could well afford to wait to see what the pope would do next.

Innocent did not leave him long in doubt. Early in January 1209 the pope ordered John to carry out the offer he had sent to Rome by the abbot of Beaulieu. If peace was not made in three months, the king would be excommunicated. The bishops of London, Ely, and Worcester were directed to publish the sentence if John did not comply with the pope's demands.[122] This threat does not seem to have disturbed John, but it worried his servants. If the king were excommunicated, they would incur the church's censure for serving him. Hence a group of John's intimates urged him to make peace before the new blow fell. Their leader was Geoffrey fitz Peter and he was supported by the bishops of Winchester and Bath and the latter's brother, Hugh de Welles, who was bearing the title of bishop-elect of Lincoln.[123] Besides his general interest in the welfare of John and his realm Geoffrey had personal reasons for wanting to be on good terms with the pope. He had long been a sworn crusader and had avoided going to the Holy Land by obtaining a series of papal dispensations.[124] Peter des Roches and Jocelin de Welles could hardly relish the prospect of being at once successors of the apostles and intimates of an excommunicate while Hugh de Welles was naturally anxious to be confirmed in the rich see to which he had been elected. John listened to his friends' plea to the extent of reopening negotiations.

---

[120] *Rot. pat.*, p. 85.
[121] *Ibid.*, p. 86.
[122] Gervase of Canterbury, II, xcviii-c.
[123] *Ibid.*, p. ci.
[124] Migne, *Patrologia*, ccxiv, 1088-1090; ccxv, 745-746.

On March 23, 1209, a conduct was issued for Simon Langton to journey to London to talk with the justiciar and the two bishops.[125] If this conference took place, it accomplished nothing.

The royal officials did not give up hope and by July they had persuaded John to try again. On July 13 the king addressed a letter to the three bishops who were serving as Innocent's agents. On the advice of the justiciar, the bishops of Winchester and Bath, and the elect of Lincoln he had decided to satisfy the church. The three bishops were to cross to Dover. There they would be met by the group already mentioned reinforced by the earls of Arundel and Oxford, William Brewer, the abbot of Beaulieu, Henry, archdeacon of Stafford, and William de Cornhill, archdeacon of Huntingdon. The bishops were to bring with them the "*privilegium domini papae quod de indempnitate nostra conservanda impetratum est et repositum apud Clarum Mariscum.*" If they could not get the bull itself, they were to bring a copy. At about the same time Geoffrey fitz Peter wrote to the bishops asking them to hasten their crossing.[126]

It is not known exactly when this conference began. On July 26, 1209, King John sent a messenger to his representatives at Dover and by August 10 the meeting was over.[127] The appendix to the Canterbury chronicle printed in the rolls series edition of Gervase of Canterbury contains a document purporting to state the terms offered by the pope's agents and agreed to by John's.[128] Stephen Langton was to receive the see of Canterbury as Hubert Walter held it the day he died. The bishops of London, Ely, Worcester, and Hereford were to have their lands as they were when the interdict was declared. Thus Giles de Briouse whose expulsion was the result of the purely secular quarrel between his father and John had found refuge behind the broad skirts of the Mother Church. The monks of Canterbury were also to regain their estates. All the money that John had taken from the clergy of England because of his controversy with the pope was to be re-

---

[125] *Rot. pat.*, p. 90.
[126] Gervase of Canterbury, II, c-ci.
[127] *Rot. liberate*, p. 123; Gervase of Canterbury, II, cii.
[128] Gervase of Canterbury, II, ci-ciii.

turned within three weeks after the feast of St. Lawrence, August 10. This clause was carefully worded. John was to return all money that he would not have taken "if the church had been in good peace and full liberty." As the clergy headed by Geoffrey of York had protested the levying of the thirteenth of 1207, the money obtained from them by this tax could be included in the sum to be made good. John was to receive Stephen as archbishop and give a guarantee of safety to him and the four exiled bishops "by his own mouth before his magnates." A group of bishops and barons to be named by Stephen would issue letters patent guaranteeing the safety of the exiles. When Stephen reached England, he would receive the regalia and swear fidelity to John. The three bishops and Simon Langton promised that they would in so far as they could preserve John's rights and privileges and see that the royal prerogative did not suffer as a result of the agreement.

According to the document we have been following, John's agents accepted these terms. It seems more likely that they simply agreed to carry them to their master. The pope's representatives on their part postponed the publication of the sentence of excommunication against the king until five weeks after August 10.[129] The terms were unsatisfactory to John, and on August 23 he wrote to the bishops of London, Ely, and Worcester to meet him at Northampton.[130] But the three bishops refused. They feared apparently that John might seek to delay the publication of his excommunication by seizing them. They wrote to the bishop of Winchester pointing out that John's letters granting them safe-conduct to Northampton were letters close and not letters patent, and they doubted their validity. Moreover no move had been made to restore the money taken from the clergy. Finally the letters of conduct to go to Northampton did not include Simon Langton and they could not negotiate without him.[131] Once more Geoffrey fitz Peter intervened. With the assistance of the bishops of Rochester, Salisbury, and Bath, Hugh de Welles, and Walter de Grey he persuaded the bishops to postpone the publication of the excommunication until October 7.[132]

[129] *Ibid.*, ciii.
[130] *Ibid.*
[131] *Ibid.*, p. civ.
[132] *Ibid.*, p. cvi.

Meanwhile Stephen Langton had received optimistic reports of the progress of the negotiations and sent his seneschal to John's court. The king received him well and expressed a desire to confer with the archbishop. After receiving adequate guarantees of his personal safety, Stephen crossed to Dover early in October.[133] John went as far as the castle of Chilham in Kent and sent the justiciar and Peter des Roches to treat with Stephen, but they could come to no agreement and the archbishop returned to the continent without seeing the king.[134] Geoffrey fitz Peter paid the archbishop and the three bishops 400 marks presumably to cover the costs of their visit though it may have been intended as a first payment on their lost revenues.[135] Another effort was made in the spring of 1210. John sent the abbot of Stratford and the prior of Holy Trinity, London, to invite Stephen to cross to talk with him at Dover.[136] But the archbishop discovered that the king was still unwilling to accept his terms and did not cross the channel.

While it is comparatively easy to construct a narrative account of these prolonged negotiations, it is extremely difficult to discover the issue or issues that made them fruitless. The contemporary sources contain two explanations and it seems likely that both the issues mentioned played some part in preventing the conclusion of peace. According to the Waverley annalist when John sent Geoffrey fitz Peter to meet the pope's emissaries at Dover in July 1209, he authorized him to offer the archbishop and each of the three bishops £100 as full payment for the revenues they had lost. The king absolutely refused to consider the full restitution demanded by the papal terms of peace.[137] This may well have been one of the vital issues. As the pope's terms were worded in the document we have the clergy could have demanded the restoration of practically any payments they had made to the crown since Stephen's consecration. While one may doubt that John really hoped to settle for £100 a piece to four prelates, he may well have

[133] *Annals of Waverley*, p. 263; Gervase of Canterbury, II, 104.
[134] *Ibid.*
[135] Pipe roll 11 John, Public Record Office.
[136] Gervase of Canterbury, II, cvi-cvii, cx-cxii, 105-106; *Annals of Waverley*, p. 264.
[137] *Ibid.*, pp. 262-263.

been determined to offer nothing but a lump sum. But the letters in the appendix of the Canterbury chronicle make no reference to this question. They make the central issue the safeguarding of John's prerogative. The three bishops and Simon Langton had promised to do their best to see that John's rights were not impaired. Stephen had made the same promise when he landed at Dover. He was ready to repeat it in May 1210.[138] But John wanted something more solid.

When John notified his subjects of the failure of his conference with Simon Langton in March 1208 he said " and when we spoke with him about safeguarding our dignity in this matter, he said to us that he would do nothing for us in that respect unless we placed ourself entirely at his mercy." [139] John then sent the abbot of Beaulieu to Rome to discuss the matter with the pope and Simon went to the papal court at about the same time. Innocent then wrote to the three bishops directing them to accept John's offer and sent Beaulieu and Simon north once more.[140] They seem to have carried with them the pope's detailed terms. They also seem to have borne the letters mentioned in John's letter to the three bishops in July 1209—the *" privilegium domini papae quod . . . de intempnitate nostra conservanda . . ."* Beaulieu had obtained these letters from the pope and they had been deposited in a French abbey. John wanted to see them or at least a copy of them. Stephen, Simon, and the three bishops maintained that they could obtain them only by a special papal order. The king clearly did not believe this and repeated his demands while his opponents repeated their refusal.[141]

There seems to me to be only one hypothesis that can explain all this. John wanted a definite guarantee that his acceptance of Stephen who had been consecrated without his consent could not be used as a precedent in other cases. Simon Langton had neither the power nor the desire to give such a guarantee. The abbot of

---

[138] Gervase of Canterbury, II, cx-cxii.
[139] *Rot. pat.*, p. 80.
[140] Gervase of Canterbury, II, xc-xci; Migne, *Patrologia*, ccxv, 1422-1423.
[141] Gervase of Canterbury, II, c, cx, cxii.

Beaulieu was instructed to tell the pope that John would accept Stephen if Innocent would issue a bull to cover this matter. In all probability Simon argued against the issuing of such a bull. Innocent's solution was to issue it and give it to Simon with orders to deposit it in a French monastery until the pope himself should release it. He could then write to the three bishops stating that he had accepted John's terms. The king knew of the existence of the bull from the report of the abbot of Beaulieu, but he had no intention of making peace until he knew its exact contents. When he learned that the pope's orders forbade him to be shown either the document itself or a copy of it, he naturally suspected that it would not prove satisfactory. In short John's demands may have been unreasonable, but he stuck to them consistently. It was Innocent's very dubious device that made the negotiations fruitless. I suspect that John did not care very much whether or not peace was made. At the same time it is unfair to state that he refused to carry out the terms he had offered through the abbot of Beaulieu.

In June 20, 1209, Innocent had ordered the bishop of Arras and the abbot of St. Vast of Arras to assist the bishops of London, Ely, and Worcester in publishing John's excommunication whenever Stephen Langton should request them to do so.[142] The publication seems to have taken place in November. The exact effect of this on John's status is not clear. Englishmen could argue that they were not bound by a decree proclaimed on the continent, and there is evidence that Innocent either actually suspended its operation or at least regarded the publication to be of doubtful validity. But it did deprive John of most of his supporters among the episcopate. Herbert Poor of Salisbury and Gilbert de Glanvill of Rochester retired to Scotland while Jocelin of Bath crossed to France.[143] With Jocelin went his brother, Hugh de Welles, to seek consecration as bishop of Lincoln from Stephen Langton.[144] Geoffrey of York was still in exile because of his opposition to the

[142] Migne, *Patrologia,* ccxvi, 64.
[143] Gervase of Canterbury places the retreat to Scotland in 1207, but the bishops of Rochester, Salisbury, and Bath were clearly in England in 1209. Gervase of Canterbury II, cvi, 100. The bishop of Bath was in France by 1211. *Ibid.,* p. cxiv.
[144] *Ibid.*

thirteenth of 1207. As the sees of Chichester, Durham, Exeter, Lichfield, and Lincoln were vacant, the bishops of Winchester and Norwich were the only ones left at John's side. And John de Grey had been sent to Ireland in February 1208 to succeed Meiler fitz Henry as justiciar.[145] Hence the only bishop in England by the end of 1209 was Peter des Roches.

Before reaching the final scenes of King John's quarrel with Innocent III over the Canterbury succession it seems well to glance at a few other aspects of his relations with the church during this period. By far the most interesting of these, at least from John's point of view, was the extorting of money from the English clergy. Unfortunately little is known about the details of this highly successful financial operation. What evidence there is suggests that the usual procedure was for the king to make a barefaced demand for a large sum of money. Before the interdict was proclaimed, an exchequer clerk, William de Neckton, seems to have been the collector of "the gifts of the prelates," but it is not clear whether these early gifts were the result of outright extortion or simply the payments made in lieu of the thirteenth.[146] By 1208 Richard Marsh seems to have become John's chief agent in drawing money from the clergy.[147] In addition to fines and gifts the king was enjoying a large part of the revenues of the English church. The *Red book of the exchequer* contains an account of the "receipts of King John from bishops, abbots, and other clerks of England in the time of the interdict for Stephen, archbishop of Canterbury."[148] It shows a total of over 58,000 marks received from the baronies of the exiled prelates—the two archbishops and the bishops of London, Salisbury, Lincoln, Worcester, Bath, Ely, and Hereford. Then there was a sum of over 16,000 marks from the clergy of eleven dioceses. In addition, nearly 40,000 marks were received from monastic houses. The grand total of this account comes to some 110,000 marks. Unfortunately it is difficult to discover just what the account covered. There is no record of

---

[145] *Annals of Dunstaple*, p. 30.   [146] *Rot. claus.*, I, 103.
[147] William of Newburgh, p. 512, *Chronica monasterii de Melsa* (ed. Edward A. Bond, Rolls series), I, 326.
[148] *Red book of the exchequer*, II, 772-773.

receipts from the clergy of four dioceses—Ely, Hereford, Lichfield, and Rochester. In short even as a record of the money "that would not have been received if the church had been in peace" the account is clearly incomplete. And it does not pretend to include the revenues that were less directly the result of the interdict. The bishops of Exeter and Lincoln died in 1206, the bishop of Chichester in 1207, and those of Durham and Lichfield in 1208. Ordinarily these prelates would have been replaced within a year or so, but as a result of his quarrel with Rome John enjoyed their baronies until 1213. This was also true of a number of abbeys including some of the richest in England. I suspect that John's total profits from the struggle with Innocent reached £100,000 and may well have exceeded that sum. The steady flow of cash into the royal coffers must never be underestimated as a reason for the king's lack of any burning desire to make peace with the Holy See.

English kings were ordinarily inclined to let sees lie vacant while they enjoyed the revenues, and the quarrel with Innocent III gave John an unusually good excuse for following this policy. But the pope had no intention of allowing him to do so without a contest. Early in January 1209 he wrote to the priors and convents of Coventry and Durham and the deans and chapters of Chichester, Exeter, and Lincoln instructing them to hold elections. If they did not choose successors to their late bishops, the pope himself would fill the vacancies by appointment.[149] These papal letters moved John to take the obvious course—fill the vacancies with his servants. As the clergy were completely at his mercy, the chapters could give him no trouble. The bearer of the royal seal, Hugh de Welles, was elected bishop of Lincoln, Walter de Grey, the chancellor, bishop of Lichfield, Coventry, and Chester, Henry of London, archdeacon of Stafford, bishop of Exeter, and Master Gilbert de Laigle, bishop of Chichester.[150] Three of these men

---

[149] Migne, *Patrologia*, ccvx, 1528-1529.

[150] *Annals of Osney* (ed. H. R. Luard in *Annales monastici*, IV, Rolls series), p. 54; *Annals of Tewksbury* in ibid., I, 59; *Annals of Dunstaple* p. 31. The elect of Chichester is variously called Richard and Nicholas de Laigle, but it is clear that Gilbert must have been the man meant. *Ibid.*, p. 40.

were well known as royal servants. Gilbert de Laigle had been a friend of Hubert Walter and had received his final confession, but he had joined the king's party in the quarrel with the pope. In 1211 Stephen Langton declared void the elections of Walter de Grey, Henry of London, and probably that of Gilbert de Laigle.[151] They had all incurred the censure of the church by standing by John after his excommunication. The outcome of the election of Hugh de Welles deserves a separate paragraph.

There is no evidence that Innocent III paid any attention to the election to the episcopate of Walter de Grey, Henry of London, or Gilbert de Laigle, but on June 21, 1209, he addressed a letter to Stephen Langton about the election of Hugh de Welles. Perhaps the influence of his mitre-crowned brother placed Hugh in a special category. The pope had received the king's letters patent certifying that the dean and chapter of Lincoln had elected Hugh and that he had given his assent. But the pope feared that the state of the English church might have led to an uncanonical election. While the king had the privilege of giving his assent to an election after it was made, it was highly improper for him to suggest in advance the name of the man to whose election he would assent. Stephen was to consult at least three canons of Lincoln who had been present at the election to make sure that there had been no such abuse of the church's freedom. One can only conclude that Innocent was here being intentionally naïve. There was no need for John to express formally his choice for the vacant see —Hugh de Welles was himself a canon of Lincoln and the chapter was well packed with such other royal servants as William of Ely, the treasurer. The pope then directed Stephen to investigate Hugh's suitability for high ecclesiastical office. As senior clerk of the chancery and bearer of the seal he had sealed royal letters directing the seizure of church property. He had also had intercourse with those who had been excommunicated for expelling the monks of Canterbury. On the other hand the pope pointed out that even bishops were often royal chancellors and they could not be held responsible for all the wrongs authorized by the letters they

---

[151] *Annals of Worcester* (ed. H. R. Luard in *Annales monastici*, IV, Rolls series), p. 399.

sealed. It would be very difficult to prove that Hugh had had intercourse with the excommunicants. There was, however, another difficulty. Hugh was suspected of incontinence as he had daughters born in matrimony. But if the children were not so young as to show that the incontinence had been recent, this need not bar him from the episcopal office. In short Innocent gave Langton a free hand to do what he thought best.[152] We can only speculate as to just what happened. Hugh de Welles was one of the group sent to confer with the bishops of London, Ely, and Worcester in July 1209 and he also took part in the negotiations with Langton in early October of that year. Presumably Stephen offered him confirmation of his election if he would desert John's cause. At any rate Hugh crossed to the continent and was consecrated by the archbishop on December 20.

In the spring of 1211 Pope Innocent decided to send another embassy to England. For this delicate task he chose Pandulf, a cardinal sub-deacon, and Durand, a knight of the Temple.[153] On August 30 the two emissaries met John at Northampton. The *Annals of Burton* contain a long account of the conversation between the king and the papal envoys and Roger of Wendover gives a brief summary of the negotiations.[154] Wendover states that the king was willing to accept Langton, but refused to restore the money he had taken from the church. While it seems most unlikely that John was unwilling to make any restoration, it is quite probable that he declined to make it as complete as the pope required. This may well have been one of the issues that led to the failure of the conference. The passage in the *Annals of Burton* cannot be taken very seriously as an account of this interview. It is rather a dramatically written resumé of the whole series of negotiations between the king and the pope. John starts by saying that he will hang Stephen if he sets foot in England, then suggests that he resign Canterbury and accept another English see, and finally agrees to receive him as archbisop if his royal rights are

[152] Migne, *Patrologia,* ccxvi, 62-64.
[153] Gervase of Canterbury, II, cxiii.
[154] *Annals of Burton* (ed. H. R. Luard in *Annales monastici,* I, Rolls series), pp. 209-217; *Annals of Waverley,* pp. 268-271; Wendover, II, 58

safeguarded for the future. The pope's ambassadors refuse to compromise, solemnly announce John's excommunication, and release his subjects from their oaths of fidelity to him. According to the annals John's excommunication had been suspended up to this time and was put into effect by Pandulf and Durand. Now it seems unlikely that this was true in any strictly legal sense. John had been excommunicated by the pope and the sentence had been published in France. But it had not been published in England and Pandulf and Durand may have done this. They certainly did not release John's subjects from their oaths of fidelity. The papal letter directing them to proceed to England gave them no authority to take any such action. On the other hand most of Innocent's letters to John speak vaguely of more severe penalties to follow if he remained contumacious and it is very probable that Pandulf made these threats precise. Two English chroniclers state that Pandulf released the English from their oaths of fidelity, another says that he threatened that Innocent would do so, and a fourth asserts that the pope took this action when he learned of the failure of Pandulf's mission.[155] Solemn letters patent issued by the barons of Ireland state that the pope proposed to release John's subjects from their obligations to him.[156] In the light of this evidence it seems impossible to escape the conclusion that Pandulf must have uttered a threat of this sort.

John rejected the demands of Pandulf and Durand in the summer of 1211, but that year and the next saw the development of new circumstances that were to oblige him to make peace with the pope. Perhaps the most serious of these was a diplomatic revolution among the powers of western Europe. On October 4, 1209, while his envoys were negotiating with John in Kent, Pope Innocent crowned Otto of Brunswick as Holy Roman Emperor. Unfortunately Otto proved intractable. Within a year he was excommunicate, and the pope was supporting the imperial preten-

---

[155] *Annals of Burton*, p. 215; *Annals of Waverley*, p. 270; Wendover, II, 59; Geoffrey de Coldingham (ed. James Raine in *Historiae Dunelmensis scriptores tres*, Surtees Society, IX [1839]), pp. 26-27.

[156] *Calendar of documents relating to Ireland* (Rolls series), no. 448; Painter, *William Marshal*, pp. 172-174.

sions of young Frederick of Hohenstaufen, king of Sicily. This change in papal policy brought Innocent into the same camp as Philip Augustus who had been a consistent supporter of the house of Hohenstaufen. It also deprived John of his most powerful ally in the papal party. Finally it made available to Innocent a secular power so situated that it could act against England. Philip Augustus had long toyed with the idea of invading John's island realm. It would not be hard to persuade him to do so as the pope's agent— as a crusader.

The prospect of an attack by Philip of France would not of itself have disturbed John very much. His nephew, the count of Toulouse, was at odds with both Philip and the pope, and many of the knights of France were engaged in the Albigensian crusade. Moreover the counts of Boulogne and Flanders were disaffected and in the spring of 1212 both formed alliances with John. There were other French nobles who were not adverse to listening to treasonable proposals supported by pounds sterling. Otto was still master of northern Germany. While Philip dreamed of invading England, John planned a campaign in which an English army supported by the count of Toulouse should move northwards from Aquitaine to meet Otto and the counts of Boulogne and Flanders. France would be crushed in a vise.

The only thing that really troubled King John was the situation at home. The Welsh gave continual trouble in 1211 and 1212 and there was reason for suspecting that they were allied with King Philip.[157] The king of Scotland had been forced to make a humiliating peace in 1211, but there was little doubt that he would cheerfully break it if a really good opportunity arose. But most serious of all was the temper of the English baronage. This is not the place to discuss the beginnings of John's final quarrel with his barons. Suffice it to say that William de Briouse had fled to France in 1210 and King Philip was negotiating with English barons. When the plot of Robert fitz Walter was discovered in the summer of 1212, that baron promptly crossed to France. Moreover it is clear that while few if any English barons were inclined to desert the king for the pope, many were growing restive

[157] *Layettes du trésor de chartes*, I, 386-387.

under the interdict. It was Geoffrey fitz Peter who had urged
John to negotiate in 1209 and he seems to have taken the lead in
the renewed effort in 1210. In 1212 William Marshal wrote from
Ireland to beg John to make peace with the church.[158] When he
thought of Innocent III, Philip Augustus, the Scots, the Welsh,
and his disaffected barons, King John might well conclude that
he had too many foes. The cheapest of these to buy off and the
most effective ally when bought was obviously Pope Innocent.

By November 1212 John had decided to make peace with the
pope on the latter's terms. He therefore despatched to Rome an
embassy consisting of the abbot of Beaulieu, Alan Martel, a
Templar, Master Richard de Tiring, Thomas de Eardington,
Philip of Worcester, and one other.[159] The abbot and Alan Martel
acting with three others were given authority to negotiate in
John's name and to pledge his acceptance of the terms agreed
upon.[160] Unfortunately Thomas de Eardington, Philip of Worcester, and Richard de Tiring were captured while crossing the
domains of John's enemies.[161] Presumably no one dared seize a
Cistercian abbot and a Templar. Hence the delegation arrived at
Rome lacking a quorum. Finally, however, the abbot and Alan
Martel agreed to promise that John would accept the terms that
would be offered him by Pandulf and Durand. On February 27,
1213, the pope informed King John of these negotiations and sent
him a copy of the terms.[162]

John was to swear before the pope's agents to obey Innocent's
commands in respect to all the offenses for which he had been
excommunicated. He was to receive in his realm Archbishop
Stephen, the exiled bishops, the monks of Canterbury, Robert fitz
Walter, Eustace de Vesci, and all clerks and laymen who had been
exiled during the controversy. The archbishop and bishops were
to choose a group of bishops and barons who were to issue letters
guaranteeing their safety. If John violated these guarantees, he

---

[158] *Calendar of documents relating to Ireland,* no. 448.
[159] *Rot. claus.,* I, 125.
[160] Migne, *Patrologia,* ccxvi, 772-773.
[161] " Rotulus misae 14 John," p. 256.
[162] Migne, *Patrologia,* ccxvi, 772-775.

was to lose forever his rights of patronage over the English church. If the king wanted to, he might oblige the archbishop and his colleagues to swear that they would do nothing against his person or his crown. All the money taken by John from the church was to be restored. As soon as the pope's agent sent to absolve the king arrived in England, John was to pay £8,000 to the exiles. He was also to swear never again to presume to outlaw clerks. The outlawry of the laymen involved in Robert fitz Walter's plot was to be revoked. Except for the references to Robert fitz Walter, Eustace de Vesci, and their accomplices who had managed to persuade the pope's agents that they had suffered exile for their love of the church these terms were essentially the same as those offered many times before.

Before John's emissaries had arrived in Rome, Stephen Langton and the bishops of London and Ely had visited the papal court.[163] The bishop of Worcester had died during the previous summer. They told Innocent a horrifying story of John's treatment of the English clergy.[164] Moved by their pleas the pope issued letters deposing John and calling on Philip Augustus to conquer the English realm.[165] These letters were given to Langton, and the three bishops started north arriving in France in January 1213. They found King Philip in a highly receptive mood. He had been negotiating with the dissident English barons for at least four years. He undoubtedly knew that John was in league with his foes among the baronage of France and had formed an alliance with Otto to crush the French realm. Even without papal encouragement he might well have decided to take the offensive before John was ready. Innocent's letters and Langton's pleas were decisive. On April 8 the pope's letters were read before an assembly of the baronage of France at Soissons, and King Philip summoned his host to muster at Rouen on April 21.[166] But shortly after the council at Soissons Pandulf arrived in France bearing the news that

---

[163] Coggeshall, pp. 165-166; Coventry, II, 209; Wendover, II, 63.
[164] *Ibid.*
[165] *Ibid.;* Coventry, II, 209.
[166] Wendover, II, 65.

King John had agreed to accept the pope's terms and that he was to conclude the negotiations.[167]

The events that occurred between the arrival of Stephen Langton and his fellow bishops in Rome in the autumn of 1212 and the appearance in France of Pandulf in the spring of 1213 have been the subject of much controversy among historians.[168] While I believe that the account given in the previous paragraph is essentially correct, a number of interesting questions cannot be answered with any assurance. As the papal letters deposing John and calling on King Philip to invade England have not been preserved, their exact terms are unknown. Moreover while it seems clear that the contents of these letters were communicated to King Philip and his barons at the council of Soissons, they may not have been formally published.[169] In short it is impossible to say whether or not John was deposed by the pope. Then there is no definite evidence as to when the English embassy arrived in Rome. If Innocent III allowed Langton to leave for France with his letters deposing John after the pope learned that the English king had offered to submit, he was, as Wendover suggests, guilty of un-

---

[167] Wendover and Coggeshall believed that Pandulf had gone to France with Langton. Wendover II, 64; Coggeshall, pp. 165-166. But Coventry states clearly that Pandulf arrived later with John's returning embassy. Coventry, II, 209. As Langton reached France in January and Pandulf did not leave Rome until February 27, Coventry is clearly right. Wendover, II, 65. Migne, *Patrologia*, ccxvi, 772-775.

[168] For a detailed discussion see C. R. Cheney, " The alleged deposition of King John," in *Studies in medieval history presented to Frederick Maurice Powicke* (Oxford, 1948), pp. 100-116. While I am unable to accept a number of Professor Cheney's conclusions, his article has enabled me to correct several serious errors in my own account.

[169] Professor Cheney does not believe that Innocent asked Philip to invade England. To me the evidence on this point seems very strong. A number of chronicles state definitely that he did. *Annals of Waverley*, p. 274; *Annals of Winchester*, p. 82; Coventry, II, 209; Wendover, II, 63-65; William of Andres, *Chronica (Monumenta Germaniae historica, Scriptores)*, XXIV, 754. Other chronicles without definitely mentioning the papal request seem to me to assume that it was made. Guillaume le Breton, *Gesta Philippi Augusti* (ed. H. F. Delaborde in *Oeuvres de Rigord et de Guillaume le Breton*, Société de l'histoire de France), I, 253; *ibid., Philippidos* in *ibid.*, II, 255; Coggeshall, pp. 165-166; *Histoire de Guillaume le Maréchal*, II, lines 14494-14498.

worthy subterfuge. But this seems most unlikely. The English envoys started for Rome in November.[170] Wendover states that Langton reached France in January.[171] The papal letters to John accepting his offer of submission are dated February 26.[172] If this chronology is correct, Innocent acted with perfect propriety. When he gave Langton the letters deposing John and calling on Philip to invade England, the English king was, as far as he knew, completely contumacious. As soon as John's offer of submission arrived, the pope despatched Pandulf to give him an opportunity to make peace before the letters borne by Langton came into full operation.

Early in May while King Philip's host was poised on the coast of France Pandulf sent two Templars to England to inquire whether or not John was still willing to make peace with the church. The king received them well and invited Pandulf to England.[173] On May 13 John issued letters patent stating that four of his barons had sworn in his behalf that he would accept the pope's terms and reciting the terms contained in Innocent's letters.[174] One would expect that the four barons chosen would have come from the ranks of the greatest English earls—especially those who had counseled the king to make peace. But actually only one, Earl William de Warren, was a baron of the first rank. The others were the king's half-brother, Earl William of Salisbury, William de Ferrers, earl of Derby, and the French renegade, Count Reginald of Boulogne. These names may have no particular significance. Perhaps they were the lords at hand when the oaths were to be taken. Still one cannot help wondering whether such comparatively conscientious barons as Geoffrey fitz Peter and William Marshal knew their master too well to be willing to pledge their word that he would carry out a treaty.

From John's point of view merely making peace with the church would yield him only small benefits. Neither interdict nor excommunication had troubled him much. The peace would deprive King Philip of an excuse for invading England and might force

---

[170] *Rot. claus.*, I, 126.
[171] Wendover, II, 65.
[172] Migne, *Patrologia*, ccxvi, 772-775.
[173] Wendover, II, 68-69.
[174] *Ibid.*, pp. 70-73.

King John and the Church

him to give up his plans. It would also stop John's disaffected barons from using his quarrel with the pope as justification for plots against him. On the other hand it would cost him a lot of money. John well knew that Philip had been for years thinking of an invasion of England, and that his barons' real grievances had nothing to do with his excommunication. If he were to carry out his cherished plan of crushing King Philip in concert with Otto of Brunswick, he needed more than the pope's forgiveness—he needed active support. Out of thoughts such as these came a brilliant idea—a true stroke of genius. If he formally surrendered his realm to the pope and received it back as a fief, he would gain the active friendship of Innocent and his support against all his foes. One of Innocent's prime concerns was to increase the prestige and dignity of himself and his see in both ecclesiastical and secular affairs. He was bound to be deeply gratified if the powerful English king became his vassal. Moreover Innocent would be given an interest in that royal prerogative that John had been defending so vigorously against him. If in the future the bishops of England infringed on the king's rights, they would be indirectly injuring the pope. All this would cost John little. He would promise an annual tribute that he would pay when convenient. The obligations involved in homage and fidelity were not likely to worry King John.

On May 15, John issued a charter putting this scheme into effect. He had gravely offended God and Holy Mother Church in many ways and was unworthy of divine mercy. He could think of no suitable way of giving satisfaction except by surrendering his kingdom to God and the apostles Peter and Paul in the person of Pope Innocent. He did this voluntarily with advice of his barons. The realms of England and Ireland were placed in Pandulf's hands as the pope's agent. John would do liege homage to the pope in person if he could get to Rome and his heirs would do the same to his successors. The feudal service due from the king of England to his suzerain would consist of a tribute of 1,000 marks a year—700 marks for England and 300 for Ireland.[175] This remarkable document was attested by Henry of London, who had become

[175] Wendover, II, 74-76.

archbishop of Dublin, John de Grey, bishop of Norwich, Geoffrey fitz Peter, Earl William of Salisbury, Earl William Marshal, Count Reginald of Boulogne, Earl William de Warren, Saher de Quency, earl of Winchester, William, earl of Arundel, William des Ferrers, earl of Derby, William Brewer, Peter fitz Herbert, and Warin fitz Gerold. Even if these were the only lords who approved the transaction, John could say that he had acted with the consent of the great barons of his realm.

Before a century had passed historians were criticizing John for this surrender of his realm to papal suzerainty. During the middle years of the thirteenth century the pope's efforts to raise money in England to support his long struggle against the house of Hohenstaufen bred strong anti-papal feeling. Then as English national feeling developed, it became more and more inconceivable that an English king would surrender his kingdom to a foreign potentate. But there is no evidence whatever that any such sentiment existed in John's time. No contemporary chronicler criticized the king for his action. A group of the greatest lords of the realm witnessed the formal charter of surrender. Moreover it was no disgrace to be a vassal of the Holy See. Frederick of Hohenstaufen, Holy Roman Emperor, was himself the pope's vassal for his kingdom of Sicily and several other secular princes were in the same position. I suspect that John's barons fully understood his motives and considered the surrender a brilliant maneuver. Immediate aid was bought with promises.

The non-financial terms of the peace were quickly executed. On May 24 the three bishops, seven earls, and five barons chosen for the purpose by Stephen Langton issued letters patent guaranteeing the safety of the exiles when they returned.[176] On May 31 and June 1 the baronies of the exiled prelates were placed in the custody of their agents.[177] On July 1 the archbishop of Dublin, the bishop of Norwich, the earl of Arundel, Matthew fitz Herbert, and William de Cornhill, archdeacon of Huntingdon, were despatched to hasten the return of the exiles.[178] They finally landed on July 16 and met John at Winchester on July 20.[179] On July 18 the king

[176] *Rot. pat.*, pp. 98-99, 114.
[177] *Ibid.*, p. 99. *Rot. claus.*, I, 145.
[178] *Ibid.*, p. 164.
[179] Wendover, II, 80-81.

issued a charter stating that he had sworn before Stephen to obey the terms of the peace and had paid the exiles £8,000 as a first installment of the money due them.[180] Meanwhile the pope had received word of the conclusion of peace. On July 6 he despatched a group of letters to England announcing to the king, the clergy of the realm, the former exiles, and the barons that he was sending Nicholas, cardinal-bishop of Tusculum, "like an angel of peace and safety" to supervise the execution of the agreement.[181]

The determination of the amount of money that John should pay the English clergy was an extremely complicated matter. In the summer of 1212 when the king realized that he would be forced to accept the pope's terms, he began his preparations for reducing the sum of money to be restored. The chancery prepared form letters to be issued by religious houses. "Know all that when our lord, John by God's grace king of England, lord of Ireland, duke of Normandy and Aquitaine and count of Anjou, was ready to restore to us all the money that he had received from our house from his first coronation to the feast of the Nativity of the Blessed Virgin Mary in the fourteenth year of the lord king's reign [September 8, 1212], we in good spirit and entirely of our free will gave him that money." The letters go on to state that they were issued for fear someone might call these sums "exactions or extortions."[182] As the clergy of England were entirely at the king's mercy in 1212, it seems likely that he had little difficulty persuading them to issue letters in this form. When Stephen Langton went to Rome in the winter of 1212-1213, he told the pope of John's ingenious device, and the papal terms of peace specifically provided that such letters were to be deemed invalid.[183] On October 30, 1213, Innocent ordered Nicholas of Tusculum to see that the sums covered by such letters were restored. If the houses refused to accept the money, it was to be given to the Templars and the Hospitallers to be used for the crusade.[184] But John was not to be out-maneuvered so easily. He simply had his chancery concoct

---

[180] *Rot. chart.*, pp. 193-194.
[181] Migne, *Patrologia*, ccxvi, 881-884.
[182] *Rot. chart.*, pp. 191-192.
[183] Migne, *Patrologia*, ccxvi, 775, 780.
[184] *Ibid.*, columns 927-928.

different letters. "We wish it to be known to all of you that our lord, John, by God's grace king etc. has fully satisfied us and our church in respect to all that was received by him or any of his men from the goods of our house from the beginning of the interdict to such and such a day."[185] We have ample evidence of the none too subtle methods by which John persuaded religious houses to issue letters in this form.[186]

It was agreed that a general investigation would be made to determine the sum that had been taken from ecclesiastics. The machinery for this was set in motion on August 31, 1213. Two or three royal agents were sent into each diocese to sit with the local ecclesiastical authorities and clerks sent by Langton for the purpose. They were to summon before them all those who had had custody of ecclesiastical property.[187] But an investigation of this sort was bound to be a long process—especially if the royal agents were in no hurry. When Nicholas of Tusculum arrived in England in the autumn, he set to work to negotiate a quick settlement so that the interdict could be lifted. At a conference held in London the king agreed to pay 100,000 marks. If the investigations showed that a larger sum was due, he would make it up later. The legate was all for accepting this offer, but the bishops preferred to wait until the inquiries were finished and they could get all their money at once.[188] Presumably they suspected that once the interdict was lifted, they would have trouble collecting future payments. Apparently, however, the legate transmitted this offer to the pope who accepted it. In letters dated January 23, 1214, he directed the legate to relax the interdict when the 100,000 marks had been paid.[189]

It seems doubtful that John ever really intended to pay 100,000 marks in cash on the spot. He was hard at work on his plans for an invasion of France, and so large a payment would have seri-

---

[185] *Rot. pat.*, pp. 140-141.
[186] *Ibid. Rot. oblatis*, p. 559; "Cronica de electione Hugonis abbatis" in *Memorials of St. Edmund's abbey* (ed. Thomas Arnold, Rolls series), II, 105-113; *Annals of Waverley*, p. 268; Coggeshall, p. 165.
[187] Rymer, *Foedera*, I, 114; *Rot. claus.*, I, 164.
[188] Wendover, II, 94.
[189] Migne, *Patrologia*, ccxvi, 953-954.

ously drained his war-chest. At any rate he despatched an embassy to Rome to seek better terms. This resulted in another papal letter to the legate. The bishop of Norwich, Richard Marsh, archdeacon of Northumberland, Thomas de Eardington, and Alan Martel had conferred before the pope with Simon Langton and two of his clerks. John was to pay 40,000 marks before the interdict was relaxed—this 40,000 marks to include all payments already made. Then he was to pay 12,000 marks a year until he had restored the full amount set by the inquisitions. The bishops of Winchester and Norwich, the earls of Chester, Winchester, and Pembroke, and William Brewer were to guarantee that these payments would be made.[190] It is not too difficult to guess at the arguments advanced by John de Grey and Richard Marsh. King John owed the pope £1,000 marks a year. Innocent was again pressing him to do something about Berengeria's dowry.[191] The king could not pay 100,000 marks at once. Actually John did not even pay the 40,000 marks. Nicholas of Tusculum allowed him to postpone payment of 13,000 marks on the guarantee of the bishops of Winchester and Norwich.[192] As the civil war broke out in the following year, it is most unlikely that John made many further payments.[193] His quarrel with the church had resulted in a splendid profit for his treasury.

John's emissaries to Rome were not there solely on the king's business. Innocent had ordered that all English ecclesiastics who had aided or counselled John during the quarrel with the church, who had accepted benefices from him during that period, or had communicated with him while he was excommunicate should travel to Rome in person to seek absolution.[194] While the pope did issue letters authorizing the legate to absolve minor clerks who had been

[190] Wendover, II, 100-102; *Rot. chart.*, pp. 208-9. The charter roll gives "R. de Marisco" and "nobiles viri T. and A." Wendover incorrectly extends R. to Robertus. Hence I take the liberty of ignoring his Adam and extending the A to Alan Martel who had been on similar missions. See Migne, *Patrologia*, ccxvi, 922-923, and *Rot. Claus.*, I, 123.
[191] *Annals of Waverley*, p. 278.
[192] Wendover, II, 102-103.
[193] He paid 6,000 marks in October 1214. *Rot. claus.*, I, 175.
[194] Migne *Patrologia*, ccxvi, 780-782.

but slightly involved in the controversy, the king's chief ecclesiastical servants were obliged to obey the order.[195] Moreover they were expected to bring with them a letter from Langton explaining their offenses in detail. Richard Marsh had no such letter, but he was clearly a plausible arguer. He had been John's chief agent in extorting money from monastic establishments and was cordially hated by the English clergy.[196] He succeeded in persuading Innocent that he was greatly slandered. He had been in too much of a hurry to leave for Rome on the king's business to get the letters from Langton. The pope absolved him, directed the legate to see that he was not molested by his clerical foes, and took him and all his possessions under the special protection of the Holy See.[197] While there is no evidence that any of John's clerical supporters had any great difficulty in obtaining absolution, Richard Marsh did it with rare effectiveness.

King John was not disappointed in his hopes that his surrender of the kingdoms of England and Ireland to the pope would bring him active papal support. Immediateley after the king's submission Pandulf issued a declaration that "the lord king is another man by God's grace." All John's subjects were called upon to adhere faithfully to him against the king of France and all other foes.[198] In his letters of October 30, 1213, to the prelates and barons who had guaranteed the safety of the exiled bishops Innocent directed them to use their influence to suppress any movement against the king.[199] A bull was issued stating that John could not be excommunicated nor his private chapel included in an interdict without the approval of the pope himself.[200] The king's person and the persons of his heirs with all the lands they possessed were taken under the special protection of the Holy See.[201] Finally letters addressed to all the people of England emphasized the pope's interest

---

[195] *Rot. chart.*, p. 209.
[196] *Rot. pat.*, p. 140. " Electio Hugonis," pp. 105-113. William of Newburg, p. 512; *Chronica de Melsa*, I, 326.
[197] Migne, *Patrologia*, ccxvi, 961-962.
[198] Rymer, *Foedera*, I, 112.
[199] Migne, *Patrologia*, ccxvi, 925-926.
[200] *Ibid.*, columns 922-923.
[201] *Ibid.*, columns 923-924.

in the kingdoms held of him and enjoined fidelity to his vassal, John. Similar letters were sent to King William of Scotland and his son Alexander.[202] As we shall see in a later chapter, these were not empty words. John had gained a vigorous, determined, powerful, and none too discriminating ally.

As John had been obliged to accept as primate of all England a man whom he neither liked nor trusted, he was naturally particularly anxious to fill the vacant episcopal chairs with men in whom he had complete confidence. In this project he found the goodwill of Innocent and his legate peculiarly helpful. The pope directed Nicholas of Tusculum to see that the bishops and abbots elected to fill the vacancies existing in England "be not only men illustrious in way of life and learning but also men faithful to the king and useful to his realm."[203] These instructions put the legate in a difficult position. It would not be likely that Stephen Langton and the prelates who had been in exile with him would regard as men illustrious in way of life anyone whom John considered faithful to him and useful to his realm. Nicholas of Tusculum had to side with one party or the other and from the beginning he chose that of the king. There is reason for believing that in so doing he was following Innocent's intentions. Stephen and his fellow prelates protested the favor shown to John's nominees, but they were powerless before the vast authority of a legate *a latere*.[204]

By the summer of 1214 seven English sees were vacant. Exeter was given to Simon of Apulia, dean of York, to please the pope and the legate.[205] The see of Rochester was used for what looks like an attempt to buy off Stephen Langton. The archbishop was granted the patronage of the bishopric of Rochester. He was to have custody of the see when it was vacant and could invest the bishop-elect with both his temporal and spiritual powers without seeking the royal assent. The bishop of Rochester would swear fidelity and perform the service due from his barony to the archbishop.[206] Four sees went to familiars of the king. Apparently

[202] *Ibid.*, columns 926-927.
[203] *Ibid.*, column 928.
[204] Wendover, II, 96-98; Coggeshall, p. 170.
[205] *Annals of Dunstaple*, p. 41.
[206] *Rot. chart.*, p. 202; *Rot. claus.*, I, 179.

Walter de Grey and William de Cornhill were placed in Worcester and Lichfield respectively without serious difficulty. The chapter of Durham gave a little trouble. Before the legate arrived, they elected Richard Poor, dean of Salisbury, who had some years before been Peter des Roches' rival for the see of Winchester. Everyone agreed that Richard was able, pious, virtuous, and learned. Without knowing of Richard's election Innocent directed the legate to see that the chapter of Durham elected John de Grey, bishop of Norwich. Undoubtedly this was arranged by John who was then in Rome. The legate tried to bully the chapter without success and the case was carried to Rome. Innocent declared Richard's election invalid, but directed that he should get one of the two sees involved—Durham or Norwich. John de Grey was duly elected bishop of Durham, but died before he could be consecrated.[207] Richard Poor was consoled with a far more modest benefice—the see of Chichester.

Geoffrey Plantagenet, archbishop of York, died in exile on December 18, 1212. Apparently Simon Langton who was a canon of York made use of one of his visits to Rome as his brother's agent to suggest himself as a suitable candidate for the vacant chair. But Innocent refused to approve this idea and made Simon promise not to seek election. Once back in England, Simon forgot his promise. When rumors came to King John's ears that the chapter of York planned to elect Simon, he wrote the canons a stern note of warning—if they made such a choice they could never again hope for his peace and affection.[208] Nevertheless the chapter proceeded to elect him. When a delegation from the chapter appeared before the pope to seek Simon's confirmation, Innocent indignantly voided the election as one made against his express prohibition. He then called on the canons to hold another election. There was no doubt of the result. When John had given the chapter permission to hold an election, he had suggested that Walter de Grey, bishop of Worcester, was a highly suitable candidate. His agents had pressed Walter's case before the pope. All the canons had to do was to think of a good reason for choosing

[207] *Rot. chart.*, pp. 207-208.
[208] Wendover, II, 153-4; *Rot. chart.*, p. 207.

Walter whom they had previously rejected on the ground that he was completely unlearned. They solemnly assured Innocent that they chose Walter because he had remained a virgin from the day he left his mother's womb. The pope agreed that virginity was a great virtue and confirmed the election. Wendover suggests that this cost Walter £10,000.[209]

The extent of the change in Innocent III's attitude toward King John is extremely difficult to explain. John had driven his bishops into exile, outlawed and killed clerks, seized and enjoyed church property, and ignored all the spiritual weapons of the papacy. Only baronial plots and the raised sword of Philip Augustus had brought him to submission. The pope was obliged to receive a repentant sinner. It is also quite conceivable that he had no desire to increase the power of King Philip whom he knew to be fully as intractable as John. In short it is not hard to understand why Innocent accepted the belated submission of the English king. The pope's pride in becoming the suzerain of a great feudal monarch is also comprehensible. But it is hard to believe that Innocent really thought John had become a " new man " as Pandulf so blithely announced—one worthy of full papal support. The pope's affection for the king first flowered while John de Grey and Richard Marsh were in Rome. Perhaps they were able to persuade him that he had misjudged the king. In that case the pope fully deserved the name he had chosen. But one cannot help wondering whether there were not more material considerations. It is clear that a large amount of sterling money was spent in Rome during the protracted negotiations and it seems doubtful that it all went for the living expenses of John's agents.[210] Then in 1213 and 1214 new pensions were established on the English exchequer. We find on the list Gualo, a future legate to England, the nephew of the bishop of Ostia, Count Richard, the pope's brother, and Stephen his son, Simon, nephew of Nicholas of Tusculum, and a fair number of other Romans both clerks and laymen.[211] The 1,000 marks a year promised in tribute was no paltry sum. Moreover the English

---

[209] Wendover, II, 160-161.
[210] *Rot. claus.*, I, 153.
[211] *Ibid.*, pp. 153, 156, 157, 180; *Rot. pat.*, pp. 108, 111.

records show that Nicholas of Tusculum who turned so benign an eye on the repentant king was a very expensive "angel of peace and safety."[212] His way of life in England was far from niggardly. One hesitates to use the term bribery—it always cost money to get things done in the papal court. But it certainly looks as if money well spent had smoothed the way for the pope's change of heart. The ironically inclined can well speculate as to how much of the booty pillaged from the English church ended in Roman strongboxes.

---

[212] Pipe roll 13 John, Public Record Office.

Chapter VI

KING OR TYRANT

THE dominant feature of the political history of England during the second half of John's reign was the series of quarrels between the king and various groups of barons that culminated in a fairly general revolt of the feudal aristocracy. The fact that the formulation of Magna Carta was an incident of this revolt makes the study of its origins and progress of more than ordinary interest and importance. Magna Carta occupies a deservedly high place in the history of political thought. While an adequate comprehension of the document requires far more than a knowledge of its immediate background, such a knowledge is absolutely essential for its interpretation. This absorbing interest in the background of Magna Carta is bound to distort any account of the history of the period. Events that form an essential part of it take on an importance that they would not otherwise have. The historian who wants to achieve a reasonably well-balanced narrative must continually guard against neglecting events of contemporary importance because they have no apparent relevance to Magna Carta. The next few chapters will be unbalanced in the sense that events forming a part of the background of Magna Carta will be treated at greater length than they would otherwise deserve, but no important phase of the political history of the period will be intentionally neglected.

Two fairly distinct types of grievances lay behind the revolt of the feudal aristocracy against King John. In a feudal state the political power and prestige and the surplus of goods produced by the labor of farmers, merchants, and artisans were divided between the monarch and the members of the feudal class. The political history of every feudal state of western Europe is essentially an account of the efforts of each of these parties to increase its share at the expense of the other. This process had been going on in England since the Norman Conquest. William I, William II, and Henry I had vigorously developed the power of the crown and had successfully suppressed feudal rebellions. During the long contest between King Stephen and the Empress Matilda the feudal class had recovered much of what it had lost and actually gained some new ground. Henry II had restored the crown to the position it had occupied under his grandfather and developed its power still further. He too was obliged to suppress a large-scale revolt of his vassals. When Richard came to the throne, the English feudal class was still smarting from the crushing defeat inflicted on it by his father. This fact combined with Richard's military prestige and personal popularity saved him from having to face a revolt. But the behavior of the barons when they learned of Richard's death showed that they had lost neither their ambitions nor their rebellious spirit. In short any king who tried to increase the power of the crown or even maintain its position as he found it was liable to be confronted with a baronial rising.

Most of the grievances that eventually found expression in Magna Carta grew out of this fundamental contest between the crown and the feudal class. Almost all of them had existed in the reigns of Henry II and Richard if not in that of Henry I. John made a few unpopular innovations and some of his practices made old grievances more acutely felt, but the general issues between him and the feudal class were far from new. Some of John's innovations and aggravated practices have already been discussed. Others will be mentioned as we examine his government in the later years of his reign.

General grievances produce general discontent, but they have to be extremely acute before they can in themselves cause a revolt against a reasonably strong government. A rebellion requires leaders, and they are likely to have more personal reasons for their disaffection than any general dislike of the government's policy. The grievances of John's feudal vassals as a whole supplied excellent tinder, but the spark had to come from men with personal reasons for hating the king and his government. These personal grievances grew out of John's quarrels with individual barons or small groups of barons. Hence these quarrels will have an important place in my discussion of this period.

The seven or eight years preceding the outbreak of the baronial revolt saw little change in the personnel of John's government. The most important new appointment was that of Peter des Roches as justiciar to succeed Geoffrey fitz Peter.[1] Peter's elevation was deeply resented by the barons. Not only was he considered a foreign adventurer, but he was believed to be John's creature. Actually it seems doubtful that the change made much difference. While Geoffrey may well have opposed John's policies in council, he seems to have always carried them out loyally and effectively. The king's dislike for him was probably based on envy of his wealth, power, and prestige.[2]

Probably of greater significance than the advancement of Peter des Roches was the rapid rise of Richard Marsh. Richard became a member of John's court in 1205 and by 1207 had become clerk of the chamber.[3] During the course of 1209 he succeeded Hugh de Welles as senior clerk of the chancery, but he continued to act as an officer of the chamber.[4] While the interdict rested on England, he showed himself extremely adept at extorting money from the clergy and was rewarded with two archdeaconries—Northumberland and Richmond.[5] When Walter de Grey became bishop of Coventry in October 1214, Richard Marsh succeeded him as chancellor.[6] With the possible exception of John de Grey, bishop of Norwich, Richard was John's most trusted servant. When the king was in Poitou in the spring of 1214, he despatched Richard to England to supervise the conduct of the government under Peter des Roches and William Brewer.[7] Twice in 1212 and once in 1214 he watched over the sessions of the exchequer. In fact some writs ordering the payment of funds were addressed to him as well as to the treasurer and chamberlains.[8] During these periods Richard Marsh seems to have had in his hands the actual exercise of the functions of three great officers—chamberlain, chancellor, and

[1] *Rot. pat.*, p. 110.
[2] *Histoire des ducs de Normandie*, p. 116.
[3] *Rot. liberate*, pp. 274-275; *Rot. pat.*, p. 74.
[4] *Calendar of charter rolls*, IV, 7; *Rot. claus.*, I, 153.
[5] *Rot. pat.*, pp. 93, 102, 105.
[6] *Rot. chart.*, p. 202.
[7] *Rot. pat.*, p. 139.
[8] *Rot. claus.*, I, 183-185.

treasurer. Thus a fair part of the functions of government were concentrated in the hands of one highly trusted royal servant.

The same essential stability of personnel that existed in the central administration appeared also in that of the shires. The only striking innovation during this period was the appointment of mercenary captains to three shrievalties. When in 1208 John decided to curb the power of William de Briouse, he placed the two shires that bordered on William's Marcher fiefs, Herefordshire and Gloucestershire, in the care of Gerard de Athies.[9] Gerard had been a soldier in the service of the Plantagenets since Richard's reign.[10] John placed him in command of the great fortress of Loches.[11] When that castle fell to Philip Augustus, John ransomed Gerard and brought him to England. He also brought over a number of Gerard's relatives.[12] Gerard served as sheriff for only two years, but he was replaced by his kinsman Engelard de Cigogné who held the two shires until after the issuing of Magna Carta.[13] Another mercenary captain who seems to have been a relative of Gerard's, Philip Marc, became sheriff of Nottingham and Derby in 1208 and held that office for the rest of John's reign.[14] The appointment of these foreign soldiers to English shrievalties was fiercely resented by the barons, and in chapter 50 of Magna Carta John promised to remove them from office. While it is perfectly conceivable that these mercenary captains ruled their shires with an unusually heavy hand and without too fine a regard for English customs, there is little evidence that they were worse than many native sheriffs. Certainly there is no indication that they were hated by the people they ruled as cordially as was William Brewer. It seems likely that dislike of seeing foreigners in profitable offices was the chief cause for the baronial hatred for Gerard and his relatives.

The rest of the English shrievalties were held by essentially the

[9] *Rot. pat.*, pp. 78, 83.
[10] Landon, *Itinerary*, p. 132.
[11] Coggeshall, p. 146.
[12] *Rot. claus.*, I, 57, 79, 97, 104; *Rot. pat.*, pp. 56, 65.
[13] Pipe roll 11 John, Public Record Office.
[14] *Rot. pat.*, p. 86.

same group of men that had served in the early years of the reign. While sheriffs were shifted from one county to another, there was little change in the group as a whole. Some of these shifts were apparently connected with John's quarrels with his barons and will be discussed later in that connection. It is interesting to notice that nine men who held office as sheriff during this period took part in the baronial revolt against John.[15] Three of them were among the twenty-five barons chosen to enforce Magna Carta.[16] Hence John can hardly be charged with filling the shrievalties with his creatures.

Our knowledge of the activities of the royal government during the four years following the levying of the thirteenth of 1207 will always be extremely limited because of a grave lack of sources. While patent and charter rolls exist for the tenth year of John's reign, 1208-1209, the far more valuable close roll is missing. Then for three years, the eleventh, twelfth, and thirteenth, there are no chancery rolls. The only available official records are the pipe rolls, a misæ roll for the eleventh year, and a præstita roll for the twelfth. The chroniclers were primarily interested in the great struggle between John and the church and make only casual references to domestic politics. These sources show clearly that interesting things were being done, but tell us little or nothing about them.

The year 1208-1209 seems to have been devoted chiefly to organizing the administration of the vast amount of ecclesiastical property seized because of the interdict. During the following summer the government apparently turned its attention to the royal forests. Wendover states that all buildings, fences, and ditches that had been constructed within the borders of the forests were razed.[17] The *Annals of Dunstaple* suggests that in Essex at least this included structures on clearings that were so old that they were assumed to be legal. The annalist adds that eighty foresters

---

[15] Henry de Braybrook, William Malet, Hugh de Neville, Gilbert fitz Renfrew, Reginald de Cornhill the younger, William de Huntingfield, John fitz Robert, John fitz Hugh, Robert de Ropsley.
[16] William Malet, William de Huntingfield, John fitz Robert.
[17] Wendover. III, 50-51.

in Essex were imprisoned and forced to ransom themselves.[18] The pipe roll shows that the forests of Essex were in the hands of special royal custodians for several years. Except for the general statement of Wendover, there seems to be no clear evidence that the government's purge of the forests extended beyond Essex.[19]

A series of accounts on the pipe roll of 1211 indicates that John made an interesting administrative experiment, but nothing further is known about it. These show the receipts of the "custodians of the ports" from Michaelmas 1210 to mid-Lent 1211. There were five groups of custodians headed respectively by Earl William of Salisbury, Gilbert fitz Renfrew, William de Albini, Aubrey de Vere, earl of Oxford, and Hugh de Neville. All of them record sums received from a customs duty on woad. Most of the groups also received money from an "assize of grain" which was presumably a tax on the export of corn. One group seems to have collected tolls on ships entering ports.[20] The *Annals of Waverley* state than in 1211 John closed all the ports of England.[21] These groups of officials may have been intended to enforce restrictions on trade as well as to collect dues. But without additional evidence any statements about this experiment can be mere guesses.

With the coming of John's fourteenth year the chancery rolls appear once more—in fact for that year we possess the patent, close, charter, pipe, and misæ rolls. Despite this abundance of material there are but a few references to one of the most important administrative events of John's reign. On June 1, 1212, writs were issued directing the sheriffs of England to conduct an extensive inquiry into all tenements held in chief of the crown by knight service or serjeantry. They were to list all such tenements with the names of the holders and the service owed. The sheriffs were also to list all lands once held *in capite* that had lost this status through alienation. They were to report who alienated them, what consideration or service he received, and what the occasion of alienation was.[22].

[18] *Annals of Dunstaple*, p. 31.
[19] Pipe rolls 12 and 13 John, Public Record Office.
[20] Pipe roll 13 John, Public Record Office.
[21] *Annals of Waverley*, p. 266.
[22] **Red** *book of the exchequer*, II, cclxxxv; *Book of fees*, I, 52.

If this incredibly ambitious project could have been carried out exactly, it would have furnished a complete survey of the feudal organization of England in 1212 and the history of that organization up to that time. The whole process of sub-infeudation would have been laid bare before us, and we should be able to see in detail how the church built up its estates. The listing of lands given in marriage would have filled many of the gaps in our knowledge of feudal genealogy. But obviously no such survey could be made. If the records we possess are safe criteria, it was even impossible to furnish all the information desired on the contemporary situation. In most shires there are long lists of tenements labelled "service unknown."[23] In other cases the statement is made that the land in question was held as part of a certain barony.[24] Except in the returns for Lincolnshire printed in the *Book of fees* there is little information about mesne fiefs and lands given in free alms.[25]

As we have no information about this inquest beyond what is supplied by the writ that initiated it and the returns printed in the *Red book of the exchequer* and the *Book of fees,* one can only speculate as to John's purpose.[26] It seems unlikely that the government had any great interest in the baronies. Their holders were perfectly well known and their service was firmly fixed by long custom. Moreover the form of the returns make it practically impossible to use them to discover the service due from a barony. In all probability the administration's concern was centered in small holdings that were not part of a formally organized barony. They might well be escaping their obligations. The returns show that there were a large number of serjeantries held by a wide variety of services. John was undoubtedly anxious that the holders should not escape their obligations as tenants-in-chief. Henry II and Richard had been extremely lavish with their grants from the demesne of the crown and from the demesnes of escheated baronies. The government wanted to know the obligations of the holders of these

---

[23] *Ibid.*, pp. 72, 79, 81, 82, 83, 88, 90, 97, 129, 131.
[24] *Ibid.*, pp 74, 75, 83, 93, 120, 122, 123, 137.
[25] *Ibid.*, pp. 153-197.
[26] For a discussion of the returns see *ibid.*, I, 52-65.

grants. Then there was the "land of the Normans" that had been distributed by John. He may well have had little clear idea about who held these lands and what service was due from them. In short I am convinced that the royal government was primarily interested in the small tenants-in-chief. As far as the barons were concerned the chief question was what lands they held that were not covered by the service due from their barony. For instance it seems clear that Earl William Marshal had been doing no service whatever for his manor of Tidworth in Wilts. In the inquest he claimed to hold it by serjeantry as marshal of the court, but in all probability he invented this tenure for the occasion.[27] Many barons held detached fees that they could easily forget, and the government was anxious to unearth them.

Then there is the possibility that John hoped to uncover flaws in the titles of some of the barons whom he suspected of disloyalty. A few months before the inauguration of the inquest Henry de Bohun, earl of Hereford, had been summoned to the king's court to tell what service he performed for his barony of Trowbridge and to whom he gave this service. At the same time Earl William of Salisbury and his wife instituted suit against Earl Henry for this barony.[28] The origin of the barony of Trowbridge is obscure. Of the eight townships mentioned in 1212 as belonging to the barony, presumably as demesnes, two belonged at the time of *Domesday book* to Edward of Salisbury, three to Brictric, and three to three other crown tenants. The great-grandfather of Earl Henry had married the daughter of Edward of Salisbury and had undoubtedly received with her the two estates that had been Edward's in *Domesday*. It is quite possible that the other lands had passed through the hands of the house of Salisbury before they went to the Bohuns. If John's instructions to gather full information about lands given as marriage portions should be carried out, all the details of the creation of the barony of Trowbridge would come to light. Obviously Earl William of Salisbury claimed that the barony should be held of him—the inquest might support his claim.

---

[27] *Red book of the exchequer*, II, 487. This may not be actually part of the returns to this inquest.

[28] *Curia regis rolls*, VI, 270, 320.

While there is no absolute evidence that there was any connection between Earl William's suit that certainly had John's support and the decision to hold the inquest, there seems a decided possibility that there was.

Finally it seems likely that the king was interested in the source of the lands held by the various monastic establishments. When the ecclesiastical property was seized at the time of the interdict, the barons had claimed the custody of the houses founded by their predecessors.[29] The fact that the rights of patronage over houses founded by their ancestors were guaranteed to the barons by a section of Magna Carta indicates that the question was an important one.[30] Through the inquest into lands granted in free alms John could discover what lay behind baronial claims to these rights. He may also have been interested in uncovering fraudulent grants in free alms—lands given to a monastic house and then re-granted to the donor as a fief. This abuse was prohibited in an early reissue of Magna Carta.[31]

As the inquest of 1212 preceded immediately the outbreak of the conspiracy of Robert fitz Walter and Eustace de Vesci, one is tempted to connect the two events and to suggest that the inquest may have been a major reason for baronial discontent. But this seems extremely unlikely. The general policy of John was to seek every right, service, and source of revenue that he could possibly find. As part of the implementation of this policy the inquest may well have been unpopular. But I cannot see in it any serious threat to the position of the barons or any indication that extra demands for service were made on them because of it. The scutage of Poitou of 1214 was based on the same assessments that had prevailed since 1167.

The formal taxation imposed by John's government between 1207 and 1215 was extremely moderate. There was a scutage of one pound in 1209, another at two or three marks in 1210, one at two marks in 1211, and one at three marks in 1214. The first three were levied on the occasions of expeditions into Scotland, Ireland,

---

[29] *Rot. claus.*, I, 107, 109.
[30] *Magna carta*, c. 46.
[31] Charter of 1217, c. 43; Stubbs, *Select charters,* p. 397.

and Wales. While the fines imposed on those tenants-in-chief who sought to buy exemption from service in these expeditions were extremely heavy, most of the tenants performed their service.[32] As these exactions were connected with actual military operations, they were unquestionably proper. The fourth of these scutages was levied on the occasion of John's expedition against Philip Augustus. Although the rate was the highest ever asked by John, the fact that no fines were demanded made the actual financial burden on those who did not serve lighter than usual. In fact a scutage unaccompanied with fines was actually profitable for most barons.[33] The burden was borne by their mesne tenants who paid the higher rate.

Altogether too much has been made of the expedition to Poitou and the scutage connected with it as one of the reasons for the baronial revolt. Ralph of Coggeshall says that when John was about to cross to the continent in 1213 the northern barons refused to go on the ground that they owed no service outside the realm, but Wendover states that their reason for declining to leave England was that the kingdom was still under interdict.[34] According to Walter of Coventry the northern barons claimed in the autumn of 1214 that the scutage of Poitou was illegal because they owed no service outside England.[35] Now by 1213 King John was at bitter odds with several groups of barons, and it is quite conceivable that his foes advanced this argument to hamper his expedition to Poitou. It was not a new idea—the same claim had been advanced against King Richard.[36] But both Richard and John had imposed and collected scutages and fines in connection with expeditions to the continent. The argument was a feeble one, and the barons must have known that it was.

As a matter of fact if one can assume that the men who followed John to Poitou had no strong objections to the expedition, opposition to the campaign was by no means general among the

---

[32] Mitchell, *Studies in taxation,* pp. 94-118.
[33] Painter, *Feudal barony,* pp. 125-127.
[34] Coggeshall, p. 167; Wendover, III, 80.
[35] Coventry, II, 218.
[36] Jocelin de Brakelond, p. 63.

barons who were to become the leading spirits of the revolt. Of forty-four rebels mentioned by Wendover as meeting in arms in the spring of 1215 at Stamford thirteen had served in Poitou and two others had sent their sons in their places. Of the twenty-five barons chosen to enforce Magna Carta eight had been on the Poitevin expedition and two had been represented by their sons.[37] If one considers the suggestion of Coggeshall and Coventry that it was chiefly the "northern barons" who opposed the expedition, the result is even more interesting. If one includes Lincolnshire among the northern shires there are fifteen northern barons on Wendover's list of those at Stamford. Six of these had followed John to Poitou. Of the seven northern barons among the twenty-five chosen to enforce the charter three were in Poitou. The chief agitators of the revolt against John—Robert fitz Walter, Eustace de Vesci, William de Mowbray, Henry de Bohun, and Geoffrey de Mandeville—did not take part in the expedition, but they were bitter foes of John long before 1214.

Examination of another passage in Ralph de Coggeshall will illustrate further the care that must be used in connection with the statements made by the chroniclers. Ralph says that John crossed to Poitou in 1214 with few earls but with many knights of minor importance.[38] The chronicler probably meant this statement to suggest how unpopular the expedition was, and it has been used freely if not recklessly by historians. There were fifteen earls in England in 1214. Ranulf, earl of Chester, William de Ferrers, earl of Derby, Aubrey de Vere, earl of Oxford, and Henry, earl of Warwick, accompanied John.[39] William, earl of Salisbury, commanded the English contingent in the Imperial army. Roger Bigod, earl of Norfolk, and Saher de Quency, earl of Winchester, sent sons in their places and William, earl of Arundel, William, earl of Devon, and William Marshal, earl of Pembroke, sent their contingents to the host.[40] William Marshal was bound by his

[37] In general I have established the men who went to Poitou by the lists of loans made there entered on the pipe rolls. Most of the barons with John also witnessed charters issued in Poitou.
[38] Coggeshall, p. 168.
[39] *Layettes du trésor des chartes*, I, 405-406.
[40] Lists of loans on pipe roll. *Rot. claus.*, I, 206.

homage to Philip Augustus for his barony of Longueville not to serve John in France, and the earls of Norfolk and Devon were far too old for active campaigning. Richard de Clare, earl of Hertford, William de Warren, earl of Surrey, David, earl of Huntingdon, Henry de Bohun, earl of Hereford, and Geoffrey de Mandeville, earl of Essex and Gloucester, neither went in person nor sent contingents, but Geoffrey's younger brother, William de Mandeville, was in the host.[41] Thus a third of the English earls took part in the campaign in person, another third performed their service through deputies, and only a third abstained altogether. While Coggeshall's statement is correct—few earls went with John—it has little to do with the popularity of the expedition among the English earls.

In short there seems to be no sound reason for placing the expedition to Poitou and the scutage connected with it among the reasons for the baronial revolt. There is no evidence that any baron opposed the campaign who did not already hate John for other reasons and a fair number of his future enemies accompanied him.[4] Although the scutage rate of three marks was unusually high, the absence of fines meant that the burden was borne by the mesne tenants instead of by the barons. But it seems very likely that the failure of this expedition seriously weakened John's position and encouraged the disaffected. Ever since the campaign of 1206 the king had been building up his war-chest. The need for money to recover his continental lands had been the official reason for the heavy and unpopular thirteenth of 1207. John had spent vast sums subsidizing potential allies among the neighbors and discontented vassals of Philip Augustus. The plan for the campaign of 1214— two armies moving from the north and the south to catch the French royal domain in a vise—was extremely ambitious. Certainly no English or French king had ever conceived so extensive a military operation. When John left for Poitou in 1214, he had

[41] These earls received no loans and all but Richard de Clare seem to have been charged with scutage. He was acquitted and may have sent knights. *Rot. claus.*, I, 212.

[42] On July 9 John sent a letter from La Rochelle indicating a desire to make peace with any of his foes who crossed to aid his campaign. *Rot. pat.*, p. 118.

completed a series of successful campaigns. The Irish baronage had been reduced to obedience and the native kings over-awed, the Welsh had been driven into their mountain fastnesses, and the king of Scotland had been forced to give his two daughters and many nobles as hostages as well as to raise a large sum of money for peace. John was feared by all. He returned from Poitou thoroughly beaten with his brother Earl William of Salisbury a prisoner of King Philip. All he had to show for his costly expedition was a few temporary gains in Poitou and a cousin of Philip Augustus, Robert, son of Count Robert of Dreux, as a prisoner. Barons who had hesitated to beard the victor over Irish, Welsh, and Scots would be far less daunted by the king who had been defeated by the prince royal of France at the head of a fragment of the French host.

In addition to the four scutages there were a few taxes of other kinds during this period, but there is too little evidence available to enable one to discuss them with any confidence. The tallage of the Jews in 1210 has been dealt with in a previous chapter. There are a few references to an "aid to relax the interdict" levied in 1214. This tax was a tallage levied on the urban and rural royal demesne.[43] Then there were special aids that were not apparently levied on the country as a whole. In 1210 Bristol and its suburbs and Gloucester paid a very heavy "aid for the king's passage to Ireland." Bristol and its suburb of Redcliff each paid 1,000 marks while Gloucester paid 500 marks. In the same year the men of Lancashire paid £131 for repairing Lancaster castle.[44] Obviously the line between such special aids and pure extortions is rather thin. In 1211 London made the king a gift of 2,000 marks.[45] The money extracted from the clergy was called a gift or a fine pretty impartially. Thus in 1211 Brian de Lisle accounted for forty marks gift from the abbey of York, a gift of £20 from the abbey of Selby, and a fine of 300 marks from the abbey of Rufford. The clerks of Yorkshire and Lancashire made the king a gift of 3,390

---

[43] *Rot. claus.*, I, 208-209; *Rot. pat.*, p. 111; Mitchell, *Studies in taxation*, pp. 116-118.
[44] Pipe roll 12 John, Public Record Office.
[45] Pipe roll 13 John, Public Record Office.

marks.[46] All these sums were presumably included in the total of money extorted from the church that was discussed in a previous chapter.

In addition to the revenues from the shires, royal boroughs, manors of the royal demesne, scutages, tallages, aids, customs duties, and monopolies the Angevin kings drew important sums from feudal incidents, fines offered for special privileges, and penalties for offenses. The most valuable of the feudal incidents was the right of wardship. According to English custom when a vassal died leaving a minor or a female as heir, the lord had custody of the fief. After he had given the widow her dower and provided for the support of the late vassal's children, the lord could use the revenues of the fief as he saw fit. The English kings had made their rights of wardship more profitable by inventing a device called prerogative wardship. While the ordinary lord received the custody only of fiefs held from him, the king claimed custody of all fiefs held by a tenant-in-chief. Thus a baron who had a vassal holding twenty knights' fees of him and only one fee in chief from the crown, lost his right of custody over the twenty fees. It seems probable that John was the first king to extend the claim to prerogative wardship to serjeantries held in chief and that this was one of the prime reasons for the deep interest taken in such serjeantries in the inquest of 1212.[47] Obviously the right of wardship gave many opportunities for abuse. The lord was entitled to the income from the estate, but he was expected to conserve the capital—to keep up the number of stock on the manors, keep the buildings in repair, conserve the woods and other resources, and refrain from extortion of money from the tenants of all classes.[48] When, as was usual, the lord sold the custody of the fief to the highest bidder, the temptation of the latter to abuse his rights was very strong. But unfortunately it is very difficult to

---

[46] *Ibid.*

[47] Chapter 37 of Magna Carta states that a petty serjeantry held of the king shall not be the occasion for prerogative wardship. William Marshal had seen fit to secure his position as lord by a special royal charter in case of this sort.

[48] This theory of wardship is best expressed in chapters four and five of Magna Carta.

find clear evidence of such abuse. Our only material on the exercise of the royal right of wardship comes from the accounts of the custodians preserved on the pipe roll, and as we do not know what the fiefs yielded their holders, it is impossible to estimate whether or not the crown was milking them too heavily. While the sale of stock from the manors of the Stutville barony after the death of William de Stutville was so vast in scale that it is hard to believe it represented the annual increment, we do not really know that it did not. There is, however, one point that is suggestive. The royal custodians always collected a heavy tallage from a barony the first year it was in their hands.[49] But on the whole one can only say that while it is highly probable that John abused his right of wardship, it is impossible to prove it.

Closely connected with the right of wardship was that of marriage. The English kings had always maintained that their assent was necessary before a tenant-in-chief could give his daughter in marriage. While Henry I in his charter of liberties had promised not to demand money for this assent, neither he nor his successors had allowed this promise to trouble them and Henry II had in some cases at least extended this right to male heirs.[50] When a vassal died leaving a minor or a female heir, the marriage of the heir was arranged by the lord. Here too the king used his prerogative—he claimed the right to marry the heir of any tenant-in-chief no matter how much he had held of other lords. This too John clearly tried to extend to royal serjeantries. Heirs and heiresses were valuable commodities and they were used to bring in revenue and to strengthen the king's political position. They were sold at a good price to men the king wanted to favor. There was apparently little or no objection to the selling of the marriage of heirs and heiresses. The men who bought them were offering fines for privileges. There was, however, a strong feeling that the mates chosen must be suitable—that the heir or heiress must not be " disparaged." Unfortunately we do not know enough about the social distinctions prevalent in thirteenth-century England to

---

[49] For more extended discussion of the right of wardship see Painter, *Feudal barony*, pp. 64-66.
[50] Charter of liberties of Henry I, c. 3.

be certain what this meant precisely. It was clearly not improper to marry the heiress of a great earldom to a simple English knight —no one seems to have resented the marriages of William Marshal, Geoffrey fitz Peter, and Saher de Quency. It is equally clear that it would have been considered disgraceful to marry an heiress to a villain, but villains were not likely to be able to buy them. In all probability it would be disparaging to marry a woman of the feudal class to a burgher, but even here one cannot feel too certain. The line between burgher and baron could be thin. Gervase de Cornhill was a burgher of London, but his two eldest sons married the heiresses of barons.[51] Despite the obscurity of just what was meant by disparagement, it is not hard to guess what the issue was in John's reign. It seems very likely that a number of John's favorite servants, both native and foreign, were men of humble origin—especially the captains who had won their position with their swords. When John gave or sold an heiress to one of these men, it disparaged her. Unfortunately it is impossible to estimate how frequently or how flagrantly John did this because in general we do not know which of his servants were considered of unworthy birth. The marriage of Fawkes de Breauté to the daughter of Warin fitz Gerold who was the widow of Baldwin, heir to the earldom of Devon, was clearly considered outrageous. Fawkes was a foreigner of obscure origin. The marriage of Peter de Maulay to the daughter and heiress of Robert de Turnham may also have been considered disparaging, but as we know nothing of Peter's birth we cannot be certain. Actually I suspect that the men the barons had in mind when mentioning disparagement in Magna Carta were John's foreign mercenary captains. But except for Fawkes and Hugh de Vivonne, none of these men seems to have acquired an heiress of rank.

As it never occurred to anyone that young heirs and heiresses ought to have any voice in choosing their mates, they could be injured only by disparagement. But a widow was in a different position. By feudal custom she was entitled to enjoy for life a dowry from her husband's lands—usually one-third—and what-

---

[51] On this question see Painter, *Feudal barony*, pp. 66-72.

ever property she had brought into the marriage—her marriage portion or her inheritance if she were an heiress in her own right. There was a general feeling that she should be allowed to remain single if she wanted to and if she chose to wed should be permitted to choose her second husband subject to her lord's approval. Henry I had promised not to compel a widow to re-marry. While his charter does not actually say that he will exact no fine from her for obtaining possession of her dower and marriage portion, that was probably its intent.[52] But neither Henry nor his successors could resist the temptation to sell widows whether they were willing or not. There were servants to be rewarded and barons to be won over to say nothing of the money gained by the sale. When a tenant-in-chief died, his widow as a matter of course offered a fine to have her dowry and her marriage portion, to remain single if she wanted to, and if she married to choose her husband with the king's assent. In the cases of widows of barons who were not heiresses in their own rights John usually demanded from one hundred to three hundred marks.[53] When an inheritance was involved, the fines were much higher. Amabile, widow of Hugh Bardolf, and a co-heiress of the Limesi barony offered 2,000 marks.[54] Margery, widow of Robert fitz Roger, gave £1,000.[55] Beatrice, widow of Doun Bardolf, and daughter and heiress of William de Warren, lord of Wormegay, offered 3,100 marks.[56] The largest such fine during the reign was imposed on Hawise, countess of Aumale who was obliged to offer 5,000 marks.[57] To force a woman who had married three times at the king's behest to pay so enormous a sum to obtain possession of her inheritance at the death of her third husband might well seem unreasonable.

Another important feudal incident was relief. When a vassal died, his heir was obliged to pay the lord a sum of money. By the time of Henry I custom had fixed the rate of relief at £5 per

[52] Charter of Henry I, c. 3.
[53] For examples see *Pipe roll 3 John*, p. 18; *Pipe roll 4 John*, p. 126; *Pipe roll 5 John*, pp. 22, 104.
[54] *Pipe roll 7 John*, p. 34; *Rot. chart.*, p. 150.
[55] Pipe roll 16 John, Public Record Office.
[56] *Ibid.*
[57] *Rot. chart.*, p. 189.

knight's fee for mesne tenants. In his charter of liberties Henry promised not to charge tenants-in-chief all he thought they could pay, but to accept a "just and legitimate relief."[58] While Henry's charter did not specify what a just and legitimate relief was, it is clear that by Richard's reign at least £100 was generally accepted as the reasonable relief for a barony.[59] But here again the temptation was to charge all the traffic would bear. We find Richard accepting a fine of 100 marks to persuade him to accept a "reasonable relief" of £100.[60] Then it was usually easy to think of special reasons for demanding a high relief. When an heir had an unquestioned right to a barony that had been held for a long time by his ancestors under an unchallenged title, he might escape with a relief of £100. But usually a flaw could be found in the heir's position. Then his succession to his father's lands became to a greater or lesser extent an act of grace. Actually very few of the reliefs accepted by John were as low as £100 for a barony. In 1201 Robert de Tatershall paid this sum, in 1205 Robert Arsic, and in 1209 Robert de Pinkeny.[61] These were all reasonably modest baronies held by firm titles. In 1203 John de Balon paid £100, but he held a tiny barony of only one knight's fee.[62] But Norman de Arcy in 1206, William de Beauchamp in 1207, and Henry de Pomeroy in 1207 paid 600 marks each for baronies to which their title seems to have been clear.[63] Toward the end of his reign John exacted some enormous reliefs where no reasonable excuse can be found for doing so. Robert de Vere paid 1,000 marks for the lands of his brother, Earl Aubrey, and despite their comtal title the Vere barony was of very moderate value.[64] John de Lacy had to offer a relief of 7,000 marks for the lands of his father, Roger de Lacy, constable of Chester.[65] Then in 1214 William fitz Alan was

[58] Charter of Henry I, c. 2.
[59] Painter, *Feudal barony*, p. 59.
[60] *Pipe roll 10 Richard I*, p. 222.
[61] *Pipe roll 5 John*, p. 193; *Pipe roll 7 John*, p. 151; Pipe roll 11 John, Public Record Office; *Rot. oblatis*, pp. 44, 255.
[62] *Pipe roll 5 John*, p. 57.
[63] *Pipe roll 8 John*, p. 104; *Pipe roll 9 John*, pp. 77, 157.
[64] *Rot. claus.*, I, 173.
[65] *Rot. oblatis*, p. 495.

charged the incredible sum of 10,000 marks for his medium-sized barony.[66] The same relief had been imposed on Nicholas de Stutville in 1205, but his case was rather complicated.[67] His brother had owed the crown a large sum and the fine for relief included quittance of debts. The same was true of Warin de Montchesney who paid 2,000 marks for relief and quittance of his family's debts to the Jews.[68] All in all there seems to be no doubt whatever that John charged exorbitant reliefs throughout his reign and that some of those imposed in 1213 and 1214 can only be described as fantastic.

When fines offered for something within the king's gift were truly voluntary, there could be little objection to them even when they were heavy. Thus while the fine of 5,000 marks offered by William de Briouse for Limerick without its chief town seems exorbitant, there is no reason to believe that it was not the result of a free bargain.[69] The same can be said of the 5,000 marks offered by Thomas de Eardington for the custody of the fitz Alan barony.[70] Payments for ladies fall in the same class. Gerard de Canville and William de Briouse each offered £1,000 for heiresses for their sons.[71] Roger de Clifford paid the same price to marry the heiress to the barony of Ewyas.[72] By far the largest fine of this sort was the 20,000 marks offered by Geoffrey de Mandeville for Isabella, countess of Gloucester.[73] But some of the fines offered John were clearly not entirely voluntary and others can hardly be distinguished from amercements. An ancestor of Peter de Bruce had made an exchange of lands with the crown. In 1200 Peter offered £1,000 to have the original lands again. The fact that Peter issued a charter stating that John accepted this arrangement because of Peter's extreme desire for it makes me suspect that it was not voluntary.[74] Certainly it would take many years' revenue

[66] Pipe roll 16 John, Public Record Office.
[67] *Rot. claus.*, I, 45.
[68] *Rot. oblatis*, p. 514.
[69] *Ibid.*, p. 94.
[70] *Ibid.*, p. 531.
[71] *Pipe roll 2 John*, p. 87; *Pipe roll 5 John*, p. 197.
[72] *Rot. oblatis*, p. 528.
[73] *Ibid.*, p. 520.
[74] *Ibid.*, pp. 109-110; *Rot. chart.*, p. 86.

from the lands involved to equal £1,000. In that same year William de Mowbray offered 2,000 marks to receive justice in the suit made against him by William de Stutville. While the offer may have been voluntary, its acceptance by John seems rather unethical—especially as he collected the fine after William de Mowbray lost the case or at least had to make an expensive compromise. In 1207 Gerard de Furnival paid £1,000 to have a suit against him suppressed.[75]

Even less voluntary in their nature were fines offered by officials to avoid unpleasant investigations. When Philip de Lucy retired from office as clerk of the chamber, he offered 1,000 marks to be relieved from giving a full accounting.[76] When Reginald de Cornhill who had been sheriff of Kent since the beginning of the reign and chamberlain of London for considerable periods died in 1210, his son gave 10,000 marks to avoid rendering and clearing up his father's accounts.[77] It is, of course, impossible for us to judge whether or not these large fines were justified—we cannot guess how much Philip and Reginald may have been in arrears, but they certainly were not purely voluntary. Finally there were the fines for "benevolence" or "grace." In 1205 Hugh Malebisse offered 200 marks and 2 palfreys for benevolence—everything was to be as it was before the king got angry with him.[78] In 1207 Roger de Cressi married an heiress without John's leave. His and her lands were seized. Roger paid 1,200 marks and 12 palfreys for the king's benevolence and possession of their lands.[79] In 1210 Robert de Vaux offered 750 marks for benevolence for some unspecified offense. Then in 1212 he was suspected of being involved in the Fitz Walter conspiracy. He offered 2,000 marks for grace of which 500 marks was to be paid before he was released from prison.[80] As the Vaux barony was comparatively poor it is extremely difficult to guess how he could ever hope to pay these large sums.

[75] *Rot. claus.*, I, 78.
[76] *Rot. pat.*, p. 74.
[77] Pipe roll 12 John, Public Record Office.
[78] *Rot. oblatis*, p. 334.
[79] *Rot. claus.*, I, 84; *Rot. oblatis*, p. 398.
[80] Pipe rolls 12 and 14 John, Public Record Office.

Straight amercements were rarely imposed on men of importance except for such offenses as novel disseisin that were handled by the ordinary courts. When a man of rank committed a serious offense, the king preferred to seize his property and perhaps imprison him. Then he could offer a fine for the king's benevolence. It is quite possible that this was a device to avoid a limitation placed by feudal custom on the king's power. It was generally recognized that a baron could only be amerced by his peers of the *curia regis*.[81] Fines for the king's benevolence may well have been higher than amercements set by the *curia*. But lesser men were amerced severely. When Reginald de Cornhill died a number of his men received penalties ranging from 700 marks to £1,000.[82] In 1211 the men of York paid 2,727 marks—presumably part of a higher penalty. The citizens of Lincoln in the same year were amerced 2,000 marks " for their excess."[83]

A few general remarks seem necessary in connection with the subject of taxation, reliefs, fines, and amercements. Because of the nature of early English law it is very difficult to use the terms legal or illegal in connection with the crown's exactions. Let us take one of the clearest cases—the taking of fines for giving assent to the marriage of a daughter of a tenant-in-chief. Henry I had solemnly bound himself and his successors not to do this. Yet all of them had ignored the promise. Now according to the custom of the time usage was more important than legislation. When a man claimed a privilege, it was best to have both a charter granting it and proof of usage. Strictly speaking neither was valid without the other. But there was far more inclination to accept usage without a grant than a grant without usage. Hence there is grave doubt that John's actions could be called illegal while he followed the practices of his ancestors. I am inclined to think that John charged heavier reliefs than his predecessors and was more greedy in setting fines and amercements, but it is a question of degree not of nature. Some practices of his were probably innovations and

---

[81] This was stated in chapter 21 of Magna Carta and it seems to have been the usual practice under John.
[82] Pipe roll 12 John, Public Record Office.
[83] Pipe roll 13 John, Public Record Office.

hence legally dubious. Collection of scutage without actually making a campaign seems to fall in this class as does the attempt to extend the privileges of prerogative wardship and marriage to serjeantries. But in general John seems to have been careful to stay within the framework of custom set by his predecessors even though he strained it at the edges. When he planned a real innovation such as the thirteenth of 1207, he was careful to obtain in one way or another the consent of his vassals.

Furthermore, it is important to realize that the total amount of a relief or fine may not mean much. To understand this it is necessary to glance at the procedure followed in arranging them. The original figure was set in negotiations between the individual concerned and the king or one of his officials. While John probably arranged in person the relief for important baronies and the larger fines and had the right to approve or disapprove those arranged by the justiciar and other officers, the majority were clearly negotiated in the first place with the king's agents. In special matters, such as making clearings in the royal forests, the king delegated full authority to some official—in this case to Hugh de Neville. Once the fine was negotiated it was entered on the oblate roll and in due time copied on an originalia roll and sent to the exchequer. Sometimes the original negotiations simply set a lump sum, but occasionally they also arranged the rate of payment. When the rate was not set in the first place, it was arranged when the man who offered the fine or his agent appeared at the exchequer to answer for the debt. In short while the theory may have been that such fines were due at once, no one really expected them to be paid in one installment. Now the barons of England were highly practical men. It seems unlikely that the theoretical sum of their obligations to the crown worried them greatly—it was the size of the annual installments that mattered. To take an extreme example we have seen that Thomas de Eardington offered 5,000 marks for the custody of the Fitz Alan barony. As the revolt and civil war came shortly afterwards, it is unlikely that he made much out of the custody. In the reign of Henry III his son Giles still owed this very large sum, but his annual installments were so small that if his descendants had kept up their payments, the debt would have been liquidated in 1917.[84] Then the king often forgave a large part of a fine. Thus while John de Lacy was originally charged with the very heavy relief of 7,000 marks, he paid less than 2,000 marks. A thousand marks was forgiven at once. Then a year later in 1214 when John needed friends and hoped the powerful Constable of Chester might be one of them, the remaining obligation of 4,200 marks was forgiven.[85] Hence John did not actually pay more than 1,800 marks and may well have paid less—it is difficult to be certain that one has noticed every item in an account of this sort. The circumstances made this case unusual, but one can say that in general it was extremely rare for the full amount of a fine to be demanded at the exchequer.

One can only speculate as to the advantages King John hoped to gain by arranging fines that were beyond the debtors' ability to pay. But one obvious possibility comes to mind. According to feudal custom a lord could take no action against one of his vassals without a judgment by the latter's peers in the lord's feudal court. But English practice permitted the king to take strong measures to collect the debts owed him. Apparently if a baron swore at the exchequer that he would make certain definite payments and failed to keep the agreement, he could be imprisoned. John's excuse for his first armed attack on William de Briouse was that William had failed to keep his terms at the exchequer and Thomas de Moulton was imprisoned for unpaid debts.[86] If John could persuade a baron to promise definite payments at the exchequer that were too high for him to pay, he had that baron at his mercy. It was not unlike our custom of convicting gangsters of evading their income taxes.

---

[84] Painter, *Feudal barony*, pp. 187-188.
[85] *Rot. oblatis*, p. 494; *Rot. pat.*, p. 129; Pipe roll 16 John, Public Record Office.
[86] Painter, *Feudal barony*, p. 60.

Chapter VII

THE SEEDS OF REVOLT

IN DISCUSSING the reign of a king it is, of course, impossible to distinguish clearly between actions based largely on personal reasons and those that stemmed from essentially political considerations. While the last chapter was devoted primarily to the general political activities of John's government, behind these lay his personal ambitions and desires. This chapter will describe his personal quarrels with individual barons and with small groups of barons, but often general political considerations entered into these quarrels. Hence the two chapters fit closely together and must be grasped as a whole if one is to understand the period. As the nature, frequency, and seriousness of a man's personal quarrels depend largely on his character, this chapter must begin with a discussion of John as a man. The brief summary given in chapter two must be justified and supplied with sufficient illustration to make it vivid.

The central features of John's character were his pride, ambition, and jealousy. He wanted desperately everything that gave prestige to a feudal monarch—power, wealth, and military glory. He wanted to rule the greatest possible extent of territory as absolutely as possible. I am not using absolute in a technical sense. John was brought up in the feudal environment, and there is no evidence to indicate that he ever thought of the possibility of absolute rule in its modern meaning. While at least one of his clerks used expressions that would have pleased James I—the king was the rod of God's fury constituted to rule his subjects with a rod of iron and to crush the nobles in an iron hand—John seems always to have accepted the general feudal principle of limited authority.[1] He simply wanted to develop his power as king and feudal suzerain to the greatest possible extent. While it seems likely that he abused his rights as a feudal monarch more enthusi-

---

[1] Wendover, III, 53.

astically than his predecessors, he did so along the lines laid down by them and within the framework of feudal ideas.

The turning point in John's career, the event that warped his character beyond repair, was probably the loss of Normandy, Maine, Anjou, Touraine, and Brittany. It seems unlikely that before the summer of 1203 it had ever occurred to John that King Philip could conquer these great fiefs. When Richard was a prisoner in Germany, the barons of Normandy led by the seneschal William fitz Ralph, and Earl Robert of Leicester had defended the duchy against Philip with little or no help from England. With its duke at its head and English knights to aid the duchy should be impregnable. Actually no modern historian has adequately explained the conquest of Normandy by King Philip. Lot and Fawtier certainly tell part of the story in demonstrating Philip's superior financial resources.[2] But the basic cause must have been the unenthusiastic if not actually treasonable behavior of the Anglo-Norman baronage. The loss was a cruel blow to John's pride. From then on his chief preoccupation was to recover the lost lands and revenge himself on King Philip. Moreover it intensified his naturally suspicious nature and directed it against the English baronage. Finally the catastrophe dulled John's delight in his young queen.[3] It was, after all, his marriage to Isabella that gave the French king a legitimate excuse for seizing his fiefs.

History has not, I believe, fully recognized either the full scope of John's plans to recover his prestige or how near they came to fruition. He succeeded in raising a large war-chest and in obtaining a mastery of England superior to that of any of his predecessors with the possible exception of his father, Henry II. He humbled the great Anglo-Irish barons and the native chieftains and vastly increased his authority in that lordship. He held the Welsh in check and firmly established the royal power in the middle and southern Marches. A humiliating peace was imposed on the king of Scotland. The king of Man became John's vassal and moves were made to bring the Orkneys within the scope of his

[2] Lot and Fawtier, *Le premier budget de la monarchie française*, pp. 135-139.
[3] *Histoire des ducs de Normandie*, p. 104.

power. Through his relationship with Otto of Brunswick and generous subsidies he built a close alliance with the princes of eastern Germany. Three great vassals of the French crown, the counts of Flanders, Boulogne, and Toulouse were successfully seduced. A number of lesser French barons such as the count of Nevers were in John's pay. If Bouvines had been won, John would have been the dominant power in western Europe. With Philip Augustus humbled there would have been little chance that Otto's enemies could destroy his imperial power. The papacy would have to bow to the victorious cousins. And the English baronage appeased by the recovery of their continental lands would hardly have considered revolt against so powerful a monarch.

John's pride and ambition were essentially sources of strength—they impelled him to become a powerful monarch both within and without his realm. But his almost frantic jealousy was a real weakness. A feudal monarch could best control and obtain the support of his baronage through men of baronial rank who were devoted to him and whose competence, wealth, and power gave them prestige among their fellows. At the beginning of his reign John was served by at least four such men—Hubert Walter, William Marshal, Geoffrey fitz Peter, and William de Briouse. While other motives than jealousy had a part in his quarrels with William Marshal and William de Briouse, that emotion alone seems to have produced his dislike of Hubert Walter and Geoffrey fitz Peter. Moreover the chroniclers make clear that there was a general feeling among his contemporaries that John hated all men of wealth and power.[4] This undoubtedly made it difficult for him to practice the time-honored device of feudal monarchs—to play off one great baron against another. The example of William de Briouse would hardly encourage any baron to become John's intimate.

Closely allied to jealousy was John's all-pervading suspicion. There were few men indeed whom he did not suspect of disaffection or disloyalty at some time or other. Among the prominent figures of the reign Peter des Roches, William Brewer, Richard

---

[4] *Ibid.*, p. 105.

Marsh, and John and Walter de Grey are the only ones who seem never to have incurred his serious displeasure. Even such devoted royal servants as Hubert de Burgh, Brian de Lisle, John fitz Hugh, William de Cornhill, and Peter de Maulay were out of favor for varying lengths of time.[5] No one in John's realm could ever feel certain of the king's good-will. He was continually demanding hostages and castles from his barons as pledges of their good behavior. He seems even to have taken hostages from his mercenary captains who were completely dependent on his will.[6] If, as I have suggested, it was the king's suspicion of his officials that gave us the chancery rolls, the historian must be duly grateful for it, but it was a grave source of weakness for John. No one trusts a man who trusts no one.

John was a man of ideas. He was ingenious—perhaps too ingenious. As we have seen he invented complicated counter-signs and then forgot what they were. His scheme for getting the English clergy to sign declarations that all the money extorted from them had been given of their own free will was most ingenious. While it may not be true that he forged letters to confuse his enemies, it was the sort of thing a chronicler was ready to believe about him.[7] The idea of inventing counter-signs so that he could issue orders that he knew would not be obeyed was of the same variety. If, as seems probable, John himself thought of the scheme to surrender his realms to the pope and hence secure papal support against his foes, it is further evidence of the activity of his mind. Whatever John may have been he was not dull.

It is always hazardous to apply the term unscrupulous to a man who lived in a remote age because of our inadequate knowledge of the standards accepted by his contemporaries. Certainly John had no hesitation about making promises that he had no intention of keeping, and he lied whenever it seemed convenient to do so, but these are faults common to most kings if not to all governments in general. Still it seems clear that John carried this sort

[5] *Pipe roll 8 John,* p. 39; *Pipe roll 9 John,* p. 16; *Rot. oblatis,* p. 412. *Rot. chart.,* p. 190; *Annales Sancti Edmundi* (ed. Thomas Arnold in *Memorials of St. Edmund's Abbey,* II, Rolls series), p. 25.
[6] *Rot. claus.,* I, 162.
[7] Matthew Paris, *Chronica maiora,* II, 588; Coggeshall, pp. 176-177.

of thing beyond the limits allowed by the ethics of his day. He solemnly approved Magna Carta with apparently the full intention of asking the pope to declare it invalid. Yet his baronial foes refused to issue charters promising loyalty and obedience to him because they did not believe they could keep such promises.[8] And John valued highly such a charter from a baron whose loyalty he suspected. In short John's own standards in this respect were no so high as those he felt confident his vassals would adhere to. Then in the feudal environment as in later times a safe-conduct was a sacred guarantee. Yet it is clear that Stephen Langton and his fellow exiles had little confidence in those issued by John. He insisted that John's letters be supported by those of an imposing array of prelates and barons. It seems very likely that the king's untrustworthiness was a major factor in the baronial discontent. This flaw in his character was called to the attention of all by the disappearance of Arthur. Before the march to relieve Mirabeau John had promised William des Roches that if Arthur fell into his hands, he would treat him in accordance with William's advice. There seems no reason for doubting the story that the fate of Arthur was in the mind of Matilda de Briouse when she precipitated the bitter struggle between John and her family by refusing to give her sons as hostages.[9] It is doubtful that any one took very seriously purely political promises like the king's statements that he would give his barons their " rights "—all kings made such promises and forgot them. But there were promises that kings as well as other men were expected to observe. John could be trusted to keep neither variety.

While it is extremely difficult to establish the ethical standards of a remote period, it is even harder to judge its sense of humor. I can simply cite two incidents that indicate to me that John had a sense of humor. On May 27, 1212, a curious charter was issued at Wolmere. The bishops of Winchester and Norwich, the justiciar, the earls of Salisbury, Chester, Arundel, and Oxford, Richard Marsh, Henry of London, archdeacon of Stafford, William de Cornhill, archdeacon of Huntingdon, Hugh de Neville, William

---

[8] *Rot pat.,* p. 181.　　　　　　[9] Wendover, III, 48-49.

Brewer, and thirteen lesser persons both lay and ecclesiastical stated that at their request John had restored his office to Peter de Maulay. They guaranteed that he would never again oppose the king's will. If he did, they would deliver his body to the king and would not resent any action John might take against the culprit. Then four of the guarantors agreed to pay penalties if Peter failed in his duty. Earl William of Salisbury would give John all his hawks. Peter des Roches would give him twenty palfreys and William de Cantilupe two. Henry fitz Count would allow himself to be whipped.[10] When one considers that whipping was a disgraceful punishment reserved for servants and that Henry fitz Count was John's second cousin, illegitimate son of Henry I's bastard, Earl Reginald of Cornwall, I see a grim humor in the penalty demanded by John.

During the week before Christmas 1204 King John was at his castle of Marlborough in Wiltshire. Marlborough was an important royal stronghold. Its constable was Hugh de Neville, the chief forester, and it was the headquarters of the forest administration. Hugh had made preparations for the king's visit—a few days ahead he had bought two tuns of wine from John.[11] Marlborough was also a favorite residence of the queen, and she may well have been there at this time. Be that as it may on the back of the oblate roll there appears an entry that has piqued the curiosity of many historians. "The wife of Hugh de Neville gives the lord king two hundred chickens that she may lie one night with her lord, Hugh de Neville." Her pledges were Hugh de Neville himself and Thomas de Sanford, constable of the neighboring castle of Devizes.[12] The general appearance of this entry suggests that the clerk who wrote it had shared in the two tuns of wine. I fear we shall never know what it means. It has been cited as an example of John's tyranny, and it is conceivable that Joan de Neville was a hostage for her husband and needed the king's leave to enjoy her marital rights. It is also conceivable, perhaps more probable, that she was John's mistress and was buying her way out of the royal bed. Twelve years later Hugh de Neville was to surrender

[10] *Rot. chart.*, p. 191.   [11] *Rot. oblatis*, p. 237.   [12] *Ibid.*, p. 275.

this same castle to Louis of France without any attempt at resistance. Whatever the meaning or innuendo this document certainly reeks of a fine bawdy humor. Unfortunately this entry never got past the barons of the exchequer to find its way to the pipe roll so we do not know whether or not the chickens were delivered. Or perhaps the chief clerk of the chancery, Hugh de Welles, the future bishop of Lincoln, was sober when he sent the roll into the exchequer.

The contemporary chroniclers are almost unanimous in agreeing that John was lustful and adulterous.[13] As a general accusation this needs no substantiation beyond his imposing list of illegitimate children. From the apparent ages of those known to us one would judge that they were the result of infidelities to Isabella of Gloucester rather than to Isabella of Angoulême. One of the elder ones was Joan who married Llywelyn, prince of North Wales, about 1204.[14] Many years later the seduction of this lady, by then mature to say the least, resulted in the death of a grandson of William de Briouse at Llywelyn's hands. About the same age as Joan was Geoffrey who in 1205 was old enough to hold the honor of Perche and to be at least the nominal leader of a small expedition to Poitou. Geoffrey died before the end of 1205.[15] Another son named John was being supported by the custodians of the see of Lincoln in 1201. He seems to have become a clerk.[16] In June 1207 the king sent to the prior of Kenilworth Henry "who calls himself our son, but is really our nephew."[17] In 1215 Henry fitz Roy was given the Cornish lands of Robert fitz Walter.[18] Henry married a minor heiress and lived well on into the reign of Henry III fully acknowledged as Henry, the king's brother.[19] Little is known about two other sons of John, Oliver

[13] Wendover, III, 63; *Histoire des ducs de Normandie*, p. 105; William of Newburgh, p. 521; *Chronica de Melsa*, p. 394; Giraldus Cambrensis, *Opera,* VIII, 319-320.
[14] *Rot. claus.,* I, 12; *Rot. chart.*, p. 147.
[15] *Rot. claus.,* I, 3, 27, 28, 41, 59.
[16] *Rot. liberate,* p. 12; *Rot. oblatis,* p. 391. *Rot. pat.*, pp. 129, 165.
[17] *Rot. claus.,* I, 86.
[18] *Ibid.,* pp. 200, 228.
[19] *Calendar of liberate rolls* (Rolls series), I, 126; *Close rolls, 1237-1242,* p. 511.

and Osbert Giffard. The latter is peculiarly elusive because there was a contemporary of the same name.[20] The only one of John's bastards to attain baronial rank and play a part of some importance in the history of his day was Richard. Richard served as a captain during the baronial revolt. In 1214 he married Rohese of Dover, granddaughter of that Rohese who had suffered so much from the solicitude of William Brewer, and became lord of the castle and barony of Chilham in Kent.[21]

Now licentiousness was no novel accusation against an English king. It was freely brought against both Henry II and Richard though as far as we know neither could compete in number of illegitimate offspring with either Henry I or John. I know of no contemporary suggestion that the amorous activities of either Henry disturbed their vassals though the rumor that Henry II had seduced Alis of France, fianceé of his son Richard, was probably one reason for Richard's disinclination to marry her. But the barons of Aquitaine are said to have complained to Henry II of Richard's freedom with their wives and daughters and John's assaults on the virtue of the female relatives of his vassals are generally mentioned as one of the chief reasons for their disaffection. It is for this reason that the names of John's mistresses are of historical importance.

Unfortunately little can be said on this subject that is based on anything more solid than contemporary rumor and modern speculation. Richard fitz Roy was clearly John's son by a sister of Earl William de Warren.[22] The mother of Oliver fitz Roy was named Hawise and there is some reason for thinking that she was a Tracy.[23] I can find no hint as to who were the mothers of John's other bastards. The chroniclers mention a few names, but their stories do not fill one with confidence as to their reliability. According to William of Newburgh the king hated "Eustace fitz John" because he had placed a common woman instead of his wife in the royal bed.[24] The reference is clearly to Eustace de Vesci,

[20] *Rot. claus.*, I, 230, 234, 235, 238, 266, 276, 277, 326; *Rot. pat.*, p. 140.
[21] *Rot. claus.*, I, 168, 268; *Rot. pat.*, pp. 118, 186, 199.
[22] *Histoire des ducs de Normandie*, p. 200.
[23] *Rot. claus.*, I, 326, 355.
[24] William of Newburgh, p. 521.

son of William de Vesci and grandson of the baron known as Eustace fitz John. The story may well be true. It is difficult otherwise to explain Eustace's bitter enmity for John, but the chronicler's confusion of Eustace with his grandfather makes one doubtful. The *Histoire des ducs de Normandie* asserts that when Robert fitz Walter fled to France, he told King Philip that his break with John was caused by the latter's seduction of his daughter Matilda, wife of Geoffrey de Mandeville, eldest son of Geoffrey fitz Peter.[25] But the *Histoire* itself presents a different account of the origin of the quarrel and adds that Robert told Pandulf that he left England because he would not serve an excommunicate king.[26] Obviously the author of the *Histoire* doubted the story of Matilda's seduction. There is, however, a similar tale in a monastic chronicle, but its details are too melodramatic to be taken very seriously.[27]

The rolls contain a number of references to the king's mistresses, but only once is the lady named. Early in 1213 the royal tailor supplied the damoiselle Susan, the king's friend, with a tunic and super-tunic.[28] In 1212 John sent one of his mistresses a chaplet of roses from Geoffrey fitz Peter's manor of Ditton.[29] In 1209 Peter des Roches paid a royal mistress £30.[30] If more of the records of the king's chamber survived, we would probably have more such references, but they would add little to our knowledge. When a man enjoys a reputation like John's, one is inclined to be suspicious of every favor he does for a woman. Thus one's curiosity is aroused by an entry on the memoranda roll of 1 John " On St. Catherine's day came Richard de Heriet and led a woman named Hawise de Burdels. The king says to give her a pension of a penny per day." This pension was duly assigned on the revenues of Essex and Hertfordshire.[31] Then in 1205 a Bristol wine merchant was directed to give Henry Biset a dolia of good wine

[25] *Histoire des ducs de Normandie,* pp. 119-121.
[26] *Ibid.,* pp. 116-118, 124-125.
[27] Dugdale, *Monasticon,* VI, 147.
[28] " Rotulus misae 14 John," p. 267.
[29] *Ibid.,* p. 234.
[30] Pipe roll 11 John, Public Record Office.
[31] *Memoranda roll 1 John,* p. 12; *Pipe roll 5 John,* p. 123.

"which we gave his wife."[32] On July 14, 1214, Engelard de Cigogné was directed to send to the king under the escort of two knights " Alpesia, the queen's damoiselle."[33] Such instances can obviously mean anything or nothing.

In only one case do the reasons for suspicion seem fairly strong. When Hawise, countess of Aumale, died in 1213, her heir was William de Fortibus, her son by her second husband. William was in France at the time of his mother's death. On October 1, 1213, he was given a safe-conduct to come to England to negotiate for his inheritance.[34] About a year later John issued a charter granting him the possession of his mother's lands when he had married Avelina, sister of Richard de Montfichet. Moreover the residue of the enormous fine offered by his mother for her inheritance at the death of her third husband and the relief owed by William were forgiven. Finally John himself would supply the bride with a marriage portion worth forty marks a year.[35] As Hawise had lived less than a year after offering her fine of 5,000 marks, she could not have paid much of it. According to John's standards several thousand pounds would not be too high a relief for Hawise's vast barony. John gave up all this and added a gift of forty marks a year out of the royal demesne. One cannot fail to suspect that such generosity on John's part could only be a reward for distinguished service in the royal bed.

The discussion of John's mistresses and bastards leads naturally to the question of his relations with Queen Isabella. In one of his additions to the chronicle of Roger of Wendover Matthew Paris puts a vicious attack on Isabella's character into the mouth of one of John's clerks, Robert of London. It is part of the strange tale of an embassy sent by John to seek an alliance with a Moslem emir. Robert of London tells the emir that Isabella is both incestuous and adulterous—that she had been convicted of adultery many times. Matthew says that he heard this story from Robert himself.[36] Without committing myself as to whether or not such an embassy ever took place, it seems safe to assert that little reliance

---

[32] *Rot. claus.*, I, 31.
[33] *Rot. pat.*, p. 119.
[34] *Rot. pat.*, p. 104.
[35] *Rot. chart.*, p. 201.
[36] Matthew Paris, *Chronica maiora*, II, 559-564.

should be placed on what Robert said he said about Isabella. Leaving aside the fact that it is hard to conceive how Isabella could find anyone in England to commit incest with there is no evidence whatever that she was unfaithful to John or that even his suspicious mind accused her of infidelity. One chronicle states that in 1208 she was placed in custody at Corfe and in December 1213 Terric Teutonicus was ordered to take her to Gloucester and guard her in the chamber in which she bore her daughter Joan, but neither of these necessarily implies imprisonment.[37] A few months after the second incident royal writs are addressed to the queen and Terric as joint commanders of the castle. I feel sure that in both cases custody and guard should be taken in the sense of safe-guard. John was undoubtedly unfaithful to Isabella —perhaps publicly and blatantly so—but all the evidence indicates that he treated her kindly and generously. One example must suffice. A week before her eldest son, Henry, was born John wrote to Peter de Joigny, brother of the count of Joigny in France, giving him a safe-conduct to come to see his sister "who desires him much and begs us for him."[38]

One of the most reliable of the contemporary chronicles describes King John as "a very bad man—cruel toward all men and too covetous of pretty ladies."[39] I am afraid that the first charge is even more certainly established than the second. There seems to be no doubt that John ordered the murder of his nephew Arthur and the death by starvation of Matilda de Briouse and her son William de Briouse the younger.[40] The murder in prison of Geoffrey de Norwich, the justiciar of the Jews, seems equally well substantiated.[41] Peter of Pontefract was hanged with his son for prophecying the end of John's reign in 1213.[42] Honorius, archdeacon of Richmond, died in a royal prison where he had been thrown

---

[37] *Rot. pat.*, pp. 124, 143.
[38] *Ibid.*, p. 71.
[39] *Histoire des ducs de Normandie*, p. 105.
[40] Coventry, II, 196; Wendover, II, 48, 49, 57; *Annals of Margam*, pp 27, 30.
[41] Wendover, II, 52-53; Coggeshall, p. 165; *Annals of Dunstaple*, pp. 33-34.
[42] Coggeshall, p. 167; Wendover, II, 76-77.

The Seeds of Revolt

ostensibly because he owed the king money but probably actually because he had failed to persuade Pope Innocent to accept John de Grey as archbishop of Canterbury.[43] We do not know that he died violently, but it seems likely. Beyond the specific cases are the more general ones. In July 1212 John hanged twenty-eight sons of Welsh chieftains who were hostages for their parents' behavior.[44] Now the Welsh chieftains had undoubtedly broken their promises, but John's act was savage beyond the custom of the day. While the stories of the tortures used to persuade the Jews to contribute adequately to the tallage of 1211 may well be exaggerated, it is hard to believe that they are purely imaginative.[45] Then while we have no definite evidence of violence done to clerks during the interdict, the suggestions that such violence took place are too general to ignore.[46] In short the evidence seems overwhelming that John was savage and brutal when angered. In the case of Arthur he seems to have been guilty of carefully premeditated murder of a dangerous political rival.

Recent historians have shown a marked inclination to rehabilitate King John's reputation. His crimes have been questioned and his virtues exaggerated. This tendency seems to spring from a failure to distinguish between the man and the monarch. In many, perhaps in most, respects John was an excellent king. His close attention to the business of government was in decided contrast to the negligent attitude of King Richard. He was intelligent and aggressive in trying to solve the political and financial problems that faced him. He seems to have fully appreciated the value of able royal servants. We have seen he took over the entire administrative personnel of his brother with a few exceptions when it would have been easy, perhaps even conventional, to have replaced Richard's men with his own. And while John was undoubtedly jealous of Geoffrey fitz Peter, he retained him as justiciar until his death. Moreover John's own favorites were clearly men of capacity. No more proof of this is needed than the success with which they ran the government in extremely difficult circumstances

[43] *Annals of Dunstaple*, p. 31.
[44] Coggeshall, p. 207; Wendover, II, 62.
[45] *Ibid.*, pp. 54-55.
[46] Coventry, II, 200.

after the king's death. Then I can see no justification for calling John a tyrant in the political or constitutional sense. He was an innovator who sought to develop the royal power as had his predecessors—hence he was bound to arouse opposition. He found the royal revenue nearly static in a time of rising costs and rising baronial incomes, and he sought to redress the balance. No effort to obtain for a government its share of increasing profits is ever popular. It is important to remember that the fact that Magna Carta forbade a practice, does not make that practice wrong on John's part.

While John was a far better king than his brother or his son—probably as good a one as his father—little can be said in favor of his private character. He was cruel, lecherous, and deceitful. His mind was always seething with jealousy and suspicion of his servants and vassals. He was as close to irreligious as it was possible for a man of his time to be. Against these major vices such minor virtues as generosity to small nunneries can carry little weight. And, as has been suggested before, his personal vices continually hampered his political effectiveness. While the policies of John as a king may have kept his vassals in a permanent state of discontent, it was his personal quarrels that supplied leaders for the disaffected.

King John's first major quarrel with a compact group of his barons involved the lords who dominated South Wales and its Marches and Ireland. The eclipse of Hubert de Burgh after his capture in Chinon left South Wales and the southern Marches almost completely in the hands of two men—William Marshal, earl of Pembroke, and William de Briouse. William Marshal ruled his palatine shire of Pembroke in south-west Wales, the lordship of Striguil between the Wye and the Uske, and the stronghold of Castle Goodrich on the Wye. He was custodian of the royal castle of Cardigan, the king's chief fortress in southwest Wales and of the forest of Dean with its castle of St. Briavel between the Wye and the Severn. In addition he was sheriff of Gloucestershire with the custody of the castles of Gloucester and Bristol.[47] William de Briouse held as fiefs the Marcher baronies

---

[47] Painter, *William Marshal*, p. 144.

The Seeds of Revolt

of Abergavenny, Brecon, Radnor, Gower, and Kington. John had also granted him the three castles of Grosmont, Skenfrith, and Llantilio. He had the custody of the palatine shire of Glamorgan that lay between the lordship of Striguil and the county of Pembroke. He also had the custody of the heir of Baderon de Monmouth, young John de Monmouth, with his barony and of the heir of his own nephew, William de Beauchamp of Elmley, with his fief. Moreover his son Giles was master of the see of Hereford with its castles. Finally through an agreement with his son-in-law, Walter de Lacy, who was absent in Ireland, William de Briouse controlled the large Lacy barony with its castles of Ewyas and Ludlow.[48] In short there were only three important fiefs in this whole region that were not under the control of William Marshal or William de Briouse—Henry de Bohun, earl of Hereford's, share of the lands once held by Miles of Gloucester, and the baronies of Mortimer and Clifford. But Henry de Bohun was William de Briouse's first cousin once removed, Walter de Clifford was his second cousin, and Roger de Mortimer's son and heir, Hugh, was William's son-in-law.[49] As Walter de Clifford became sheriff of Herefordshire at Easter 1205, William had little to fear from that royal agent.[50]

The same group of barons were the masters of John's lordship of Ireland. William Marshal had acquired with his wife the vast lordship of Leinster. Walter de Lacy had inherited from his father the lordship of Meath. John had given Limerick to William de Briouse and had approved and confirmed the conquest of Ulster by Walter's brother, Hugh de Lacy.[51] These great baronies were practically palatinates and the king's justiciar of Ireland had little power outside Dublin and its pale and a few other royal

---

[48] *Rot. chart.*, pp. 66, 80, 160; *Calendar of charter rolls*, III, 46; *Rot. pat.*, pp. 19, 57; *Pipe roll 1 John*, p. 86; *Pipe roll 4 John*, p. 20; *Pipe roll 5 John*, pp. 58, 70.
[49] William de Briouse, Walter de Clifford, and Henry de Bohun were descended from Walter of Gloucester. Hugh de Mortimer married Annora de Briouse. *Rot. pat.*, p. 122.
[50] *Pipe roll 7 John*, p. 272.
[51] *Rot. chart.*, pp. 84, 151.

towns.[52] And while John had not granted the city of Limerick to William de Briouse, he had placed it in his custody.[53]

From a purely political point of view, without any consideration of the personalities involved, so great a concentration of power in a few hands was bound to disturb so jealous and ambitious a monarch as John. It was almost inevitable that he should seek to establish some royal control in South Wales and its Marches and to develop the authority of his justiciar in Ireland. Once he conceived suspicions of the loyalty of any of the barons involved, his desire to accomplish these ends was certain to become acute. This situation arose in the spring of 1205. William Marshal did liege homage to Philip Augustus for his Norman fiefs and had a bitter quarrel with John about it. When in June 1206 William declined to follow John to Poitou because of his oath to King Philip, a still more savage quarrel ensued and the king took the earl's eldest son as a hostage.[54]

Open hostilities between the royal government and the Marshal-Briouse-Lacy combination broke out in Ireland late in 1206, but it is impossible to say whether the initiative was taken by John or by his justiciar of Ireland, Meiler fitz Henry. Meiler, one of the last survivors of the original English conquerors of Ireland, was a turbulent and ambitious man who was anxious to extend his authority. While it is highly probable that John had directed him to weaken the great Irish barons in any way he could and quite possible that he had specifically ordered attacks on the lands of William Marshal, Meiler was perfectly capable of acting on his own initiative. At any rate Meiler attacked the Briouse lands in Limerick and seized the Marshal castle of Offaly in Leinster. Soon he was at open war with the vassals of William Marshal and William de Briouse who were supported by Walter de Lacy, lord of Meath.[55]

When the barons of Limerick and Leinster informed their lords of the justiciar's actions, William Marshal and William de Briouse

---

[52] Painter, *William Marshal*, pp. 150-51.
[53] *Rot. chart.*, p. 107.
[54] Painter, *William Marshal*, pp. 140-143.
[55] *Ibid.*, pp. 153-154; *Rot. claus.*, I, 77, 81.

protested to the king. John, apparently, hesitated to make an open break with them. Meiler was instructed to return any of William de Briouse's men he had captured and restore all booty taken, but to keep the city of Limerick if he had obtained possession of it.[56] And John granted William Marshal's request that he be allowed to go to Ireland to see to his lands. A few days later, however, John thought better of this last concession. Most of Meiler's lands were held from the lord of Leinster and the latter's presence in Ireland would seriously hamper the justiciar. The king sent a messenger after William to demand his second son and his English and Welsh castles as pledges of his loyalty. The earl gave the pledges and proceeded to Ireland. But in the autumn at Meiler's request John summoned the lord of Leinster to England. He also made generous grants of land to certain barons of Leinster who showed an inclination to desert their lord's cause. Even William's nephew, John Marshal, accepted from the king the office of marshal of Ireland, but there is no evidence that he actively aided the justiciar, and he remained on good terms with his uncle.[57]

Shortly after William Marshal's departure for Ireland, the king deprived him of the shrievalty of Gloucestershire and the custody of Cardigan and the forest of Dean.[58] Moreover William de Briouse was replaced as bailiff of Glamorgan by one of John's foreign mercenary captains, Fawkes de Bréauté.[59] Then when the lord of Leinster had returned to England in answer to John's summons, Meiler pressed with all possible vigor his attacks on Leinster. But William had left several of his ablest English knights in Ireland and they were aided by Hugh de Lacy, earl of Ulster. Meiler was no match for these forces. His lands were devastated and he himself was captured. When he learned of this, John decided that he had been going too fast with too feeble agents. The justiciar was ordered to keep the peace and a compromise agreement was worked out with William Marshal. The earl offered 300 marks for the restoration of Offaly and agreed to accept a new charter for his lordship of Leinster which somewhat limited his

[56] *Ibid.*, p. 77.
[57] Painter, *William Marshal*, pp. 146, 153-156.
[58] *Ibid.*, p. 147.
[59] *Rot. pat.*, p. 68.

rights and extended those of the crown. A month later Walter de Lacy accepted a similar charter.[60] But John was determined to have a strong hand administering the royal power in Ireland. A local man who was the vassal of one of the great lords could not rule effectively. Hence about the time of his agreement with William Marshal he dispatched John de Grey, bishop of Norwich, to take over the government of Ireland.[61]

While King John was engaged in making these arrangements with William Marshal and Walter de Lacy, he became involved in his bitter feud with the house of Briouse. There are two fairly full accounts of the origin and early stages of this quarrel. According to Roger of Wendover John feared that the proclamation of the interdict on March 24, 1208, would encourage disaffected barons to plot against him. Hence he decided to demand hostages of those he suspected. When his officers appeared at William de Briouse's stronghold, the latter's wife, Matilda, told them she would not give her sons to the man who had murdered his nephew. William himself, however, rebuked his wife and offered to submit to the judgment of John's court for any offense he might have committed. But when John heard about Matilda's remark, he sent men to arrest the whole Briouse family. Fortunately William received warning of this move and fled to Ireland with his wife and sons.[62]

The other account is furnished by King John himself. After William's escape to France and the capture of his wife and eldest son in 1210, the king issued his official account of the quarrel " so that all may know for what cause and what crime William de Briouse left our land." The truth of this statement was solemnly witnessed by the justiciar, the earls of Salisbury, Winchester, Hertford, Hereford, and Derby, Robert fitz Walter, William Brewer, Hugh de Neville, William de Albini, Adam de Port, Hugh de Gournay, and William de Mowbray. Four of these barons, the earls of Hertford, Hereford, and Derby and Adam

[60] Painter, *William Marshal,* pp .155-160.
[61] *Annals of Dunstaple,* pp. 30-31; *Rot. pat.*, p. 79; *Curia regis rolls,* V, 200.
[62] Wendover, II, 48-49.

de Port were related to William by blood or marriage. Perhaps it is worthy of remark that of the thirteen witnesses to this document six were to be among the twenty-five barons of Magna Carta. According to this statement the origin of the quarrel was purely financial—William had not kept up his payments on the 5,000 mark fine offered for Limerick. The exchequer had ordered his chattels in England distrained for this debt, but William had removed them. Hence Gerard de Athies was ordered to seize his chattels in Wales. Then Matilda de Briouse, William de Ferrers, earl of Derby, who was William de Briouse's nephew, and Adam de Port, lord of Basing, his brother-in-law, went to the king and asked for a conference. William met John at Hereford. He surrendered the castles of his Marcher baronies and gave three of his grandsons as hostages. But when Gerard de Athies summoned the royal constables of these castles to come and get the pay for their garrisons, William and his two sons attacked the castles. This led to full scale war that culminated in William's flight to Ireland with his wife and sons.[63]

Let us now examine these two stories in the light of the evidence that can be gleaned from other sources. At the very beginning of 1208 King John appears to have expected war in the southern Marches. On January 5 Richard de Mucegros who had succeeded William Marshal as sheriff of Gloucestershire was removed from office. In his place John appointed his most experienced mercenary captain—Gerard de Athies whom he had just ransomed after his capture in Loches. Gerard was supplied with large sums of money.[64] This move may have been made in contemplation of possible war with William Marshal whose barony of Striguil was thus caught between two foreign captains—Fawkes de Bréauté in Glamorgan and Gerard in Gloucestershire. But it seems far more likely that it was made in preparation for an attack on William de Briouse. Despite his suspicions of William Marshal's relations with Philip Augustus John must have known the earl of Pembroke well enough to feel pretty certain that he would not bear arms against him. Hence it looks as if John conceived his

[63] Rymer, *Foedera*, I, 107-108.
[64] *Rot. pat.*, pp. 74, 78; *Rot. claus.*, I, 99, 100, 104, 114.

plan of attacking William de Briouse earlier than Wendover indicates. Nevertheless William was at least openly in favor on March 7—Gerard was directed to give him a manor.[65] Then on March 19, the day after he began to seize the lands of the clergy, John announced that William de Briouse had delivered his son to Walter de Lacy as a hostage for his good behavior.[66] This seems to fit in with Wendover's account. When John first asked for hostages and Matilda was indiscreet, William de Briouse may well have tried to satisfy the king by such a compromise. But a month later, on April 18, an expedition under the command of Gerard de Athies was moving against William. Gerard was supported by Thomas de Eardington, sheriff of Shropshire and Staffordshire, with 500 infantry and 25 mounted serjeants.[67] This must have been the expedition described by Wendover as an attempt to capture the Briouse family and by John as an effort to seize William's chattels in Wales. This last explanation is most implausible. William de Briouse could hardly have removed all the stock from his vast English estates. The expedition seems to have taken about nine days. On April 27 Thomas de Eardington received a writ to enable him to collect the pay for the men he had led on it.[68] On April 28 Walter de Clifford, sheriff of Herefordshire, was ordered to give Giles de Briouse possession of the see of Hereford that had been seized with the other ecclesiastical property, but to keep the castles of the see.[69] The next day William de Briouse was ordered to pay Gerard de Athies 1,000 marks within four days to cover the cost of the expedition against him.[70] As one chronicler states that this payment was part of the agreement by which William gave up some of his castles and supplied the king with hostages, this confirms that part of John's account.[71] There is no evidence to corroborate John's claim that William and his sons then attacked the castles that had been surrendered, but it is clear that the peaceful settlement lasted less than a month. On May 23 Gerard de Athies was appointed sheriff of Herefordshire

[65] *Ibid.*, p. 105.
[66] *Rot. pat.*, p. 80.
[67] *Ibid.*, p. 81; *Rot. claus.*, I, 112-113.
[68] *Ibid.*, p. 113.
[69] *Ibid.*
[70] *Rot. pat.*, p. 81.
[71] *Annals of Worcester*, p. 396.

and given custody of the see of Hereford.[72] Walter de Clifford offered a fine of 1,000 marks not to have an inquiry made as to his behavior while he was sheriff.[73] While this probably refers to the cavalier manner in which Walter had been accounting for the profits of the shire, it could indicate that he was considered to have been too lenient with his Briouse cousins. Sometime during the summer John summoned William to appear before his court, and William excused himself on the ground of sickness.[74] On September 29 John confirmed an agreement between Gerard de Athies and William's vassals by which they promised not to return to William's allegiance. At about this time William fled to Ireland.[75]

William de Briouse took with him his wife and his sons, William and Reginald. Giles joined his fellow bishops who were in exile in France.[76] William de Briouse on landing in Ireland took refuge with William Marshal who had returned to Leinster. The new justiciar of Ireland, John de Grey, promptly ordered the lord of Leinster to deliver the fugitives to him. William replied that he was performing his feudal duty in harboring his lord. He knew nothing about any quarrel between William de Briouse and the king. Considering the complexity of feudal relationships, it is perfectly possible that William de Briouse was William Marshal's lord. The other statement is a little hard to accept. John in his account stated definitely that he had forbidden William Marshal to receive the fugitives. This seems unlikely. It was not William Marshal's policy to defy the king directly. But he must have known of the quarrel. His new charter for Leinster was issued on March 28—nine days after John announced that William de Briouse had freed his son to Walter de Lacy and only three weeks before Gerard's expedition. The most one can say for William Marshal's claim of ignorance was that he may have left for Ireland

[72] *Rot. pat.*, p. 83.
[73] *Pipe roll* 10 *John,* p. 191.
[74] *Curia regis rolls,* V, 152.
[75] *Rot. pat.*, p. 86; *Annales Cambriae* (ed. John Williams ab Ithel, Rolls series), p. 66.
[76] *Annals of Worcester,* p. 396; *Annals of Margam,* p. 29; *Histoire des ducs de Normandie,* p. 112.

in one of the brief truces that marked the early stages of the quarrel. Be that as it may William kept his guests for three weeks and then escorted them safely into Meath where they were welcomed by Walter de Lacy.[77] For the time they were safe. The justiciar of Ireland had no military force that could cope with the lords of Leinster, Meath, and Ulster.

One of the most puzzling questions in connection with John's feud with William and Matilda de Briouse is why he left them unmolested in Ireland for a year. There are several possible answers. The king may have hoped that he and John de Grey could persuade Walter and Hugh de Lacy to surrender the fugitives. A military expedition to Ireland would be an enormously costly venture, and the king may well have wanted to avoid it if possible. Then there was much to do in England. Llywelyn was giving trouble, and both John and the earl of Chester made expeditions against him in the spring of 1209.[78] Moreover, as we shall see, John suspected with reason that some of his barons of the north of England were disaffected. An alliance between them and the king of Scotland while he was absent in Ireland could be extremely dangerous. So in July John led his feudal host to the frontiers of Scotland and held a conference with the king of Scotland at the castle of Norham. King John accused King William of receiving and aiding his foes. As he had no army capable of resisting John's formidable force, the aged king of Scotland made a humiliating peace. He promised to pay an indemnity of 15,000 marks and gave his two legitimate daughters as hostages.[79] This treaty made John feel that the north was secure and provided funds for his expedition to Ireland. There could be no better example of John's ingenuity—getting one foe to pay the costs of suppressing another one.

In May 1210 King John mustered his host for an expedition to Ireland. In addition to the feudal levy of England he had a bodyguard of Flemish mercenary knights and several companies

---

[77] Painter, *William Marshal*, pp. 162-163.

[78] *Rot. pat.*, p. 88; *Annals of Waverley*, p. 262.

[79] *Ibid.*; Wendover, II, 50; Coventry, II, 200; *Chronica de Mailros*, p. 108.

The Seeds of Revolt

of mercenary serjeants and cross-bowmen. With the king was William Marshal, earl of Pembroke and lord of Leinster. While William might on occasion press closely on the limits of feudal propriety, he never openly crossed them and he felt obliged to obey John's summons to the host.[80] On June 3 the royal army reached Cross-on-the-Sea near Pembroke. Meanwhile William de Briouse had returned to Wales leaving his wife and sons in Ulster. According to John's official account he had obtained a safe-conduct from John de Grey to go to the king, but had not actually proceeded beyond the Marches. This seems very plausible. William may either have hoped to make peace at the last minute and so prevent the invasion of Ireland or to create a diversion in Wales that would oblige John to stay there. John's statement goes on to say that Earl William de Ferrers went to him at Pembroke and asked leave to seek out William de Briouse to ask what he intended to do. The king sent one of his trusted followers, Robert de Burgate, with the earl. Soon William de Briouse sent messengers offering a fine of 40,000 marks for benevolence. John replied that peace with William was useless while Matilda was free and independent in Ireland. In short John wanted Matilda de Briouse —a fact that supports strongly Wendover's story that her indiscreet remarks started the quarrel. Had the king been less determined, William's attempt to keep him busy in the Marches might well have succeeded. Supported by his Welsh allies he recovered a fair part of his lands. John's officers were forced to lead an army against him and shortly after his return from Ireland the king despatched Roger de Lacy with a strong force to restore order in the Marches.[81]

From Cross-on-the-Sea John crossed to Crook near Waterford. He then proceeded through the lordship of Leinster to his city of Dublin. There he was met by some vassals of Walter de Lacy who offered their lord's submission, but John refused to accept it and seized the lordship of Meath. He then marched on Ulster. Hugh

---

[80] " Praestito roll of 12 John " in *Rot. liberate,* pp. 172-244; Painter, *William Marshal,* p. 163.

[81] *Annals of Worcester,* p. 399; *Annals of Dunstaple,* p. 32; Coventry, II, 202; Pipe roll 12 John, Public Record Office.

de Lacy, earl of Ulster, ordered his men to resist the royal host, but he himself fled to Scotland with Matilda de Briouse, her sons William and Reginald, and William's wife and sons. Hugh and Reginald de Briouse made good their escape. Matilda and her family were captured by a Scots lord, Duncan of Carrick, and held for King John. With the irony that came so easily to him the king sent John de Courcy who had held Ulster before Hugh de Lacy conquered it to bring the fugitives to England. When Matilda arrived in England, she offered John 40,000 marks ransom for herself and her family and William de Briouse went to the king at Bristol and agreed to this arrangement. Then William departed to attempt to raise the money, but instead of doing so fled to France. When the first payment fell due Matilda was unable to meet it.[82] John's account of the affair stops here. Perhaps it was issued just after William's flight and Matilda's failure to pay the first installment of the ransom. Or perhaps John preferred not to mention the sequence. For the chroniclers agree that the prisoners were consigned to a royal castle where Matilda and William the younger were starved to death at John's command.[83]

John's account of his quarrel with the house of Briouse was skilfully contrived. Only one assertion—that William de Briouse had removed his chattels from his English lands—seems extremely dubious. While I rather doubt the statement that John formally forbade the Irish lords to shelter William de Briouse, I do so simply because I prefer the word of William Marshal to that of the king. For the rest John's story seems entirely accurate in all essential points. But it can hardly have convinced anyone that it was complete. It asks us to believe that John incurred the enormous expense of an expedition to Ireland to capture some defaulting debtors and punish those who harbored them. This inconsistency appears in the story itself. Before John left Pembroke William de Briouse offered a fine of 40,000 marks for the king's benevolence, but it was declined because Matilda was still free. Then the same offer was accepted when made by Matilda. In short it was worth an expedition to Ireland to get a wife to join her

---

[82] Rymer, *Foedera*, I, 107-108; *Annals of Margam*, p. 30.
[83] *Ibid.*; Wendover, II, 57; *Histoire des ducs de Normandie*, p. 114.

husband in offering a fine. This fine of 40,000 marks was, of course, a mere form—no baron could pay so enormous a sum in any reasonable time. Both parties knew perfectly well it could not be paid. By setting so high a figure John was essentially saying that he had no intention of releasing his captives, and William recognized this by fleeing the realm. All this must have been clear to those who read or heard the official story. It was fairly accurate, but it did not make sense.

The real story of the feud between John and the house of Briouse emerges fairly clearly from the available material. William de Briouse had been an energetic supporter of John's claim to the crown after Richard's death. Perhaps he had persuaded Richard to name John as his heir—he may even have concocted the story that Richard had done so. He became one of the new king's prime favorites and was generously rewarded with lands and castles. But John was always cautious. His chamberlain, Hubert de Burgh, was given a position in the Marches that would serve to check William's ambitions. Moreover John demanded a very large fine, 5,000 marks, for the grant of Limerick. He probably felt pretty certain that William would not pay it, and this default could be used against him if the occasion should ever arise. Then William de Briouse captured Arthur at Mirabeau and turned him over to the king. As Powicke has so well shown he was one of the few men who positively knew the young prince's fate. For the moment this was to his advantage—John's grants grew more and more generous. When Hubert de Burgh was captured in Chinon, William obtained his lands in the Marches. But William's power was becoming too great and was bound to disturb John. Then too the king had become suspicious of William's friend and neighbor, William Marshal. Finally Matilda de Briouse talked too much. King John decided that the Briouse family must be wiped out. William's heavy debts to the exchequer formed an excellent excuse for action against them. John pursued the family at enormous expense in money and other resources until William and Reginald were in exile and Matilda and her eldest son starved to death in prison.

The quarrel with William de Briouse and his family was the

greatest mistake John made during his reign. It should have been avoided at any cost. For one thing it made his cruelty known to all his barons. They may have suspected, as did Philip Augustus, that Arthur had been murdered, but no one knew for certain. William de Briouse made sure that Arthur's fate was known in both France and England. Then the death of Matilda and William the younger showed what John was capable of doing to his foes. This example might terrify the disaffected barons, but it did not make them fonder of John. Then there is a clear though tenuous thread linking the Briouse affair to the great baronial revolt. Two baronial leaders, Henry de Bohun, earl of Hereford, and Richard de Clare, earl of Hertford, were closely related to the Briouse family.[84] Giles de Briouse who returned after the peace between John and the church was in the baronial councils. In fact only one thing prevented this quarrel from leading to the destruction of John and perhaps the end of his dynasty—the deep essential loyalty of William Marshal. When the earl of Pembroke returned to the king's favor in 1212, he brought with him the support of the lords of the south Marches who had been alienated during the quarrel with the Briouses. During the baronial revolt the only troops John could rely on beside his mercenaries were those of the Marcher lords—Ranulf of Chester and William de Ferrers from the north and William Marshal, Walter de Lacy, John de Monmouth, and Hugh de Mortimer from the south. Except for the earl of Chester all these barons were closely connected with the house of Briouse, but they followed William Marshal into the royal camp.

After the destruction of the house of Briouse the next open break between King John and a group of his barons came in the summer of 1212 with the sudden flight from England of Robert fitz Walter and Eustace de Vesci. But even before the climax of the Briouse affair events were taking place that were either direct antecedents of the Fitz Walter-Vesci conspiracy or had an important bearing on later baronial revolts. While the quarrel with William de Briouse was one of the seeds of the great rebellion against John, other seeds were germinating during the years 1209

---

[84] William de Briouse the younger had married Earl Richard's daughter. *Rot. pat.,* p. 101.

The Seeds of Revolt

to 1212. To examine the first of these we must glance at the north of England in the year 1209—the year of John's expedition against King William of Scotland.

Under the Angevin kings the protection of England against invasions or major raids from Scotland was primarily the responsibility of four royal officers, the sheriffs of Cumberland, Westmoreland, Northumberland, and Yorkshire, and two barons, the bishop of Durham and the earl of Richmond. At Easter 1200 John appointed Robert fitz Roger sheriff of Northumberland in place of William de Stutville.[85] Robert fitz Roger was the son of Roger fitz Richard by Alice de Vere sister of Aubrey de Vere, first earl of Oxford, and widow of Robert de Essex.[86] Through his mother Robert was first cousin of the earls of Oxford and Norfolk. Roger de Lacy, constable of Chester, was the son of his half-sister, Alice de Essex. By his own marriage to the widow of Hugh de Cressi he became the stepfather of Roger de Cressi who played an important part in the baronial revolt. Robert was not originally a northern baron. The lands of his inheritance lay largely in Essex —the manor of Clavering, a demesne of the forfeited barony of Henry de Essex, and some twenty fees held as mesne tenant. But Henry II, Richard, and John had worked industriously to move the center of his power to Northumberland. He received the castle and manor of Warkworth, the barony of Walton, and four royal manors.[87] In 1204 royal letters patent appointed him hereditary constable of Newcastle-on-Tyne "as long as he serves well."[88] When one considers John's obvious distaste for hereditary officials, this strange compromise shows how greatly he valued Robert fitz Roger as one of the guardians of the north.

During the winter of 1204 and the spring of 1205 John placed the northern frontier of England in strong hands. On December 1, 1204, Roger de Lacy, constable of Chester, was appointed sheriff of Cumberland and Yorkshire.[89] In March 1205 Westmoreland was granted as a barony to Robert de Vieuxpont.[90] The same

---

[85] *Pipe roll 2 John*, p. 1.
[86] J. H. Round, *Geoffrey de Mandeville* (London, 1892), p. 392.
[87] *Rot. chart.*, pp. 6, 116, 133, 143.
[88] *Rot. pat.*, p. 42.
[89] *Ibid.*, p. 48.
[90] *Ibid.*, p. 51.

month saw the Yorkshire lands of the earldom of Richmond given to Earl Ranulf of Chester.[91] Thus Robert fitz Roger, Roger de Lacy, Robert de Vieuxpont, Philip of Poitiers, bishop of Durham, and Ranulf of Chester were established as guardians of the Scots border. Three of these men were closely connected by blood and feudal ties. As we have seen Robert fitz Roger was the uncle of Roger de Lacy who was the chief baron of Cheshire. Although Robert de Vieuxpont had inherited lands in Westmoreland, his grant of the shire as a fief was the result of his military capacity and favor with John. When the bishop of Durham died in April 1208 the military command of his castles and men was entrusted to one of John's captains, Philip de Ulecotes.[92]

While no English baron of the first rank had interests in the far north, several secondary lords did and some whose interests were purely local were powerful enough to be of considerable importance. In the first of these groups were the count of Aumale, Robert de Ros, and Eustace de Vesci. The count of Aumale held the castle and barony of Cockermouth in Cumberland, Robert de Ros the castle and barony of Wark in Northumberland, and Eustace de Vesci the stronghold of Alnwick in Northumberland with its fees. The chief barons whose interests were local in Cumberland were Richard de Lucy, lord of the barony of Copeland, and Robert de Vaux. Gilbert fitz Renfrew held in addition to his wife's inheritance in Lancashire the barony of Kendal. This region is now part of Westmoreland, but it was not included in Robert de Vieuxpont's fief. In Northumberland there were two local barons of outstanding importance—Hugh de Balliol and Richard de Umfraville. Hugh was also one of the chief vassals of the bishop of Durham from whom he held his castle, Barnard Castle. Richard de Umfraville held the fortress of Proudhoe and in addition ruled Redesdale in the Northumbrian back country from his castle of Harbottle.

There were close ties between the barons of the northern shires and the king of Scotland. King William's father had borne the

---

[91] *Ibid.*
[92] In 1211 he took credit on his account for guarding the castle of Norham for 3½ years. Pipe roll 13 John, Public Record Office.

title earl of Northumberland and his elder brother had held both Northumberland and Cumberland from the king of England. When John succeeded to the throne, King William had claimed these two shires. While he had been unsuccessful, he had not abandoned his claims. He held as John's vassal the English liberty of Tindale that bordered on Richard de Umfraville's fief of Redesdale. Moreover King William had married two of his bastard daughters to Northumbrian barons—Robert de Ros and Eustace de Vesci. Finally a number of northern barons held lands in the earldom of Huntingdon ruled by William's brother David. King William was also bound by ties of blood to several English barons. The father of Robert fitz Walter had been his first cousin and Henry de Bohun, earl of Hereford was his nephew. In short the King of Scotland was an important figure in the internal as well as the external politics of England.

There is substantial reason for believing that a conspiracy against King John was taking shape in the north of England in the year 1209. One of the registers of King Philip Augustus now in the Vatican library contains a most interesting document—a letter from the French king to "his beloved John de Lacy."[93] John had sent word to Philip by one of Philip's liege-men, Roger des Essarts, that he, his friends, and his allies planned to make war against King John both in England and in Ireland. While the letter makes the intentions of John de Lacy perfectly clear, King Philip's end of the bargain is extremely vague—perhaps intentionally so. He seems to say that when he has clear proof that John has carried out his promise he will see that he receives justice in regard to his ancestors' land in England. John de Lacy was the eldest son of Roger de Lacy, constable of Chester. I have been unable to find any claim this house had that was unsatisfied. Only one hypothesis seems to explain this letter. John de Lacy had some reason for thinking that Philip Augustus planned to invade England and wrote to ask him to promise him possession of his lands if he and his friends made war against John. If it had been written in 1212, this letter would be easy to understand. Philip

[93] *Archives des missions scientifiques et litteraires,* third series, VI, 332, 344-345.

was then preparing to invade England at the pope's behest, and John de Lacy might well have feared that the barons who had stood by their excommunicated king might suffer. But the letter is definitely dated 1209, and the reference to Ireland seems to support that date. By 1212 Ireland under William Marshal's leadership was firmly behind King John. One can only conclude that Philip was thinking of the invasion of England as early as 1209 and that Roger des Essarts either told John de Lacy or sent word to him through relatives in England. Roger des Essarts had started his career as an English knight holding land in Essex of the Earl Warren and of the Valognes barony of Benington. By 1203 he had joined King Philip and had received a fief from him. He eventually held several small fiefs in Normandy.[94] His younger brother Richard obtained the English lands of the family.[95] When Roger de Lacy, constable of Chester, died in 1211, a number of his officials headed by his seneschal, Robert Walensis, offered fines to be excused from rendering their accounts. The first name on the list after Robert Walensis was Robert des Essarts who promised the considerable sum of £100.[96] While I have no positive evidence of any relationship between this Robert des Essarts and Richard and Roger des Essarts, it seems safe to conclude that one existed. Hence it is not difficult to see how John de Lacy may have known of Philip's plans and offered his aid. This letter was cancelled on the register, but it is not quite clear what such cancellation meant. It may mean that the letter was never sent, but from similar cancelled entries it seems more likely that cancellation was simply an indication that the agreement had never taken effect and had no permanent importance as a record.

This letter raises several interesting questions, but unfortunately we have no evidence that might furnish answers to them. The reference to Ireland suggests that John de Lacy was in comunication with William de Briouse and the Irish barons who were shel-

---

[94] *Ibid.*, p. 382; *Book of fees*, I, 579; *Curia regis rolls*, I, 174, Farrer, *Honours and knights' fees*, III, 406-408; *Récueil des historiens des Gaules et de la France*, XXIII, 245, 640, 714.
[95] *Rot. claus.*, I, 328.
[96] Pipe roll 13 John, Public Record Office.

The Seeds of Revolt

tering him. In this connection it is interesting to notice that William Marshal the younger, eldest son of the earl of Pembroke, who was a hostage for his father was probably living in Newcastle-on-Tyne in the custody of Robert fitz Roger.[97] John de Lacy, William Marshal the younger, and John fitz Robert, son and heir of Robert fitz Roger, were to be important leaders of the baronial revolt. Perhaps this was a young men's conspiracy growing in the north. Beyond this it seems useless to speculate as to whom John de Lacy had in mind as his "friends and allies."

It seems likely that King John knew that this conspiracy existed and was aware that John de Lacy was involved in it. The king's actions in 1209 show that he was disturbed over the state of his realm in general and particularly in regard to the north. In addition to making his expedition against King William of Scotland he at least made gestures toward coming to terms with Stephen Langton and the papacy. Moreover in September of that year he summoned all his vassals to Marlborough to swear fidelity to him and his infant son, Henry.[98] Then sometime during the latter part of the year John deprived Roger de Lacy of both his shrievalties. In Cumberland he was replaced with the king's favorite man for troubled spots, Hugh de Neville, and in Yorkshire by Gilbert fitz Renfrew who was already sheriff of Lancashire and custodian of the honor of Lancaster.[99] Roger was not actually in disgrace—John sent him into Wales in command of a body of troops in the late summer of 1210, but the king was unwilling to leave him in charge of vital border shires. Roger de Lacy died in 1211.[100] Not until September 1213 did John make any move toward giving John de Lacy possession of his inheritance. While John may have been a minor, it seems rather unlikely. Then the conditions imposed by the king were extremely unusual and very onerous.[101] John de Lacy offered the very large fine of 7,000 marks. He was to pay 3,000

---

[97] *Rot. pat.*, p. 94.
[98] Wendover, II, 51; Coventry, II, 200; *Annals of Waverley*, p. 262; *Annals of Margam*, p. 29; Gervase of Canterbury, II, 104.
[99] Pipe roll 12 John, Public Record Office.
[100] Dugdale, *Monasticon*, VI, 315.
[101] *Rot. oblatis*, pp. 494-495.

marks the first year, 2,000 marks the second year, 1,000 marks the third year, and the final payment of 1,000 marks for the fourth year was to be forgiven. He was to swear fidelity to John and give a charter guaranteeing his loyalty. Twenty of John de Lacy's knights were to be pledges for his loyalty and the payment of the fine. Finally King John was to keep in his own hands the castles of Pontefract and Donington, but John de Lacy was to pay £40 a year for their custody. These severe terms seem to me to indicate that the king had grave doubts of the loyalty of John de Lacy.

The awe engendered by King John's expedition against Scotland in the summer of 1209 and the humiliating peace accepted by King William seems to have convinced the northern conspirators that the time for action had not yet come. The crushing of the house of Briouse in the following year must have still further dampened their ardor. As we shall see John de Lacy was a decidedly fickle man whose mind rarely held the same intention for very long. But some of these barons may well have written the letters to the pope that Pandulf and Durand spoke of in 1211. Actually, however, between 1208 and 1212 there is no evidence of the existence of any general conspiracy. What is of interest during these years are various incidents that seem to throw light on the reasons that moved particular barons to place themselves among John's foes.

Perhaps the most striking case was that of William de Mowbray. William spent at least four years in Vienna as a hostage for King Richard and may well have felt that he deserved well of the house of Anjou.[102] Yet when John came to the throne, he permitted William de Stutville to sue William de Mowbray for his entire barony on the rather specious grounds that the settlement made between Roger de Mowbray and Robert de Stutville had never received royal approval. William de Mowbray offered 2,000 marks for justice in the case, but he lost and was obliged to give William de Stutville a demesne manor and nine knights' fees.[103] Nevertheless King John insisted on the payment of the fine. In 1209 John resorted to the highly unusual device of having the exchequer collect

---

[102] *Curia regis rolls*, I, 48.
[103] *Ibid.*, pp. 380, 440; *Rot. oblatis*, p. 102; *Cartae antiquae rolls*, no. 102; Hovedon, IV, 117-118.

from William's vassals an aid to pay this debt.[104] Ironically enough the largest single sum was due from Nicholas de Stutville. Nicholas was already disaffected because of the enormous relief of 10,000 marks that he had been required to pay for his brother's lands and the withholding from him of the barony of Knaresborough.[105] Certainly this royal maneuver did not increase his love for John. The next heaviest obligation fell on Eustace de Vesci who also held from William de Mowbray. William himself must have deeply resented this royal procedure, and William was one of the most powerful barons of the realm. His influence was great in Yorkshire, Leicestershire, Warwickshire, and Lincolnshire. His mother was a Clare, probably a sister of the earl of Hertford, and the great Lincolnshire baron Gilbert de Ghent was his cousin.[106] Nicholas de Stutville was Gilbert de Ghent's stepfather.[107] Thus we see the group later to be called the "northerners" built up by King John's policy.

During these years the king seemed determined to alienate his barons as rapidly as possible. In 1210 the two chief barons of Cumberland, Robert de Vaux and Richard de Lucy, felt obliged to offer fines of 750 marks and £100 respectively for his benevolence. Their offenses were not, apparently, political. Robert de Vaux was in trouble over someone's wife—in addition to the fine for benevolence he offered five palfreys to have the king "keep quiet" about the lady. Richard de Lucy was hereditary forester of Cumberland and his fine was nominally offered to clear himself from the charge of poor custody of the forest.[108] Yet the year 1210 seems a poor time to offend these two lords. Then in 1211 Gilbert de Ghent and Saher de Quency, earl of Winchester, were pressed about their debts to the crown. Gilbert was ordered to pay the

[104] Pipe roll 11 John, Public Record Office.
[105] *Rot. claus.*, I, 45.
[106] A monastic account calls William's mother daughter of Edmond, earl of Clare. There was no such person, but as she held Banstead, Surrey, a Clare manor, she was probably a sister or daughter of Earl Richard. Dugdale, *Monasticon*, VI, 320. *Curia regis rolls*, I, 368, V, 205. William's grandfather, Roger de Mowbray, married Alice de Ghent, aunt of Gilbert.
[107] He married Gunnora daughter of Ralph de Albini and widow of Robert de Ghent.
[108] Pipe roll 12 John, Public Record Office.

large sum of 1,200 marks in two years. Saher was to reduce his obligation of £1,276 at the rate of 200 marks a year.[109] Lesser men were being imprisoned and forced to buy their way out—Robert de Castlecarrock, Roger Bacon, and Walter de Stoke.[110] In 1211 Eustace de Vesci lost a plea in the king's court. The decision may have been in accord with the law, but as one reads the case one can easily see why Eustace might have considered the decision outrageous. To add to the injury the roll bears a note that Eustace was to be summoned to answer for his debts to the Jews.[111] All these actions of John's government may have been justified, but they did not earn the good-will of the barons concerned.

By the spring of 1210 King John was openly at odds with the lords of the southern Marches of Wales—William de Briouse, William Marshal, Walter and Hugh de Lacy, and their friends, relatives, and vassals. He was on extremely bad terms with an important group of northern lords—William de Mowbray, Eustace de Vesci, Nicholas de Stutville, and John de Lacy who was soon to be lord of Pontefract. Then in the course of that year he became involved in a bitter quarrel with an even more dangerous group of barons headed by Robert fitz Walter, Henry de Bohun, earl of Hereford, and the two sons of Geoffrey fitz Peter, Geoffrey and William de Mandeville. These men were bound closely together by marriage alliances. Geoffrey and William de Mandeville were married to the two daughters of Robert fitz Walter.[112] Henry de Bohun's wife, Matilda, was the daughter of Geoffrey fitz Peter and the sister of the two Mandevilles. It seems likely that Robert fitz Walter and Henry de Bohun were moderately disaffected before 1210. As we have seen in an earlier chapter John had created Henry de Bohun earl of Hereford on the condition that he give up his claim to the generous grants made to his father by Henry II. While Henry may have felt it necessary to accept this compromise, it can hardly have fully satisfied him. He may also have resented John's treatment of his Briouse cousins. Robert fitz Walter

[109] Pipe roll 13 John, Public Record Office.
[110] Pipe rolls 12 and 13 John, Public Record Office.
[111] *Curia regis rolls,* VI, 136.
[112] *Histoire des ducs de Normandie,* pp. 115, 118.

probably betrayed John when he surrendered Vaudreuil to Philip Augustus. Whatever reasons moved him to that probably still existed. Moreover it was well known that John never forgot nor forgave an injury but simply awaited the time for revenge.

The first open break between King John and Robert fitz Walter grew out of long-standing ill-feeling between Robert and the abbey of St. Albans. Early in John's reign Robert and the abbey had quarreled over the possession of a wood. Robert based his claim on a charter that according to the abbey's chronicler he had bribed a monk to forge for him. In 1201 the dispute was compromised. Robert gave up the wood in exchange for land worth £10 a year.[113] Then some years later Robert and the abbot of St. Albans disagreed over the latter's rights in the priory of Binham, a cell of St. Albans, that had been founded by the ancestors of Robert's wife. According to Robert the abbot brought too large a retinue when he visited Binham, put too many monks in the priory, and took too much of its revenue for the mother house. Then while Robert was with the king in Ireland, the abbot replaced the prior of Binham with a man of his own choice. Robert claimed that the foundation charter of the priory limited the abbot's retinue on visits, the monks he could place in the house, and the revenue he could draw from it. He also maintained that the abbot could not appoint or remove a prior without the consent of the patron of the priory.[114] The abbey chronicler states that the charter shown by Robert in support of these claims was another forgery, but the abbot does not seem to have made any such charge—he simply argued that Robert was not the heir of the founder, Robert de Valognes.[115] As Robert fitz Walter's wife was still alive, this argument was extremely feeble for she was the unquestioned heiress of the Valognes lords of Benington. But Robert was a proud and arrogant baron. When he returned from Ireland to find a new prior at Binham, he resorted to force instead of to the law. He laid siege to the priory and plundered its possessions. The abbot appealed to King John.

---

[113] *Annals of Dunstaple*, p. 28; Thomas Walsingham, *Gesta abbatum monasterii Sancti Albani* (ed. H. R. Riley, Rolls series), I, 220-225.
[114] *Curia regis rolls*, VI, 56.
[115] *Ibid.*; *Gesta Sancti Albani*, I, 226.

According to the chronicler the king was shocked at the story " Ho, by the feet of God, who ever heard of such a thing in time of peace in a Christian land." John promptly despatched troops to Binham, but they found that Robert and his men had retired. Shortly after this Robert fitz Walter and his wife brought their case against the abbot of St. Albans to the king's court.[116] Having failed to win by violence, they tried their luck at law. Unfortunately there is no record of the disposition of the case, but it seems unlikely that John would decide in Robert's favor under the circumstances.

The story of Robert fitz Walter's contest with the abbot of St. Albans over the priory of Binham is well established—the chronicle account is in general confirmed by the *Curia regis rolls*. For his next quarrel with King John we have only one unsupported source albeit a good one—the *Histoire des ducs de Normandie*. One day the king and his court were travelling toward Marlborough. Geoffrey de Mandeville sent a servant ahead to reserve quarters for him. The servant secured the quarters, but was soon ejected by men looking for lodgings for William Brewer. When Geoffrey arrived on the scene, he ordered William's men to leave and a brief fight ensued in which he killed one of them. William Brewer complained to the king who swore he would hang Geoffrey. Meanwhile Geoffrey had gone to his father-in-law, Robert fitz Walter. Although Robert was annoyed at Geoffrey for getting into such a scrape, he went to John and asked him to pardon him. John insisted he would hang the culprit. Robert was indignant. "You would hang my son-in-law! By God's body you will not. You will see 2,000 laced helms in your land before you hang him." Robert did, however, promise to produce Geoffrey for trial before the royal court, but he had his doubts of the impartiality of that body and arrived at the session with 500 fully armed knights. The trial was postponed, and Robert repeated his performance. A little later Robert and his family fled to France to escape John's wrath.[117]

While the *Histoire des ducs de Normandie* is generally reliable as chronicles go, this story presents several difficulties. As the

[116] *Ibid.*, pp. 226-228.
[117] *Histoire des ducs de Normandie*, pp. 116-118.

events described must have taken place before the summer of 1212 when Robert fled, Geoffrey de Mandeville's father, Geoffrey fitz Peter, was still alive. Why did not Geoffrey seek his aid? Then there is no evidence whatever that Geoffrey de Mandeville was seriously at odds with John before the spring of 1215. There is no indication that any action was taken against him at the time of Robert's flight, and when his father died he was given possession of most of his vast lands.[118] The tale of the escort of 500 knights sounds more like a *chanson du geste* than history—certainly Robert could muster no such force. I am inclined to think that the incident described actually took place, and that Robert and probably Geoffrey fitz Peter as well procured Geoffrey's pardon. The affair may well have aggravated the mutual hatred of John and Robert fitz Walter. But it seems very doubtful that it resulted in an open break and led directly to Robert's flight. As we have it in the *Histoire* the story is clearly distorted and exaggerated.

As I have indicated in discussing John's character, the story of the seduction of Robert fitz Walter's daughter by the king rests on very feeble evidence. The *Histoire des ducs de Normandie* mentions it as a tale told to King Philip—presumably because Philip would have been inclined to sympathize with John in the affair of Geoffrey de Mandeville and the serjeant.[119] The other source is a chronicle of Dunmow priory printed in the *Monasticon*.[120] According to this account John had Matilda poisoned. It sounds like a wild tale of no credibility. Matilda did die about that time, but it seems unlikely that John poisoned her. I suspect that the stories of King John's seduction of Matilda fitz Walter and his attempted violation of the wife of Eustace de Vesci arose to fill a need—to explain why those particular barons were the leaders in the revolt against John.

It is extremely difficult to work up much sympathy for Robert fitz Walter. It seems fairly certain that he betrayed Vaudreuil to Philip Augustus. While his arguments against the abbot of St. Albans may well have been sound, he chose to settle the question by

---

[118] *Rot. oblatis,* pp. 502-503.
[119] *Histoire des ducs de Normandie,* p. 118.
[120] Dugdale, *Monasticon,* VI, 147.

force instead of by law. In the case of Geoffrey de Mandeville's difficulties, he was obstructing the ordinary course of justice. From the feudal point of view he was acting like a proud and high-spirited baron. But no king worth his salt could have permitted such high-handed actions to go unpunished. It was probably the realization of this that made Robert one of the chief conspirators against John.

The *Histoire des ducs de Normandie* states that at about the same time as the affair of Geoffrey de Mandeville John quarreled with Geoffrey fitz Peter and forced him to offer a large fine for his good-will.[121] While there is no evidence to confirm this statement, it is perfectly plausible. Certainly in the spring of 1212 the king was conducting an indirect campaign against Geoffrey and his son-in-law, Henry de Bohun. Late in April of that year Earl William of Salisbury and Ela his wife instituted suit in the king's court against Henry de Bohun for the entire barony of Trowbridge, Henry's chief fief.[122] On the same day Geoffrey de Say reopened his old claim against Geoffrey fitz Peter for the Mandeville barony.[123] Neither of these suits could have been brought against John's will, and he actively assisted Earl William's case. Henry de Bohun was summoned to court to explain to whom he did service for the barony. Henry sent word that he was sick and could not come to court and four knights were sent to "view" him at his castle of Caldecot in the Marches. They found him sick and "gave him a day" at the Tower of London on June 2, 1213. But the court ruled that an "essoin" or excuse for absence could not be presented in the summons to explain to whom he did service, and the barony was taken into the king's hand.[124] Some time later Henry tried to recover his lands by replevin, but he apparently did not succeed as they were still in the king's hands in August 1214.[125] In fact there is some reason for thinking that Earl William had actual possession of the barony although the suit had never been decided.[126] The suit of Geoffrey de Say against Geof-

---

[121] *Histoire des ducs de Normandie*, p. 116.
[122] *Curia regis rolls*, VI, 270.
[123] *Ibid.*
[124] *Ibid.*, p. 320.
[125] *Ibid.*, p. 344; *Rot. claus.*, I, 210.
[126] *Ibid.*, p. 210.

frey fitz Peter was not heard until after the latter's death when it was pressed against his heir Geoffrey de Mandeville. It came up in court at a time when John was trying to win Geoffrey away from his foes and was dismissed on a technicality. Geoffrey de Say had sued for the barony held by Geoffrey and William de Mandeville under Henry II, and Geoffrey de Mandeville did not hold all that fief.[127]

Now both these suits had a sound basis in law. When Earl William de Mandeville died in 1189, his nearest relative was his aunt, Beatrice, widow of William de Say, lord of Kimbolton. But no king was likely to take seriously the claims of an elderly widow to the great Mandeville barony. Beatrice had two sons—William and Geoffrey de Say. William had died in 1177 leaving two daughters the elder of which was the wife of Geoffrey fitz Peter. Thus the succession to the Mandeville lands lay between Geoffrey fitz Peter and Geoffrey de Say. Geoffrey de Say offered Richard a large fine and had seisin of the barony for a short time, but he had trouble paying the fine and with Richard absent on the crusade he could not cope with the political power of Geoffrey fitz Peter who was one of the board of justices ruling the realm. The main basis for Geoffrey's suits in later years was his brief seisin. It is interesting to notice that his claim to the Mandeville barony resembled that of John to the English crown—that of a younger brother against the child of a dead elder brother. As we have seen the barony of Trowbridge was partially, perhaps entirely, composed of lands given by Edward of Salisbury to Humphrey de Bohun in marriage with his daughter. By the custom of the realm no homage was due for such a gift for three generations. Earl William of Salisbury had a good claim to the homage and service of Henry de Bohun for any lands of the honor that had once belonged to Edward of Salisbury, his wife's great-great-grandfather. He had no sound right to actual possession of the barony.

What is difficult to explain is why King John permitted these two suits to be started in the spring of 1212. His quarrel with the papacy had reached a crucial stage, and he was at odds with

[127] *Ibid.*, p. 168; *Curia regis rolls,* VII, 110-111.

several important groups of barons. Why offend one of the chief props of his realm, Geoffrey fitz Peter, and another powerful baron closely related to him who had on the whole been steadily loyal? There are several possible explanations. In the case of Geoffrey de Say's suit he may have hoped to frighten Geoffrey fitz Peter and his sons enough to make sure that they did not ally with his enemy Robert fitz Walter—just a reminder to Geoffrey that his position was none too secure. The case against Henry de Bohun may have been meant to serve the same purpose, but it is also possible that it was an effort to satisfy the ambitions of William Longsword. With so many barons disaffected John would be anxious to make sure of the loyalty of those he could trust. Earl William had never been satisfied with his position. Although he held the title of earl, his fief was not large and he had received meagre gifts from the crown. John gave him a pension, but the king had successfully resisted his attempt to be recognized as hereditary sheriff of Wiltshire and hereditary constable of Salisbury castle. William may well have felt that his position as a royal bastard entitled him to more generous treatment. By allowing and even encouraging the suit against Henry de Bohun John could please William at no cost to himself.

The years 1209 to 1212 were ones of almost continuous military activity. In 1209 John made an expedition against the Welsh and led his host to the borders of Scotland. In 1210 while the king invaded Ireland, the justiciar waged war on William de Briouse and his Welsh allies. In 1211 there was a major expedition against Wales that obliged Llywelyn and his fellow chieftains to sue for peace and give hostages. February 1212 saw Saher de Quency leading a mercenary force to Scotland to help King William suppress a revolt there.[128] As the Welsh showed no inclination to keep their promises, the spring and early summer of 1212 were spent in preparing a really large scale invasion of their land. Hence military preparations such as the hiring of additional mercenary troops and extensive building programs at the great royal fortresses

---

[128] Coventry, II, 206; *Curia regis rolls,* VI, 290; Saher had apparently also led a force to Scotland in the early spring of 1211. " Praestito roll 12 John," *Rot. liberate,* p. 240. Pipe roll 13 John, Public Record Office.

do not necessarily imply that John feared a baronial revolt. Still it is interesting to notice what castles received most attention. Hanley, a new castle on lands belonging to the honor of Gloucester in Worcestershire, was completed, St. Briavel's in the forest of Dean extensively improved, and small sums were spent on Ludlow and other Marcher fortresses. These could be intended to check danger from Wales. The very large sum of £645 was spent on the bishop of Durham's fortress of Norham on the Scots border and over £100 each on Bamborough and Newcastle, the chief castles of Northumberland. These works could be a further precaution against an invasion from Scotland or measures of security in case of trouble with the Northumbrian barons. Then nearly £2,000 were used to improve the fortifications of Scarborough and £440 on those of Sauvey. Knaresborough was strengthened at a cost of £140 and Rockingham at a cost of £126.[129] These fortresses did not guard England from foreign foes. The expenditure of such large sums on them must mean that John feared a baronial rising.

Ever since his expulsion from Normandy John had kept some mercenary troops in England under such captains as Gerard de Athies, Engelard de Cigogné, Philip Marc, and Fawkes de Bréauté. By 1209 he had a group of Flemish knights more or less permanently in his service and on the Irish campaign they seem to have formed a special service corps.[130] While it is impossible to form any reliable estimate of the mercenary knights and serjeants employed during these years, it seems unlikely that they were very numerous. But in June 1212 an energetic campaign was undertaken to enlist more troops from Flanders. Count Reginald of Boulogne who had done homage to John early in May, Hugh de Boves, and Adam de Keret, castellan of Bruges, were instructed to raise as many men as possible.[131] Of course this may have been simply part of the preparations for the expedition into Wales, but it seems rather unlikely that it was. Flemish knights were ex-

---

[129] Pipe rolls 12, 13, and 14 John, Public Record Office.
[130] *Rot. liberate*, pp. 124-126, 177, 182-185, 185-187, 189-191, 197-202. John's Flemish corps in Ireland numbered thirty-three knights—or rather that number received loans.
[131] *Rot. pat.*, p. 93.

pensive luxuries—they expected to be given generous money fiefs to be enjoyed in both peace and war. The feudal levy of England was more than able to cope with the Welsh. One is forced to conclude that in June 1212 John felt the need of foreign troops to guard against internal troubles.

King John devoted June and July of the year 1212 to preparations for a great invasion of Llywelyn's lands in North Wales. Large amounts of supplies of all kinds were gathered from the whole realm.[132] All men who held of the crown by knight service or serjeantry were summoned to the host.[133] John de Grey, bishop of Norwich and justiciar of Ireland, and William Marshal were ordered to be at the rendezvous with 200 knights and as many serjeants as could be spared from the defense of Ireland itself.[134] Agents were sent to Flanders to recruit mercenary knights and serjeants, and Alan of Galway, constable of Scotland, was directed to hire 1,000 Scots for John's service.[135] The towns of England were ordered to supply about 800 armed serjeants.[136] Sheriffs and custodians of lands in the hands of the crown were instructed to send over 8,000 laborers for building fortresses.[137] John had completed his system of alliances against Philip Augustus and the Welsh were the only external foes who could threaten England while he conducted his long-planned expedition to the continent. He was determined to crush them—and to have mercenaries on hand in case of baronial revolt.

The host had been summoned to muster at Chester on August 19.[138] On the fourteenth John hanged at Nottingham twenty-eight Welsh boys, sons of chieftains, who had been given to him as hostages the previous summer.[139] Clearly he planned a real attempt to break Llywelyn's power rather than the usual parade into Wales followed by a negotiated peace. But soon rumors came to the king

---

[132] Pipe rolls 13 and 14 John, Public Record Office; *Rot. claus.*, I, 121.
[133] " Rotulus misae 14 John," pp. 235-236; *Rot. claus.*, I, 131.
[134] *Ibid.*
[135] *Ibid. Rot. pat.*, p. 93.
[136] *Rot. claus.*, I, 130-131.
[137] *Ibid.*, p. 131.
[138] *Ibid.*, p. 131.
[139] Wendover, II, 61; Coventry, II, 207.

of a baronial plot. While the campaign was in progress, he was to be either murdered or handed over to his Welsh foes.[140] Wendover states that this news was carried by letters from his daughter, Joan, wife of Llywelyn, and from the king of Scotland. While this seems perfectly possible, it is equally likely that similar rumors were picked up by members of the king's household among the gathering host. Nottingham seems to have buzzed with wild reports. The barons were ready to depose John and replace him with Simon de Montfort.[141] The queen had been raped; Prince Richard, the king's second son, had been murdered; the king's treasury at Gloucester had been plundered.[142] Whatever tales he heard were enough to convince John that the danger was real. On August 16 he called off his muster against the Welsh and directed his knights, serjeants, and workmen who had started for the meeting place to return to their homes.[143] On the same day he ordered Stephen de Turnham to allow no one to see Henry, his eldest son and heir, who did not bear special letters authorizing the visit.[144] John then despatched messengers to the barons whom he suspected of being involved in the plot to demand hostages for their good behavior.[145] The recent fate of the Welsh boys would guarantee that this request would not be considered a mere formality.

The abandonment of the Welsh expedition and the demand for hostages had a dramatic result—Robert fitz Walter and Eustace de Vesci fled from England with their families and households. Robert crossed to France to join the exiled bishops and pose as a martyr to John's hatred for conscientious Christians while Eustace retired to the lands of his father-in-law, King William of Scotland.[146] Two other barons against whom John's suspicions turned very strongly gave him full satisfaction. Richard de Umfraville agreed to surrender his castle of Prudhoe and to give four sons as hostages. If it were proved that he had been in the conspiracy, he

---

[140] Wendover, II, 62; *Annals of St. Edmunds*, p. 24.
[141] *Annals of Dunstaple*, p. 33.
[142] *Annals of St. Edmunds*, p. 23.   [144] *Rot. claus.*, I, 121.
[143] *Rot. pat.*, p. 94.   [145] Wendover, II, 62.
[146] *Ibid.*, p. 62; Coggeshall, p. 165; Coventry, p. 207; *Histoire des ducs de Normandie*, p. 118; *Annals of Dunstaple*, p. 35; *Annals of St. Edmunds*, p. 25.

would lose his sons and castle and suffer as a traitor.[147] David, earl of Huntingdon, immediately gave his second son as a hostage, but seems to have hesitated to surrender his castle of Fotheringay. Hugh de Neville was despatched to take it by force if necessary. Henry de Braybrook, who was under-sheriff of Northamptonshire for his father Robert, Simon de Pattishall, Walter de Preston, and the citizens of Northampton were ordered to aid Hugh if Earl David tried to resist.[148] Alice Peche, widow of Gilbert Peche and sister of Robert fitz Walter, gave hostages for her loyalty, and John placed her late husband's lands in the custody of the Flemish captain Hugh de Boves.[149] It seems likely that Earl Richard de Clare and Richard de Lucy of Egremont gave hostages at this time.[150] In all probability there were other barons who were obliged to give hostages. It is hard to believe that John's suspicions with such excellent fuel to feed them would have operated in a narrow range.

The treason of Eustace de Vesci and his strong suspicions of the loyalty of Richard de Umfraville made John fear for the safety of the vital border shire of Northumberland. While it is clear that the king did not suspect Robert fitz Roger of being involved in the conspiracy, he was the great uncle of young John de Lacy about whose reliability John had grave doubts. Hence he seemed hardly the man to leave in so crucial a post. A man in whom John had complete confidence, Philip de Ulecotes, custodian of the see of Durham, was on hand in the north and could easily take over Robert's shrievalty, but he was a man of no feudal position, and the king felt that the prestige of a great baron was needed in the troubled shire. Only two English earls had interests in the north, and one of these Ranulf of Chester, was at the moment fully occupied with the Welsh. The other was William de Warren, lord of Conisborough in Yorkshire. Earl William gave pledges that he had known nothing of the plot and was sent north to watch over Northumberland with Philip de Ulecotes and Aimery, archdeacon of Durham.[151] The earl does not seem to have been ap-

[147] *Rot. claus.*, I, 122.
[148] *Ibid.; Rot. pat.*, p. 94.
[149] *Ibid.*, pp. 94, 101.
[150] *Ibid.*, pp. 96, 101.
[151] *Ibid.*, p. 94.

pointed sheriff and as soon as the emergency was over, he was withdrawn leaving Philip and Aimery as joint sheriffs.[152] Apparently Philip was a choice cut-throat whom John was unwilling to leave in full command despite his undoubted loyalty and ability as a captain. There is some indication that John was worried about other critical commands. John fitz Hugh was replaced as castellan of Hertford, a castle surrounded by vassals of Robert fitz Walter, by John de Bassingbourn.[153] While I know of no reason why the king should suspect John fitz Hugh, he was for a time deprived of most of his offices, and he was one of the few intimate servants of John who later joined the baronial rebellion.[154] The replacement of Alexander de Pointon by Hugh de Boves as custodian of the Peche barony seems to have had a similar motive. But Robert fitz Roger retained the shrievalty of Norfolk and Suffolk.

King John moved vigorously against the two fugitive barons and their adherents. The two castles of Robert fitz Walter, Benington in Hertfordshire and Castle Baynard in London, were razed.[155] Robert and nine of his men were solemnly outlawed by the shire court of Essex.[156] Only four of these men deserve mention by name. One was William fitz Walter, archdeacon of Hereford. His name suggests that he was a brother of Robert fitz Walter. Certainly he furnishes a possible link between his bishop, Giles de Briouse, and Robert's conspiracy.[157] The other three were William, Philip, and Gervase de Houbridge. Now Gervase de Houbridge was a prominent canon of the cathedral of St. Paul in London and there were very intimate relations between the canons of St. Paul's and the officials of the royal exchequer.[158] John was fully aware of this connection. As we have seen Richard Marsh was stationed in Westminster to keep an eye on the sessions of the

---

[152] *Ibid.* [153] *Ibid.* [154] *Ibid.*, pp. 94-96.

[155] *Histoire des ducs de Normandie*, p. 118; Coventry, II, 207; Coggeshall, p. 165; Matthew Paris, *Chronica maiora*, II, 544; *Annals of Dunstaple*, p. 35.

[156] *Rot. claus.*, I, 165-166; Coggeshall, p. 165.

[157] In the court's official statement he is called simply the archdeacon of Hereford. His name appears on *Rot. pat.*, p. 101.

[158] On Gervase de Houbridge see H. J. Richardson, " Letters of the Legate Guala."

exchequer in the autumn of 1212. At least three exchequer officials, William de Cornhill, archdeacon of Huntingdon, William de Neckton, and Geoffrey de Norwich felt the weight of the king's suspicions. William de Cornhill apparently was imprisoned and forced to offer a fine for benevolence, but he was soon restored to full favor.[159] William de Neckton fled to France.[160] The fate of Geoffrey de Norwich requires more extended discussion.

The story of Geoffrey de Norwich deserves attention partly for its own sake as an account of one of King John's atrocities and partly because so eminent an authority as Mr. H. G. Richardson has called it "a stupid fable."[161] It appears in its fullest form in Roger of Wendover. This chronicler states that in 1209 when King John had been excommunicated by Innocent III but the decree had not been formally published, reports of the pope's action spread over England by word of mouth. One day at Westminster during a session of the exchequer Geoffrey, archdeacon of Norwich, began to talk with his colleagues about the sentence and remarked that it was not safe for beneficed clerks to remain longer in the service of an excommunicate king. He then started for home without asking leave. When John heard about Geoffrey's words and departure, he was gravely troubled and sent a knight named William Talbot to arrest him. William captured Geoffrey and imprisoned him in chains. A few days later a cope of lead was put on him by the king's order. Oppressed by the weight of the cope and poorly fed, Geoffrey died.[162] Ralph de Coggeshall tells what is apparently the same story in much briefer form and places it in 1212. He says that Geoffrey de Norwich who was involved in the conspiracy of Robert fitz Walter and Eustace de Vesci died after a long imprisonment.[163] The *Annals of Dunstaple* carry the tale under the date 1210, but place it after the same baronial plot. They state that Geoffrey, a faithful and innocent man, was captured near Dunstaple by the earl of Salisbury and imprisoned in

---

[159] *Annals of St. Edmunds*, p. 25.
[160] Matthew Paris, *Chronica maiora*, II, 537.
[161] Richardson, "William of Ely," pp. 51-52.
[162] Wendover, II, 52-53.
[163] Coggeshall, p. 165.

The Seeds of Revolt

Bristol castle where he died after a long and severe confinement.[164] The *Annals of St. Edmund's* place the event in 1212 after the flight of Robert fitz Walter. Geoffrey de Norwich, a noble clerk who recited the pope's letter to the barons of the exchequer, was captured at Nottingham and died in irons.[165] These various versions completely confused Matthew Paris when he composed his *Chronica Maiora*. Under 1209 he repeated Wendover's account without change.[166] Apparently he did not identify the Geoffrey de Norwich of most of the accounts with the Geoffrey, archdeacon of Norwich, of Wendover. Hence when he came to the events of 1212 he inserted the story in Wendover's text. John ordered his faithful, prudent, and elegant clerk, Geoffrey de Norwich, captured and tortured to death in Nottingham castle. This alarmed Geoffrey's associate, William de Neckton, who promptly fled to France.[167] But by the time he came to write his *Historia Anglorum* Matthew had decided that the two Geoffreys were one. The scene of Geoffrey's death is still Nottingham castle. He was a faithful and moral clerk of the exchequer who died in a leaden cope.[168]

There is no doubt that Roger of Wendover was in error both as to the date and the man involved. Geoffrey, archdeacon of Norwich, was Geoffrey de Burgh, brother of Hubert de Burgh. Geoffrey de Burgh lived to become bishop of Ely in 1225. The other accounts call the victim simply Geoffrey de Norwich—the usual name of the justice of the Jews. Geoffrey de Norwich, justiciar of the Jews, was alive on June 14, 1212, but there is no later record of him.[169] Hence he could not have been killed in 1209, but could have been after the flight of Robert fitz Walter. One feature of Wendover's version is supported by the *Annals of Dunstaple*. Wendover has Geoffrey captured by William Talbot while the *Annals* have it done by Earl William of Salisbury. Earl William was sheriff of Cambridge and Huntingdonshire and William Tal-

---

[164] *Annals of Dunstaple*, pp. 33-34.
[165] *Annals of St. Edmunds*, p. 25.
[166] Matthew Paris, *Chronica maiora*, II, 557.
[167] *Ibid.*, pp. 537-538.
[168] Matthew Paris. *Historia Anglorum* (ed. Sir Frederic Madden, Rolls series), II, 126.
[169] *Rot. chart.*, p. 187.

bot was one of his favorite knights.[170] In short Roger of Wendover was in this case as in many others highly inaccurate, but his mistakes do not justify one in rejecting Ralph de Coggeshall and the *Annals of Dunstaple*—especially as Geoffrey de Norwich, justice of the Jews, did disappear at the time the chronicles indicate.

It seems clear that shortly after the flight of Robert fitz Walter Geoffrey de Norwich left Westminster and was captured at John's command by either Earl William of Salisbury or his knight, William Talbot. He was imprisoned in a royal castle where he died of mistreatment. Whether his offense was being involved in Robert fitz Walter's conspiracy or making remarks about serving an excommunicate king, what castle he died in, and just how he died cannot be determined conclusively. It is, however, quite conceivable that even if Geoffrey did suffer because of being involved in the conspiracy, his friends would concoct the other tale. It is far nobler to die as a martyr than as a traitor. And Robert fitz Walter himself is said to have told Pandulf that he fled England because he would not serve an excommunicate king.

Robert fitz Walter, Eustace de Vesci, and their adherents were included in the peace between John and Innocent III.[171] On May 27, 1213, letters patent of safe conduct were issued to enable them to return to England.[172] But John could not resist the temptation to strike one last blow. On the same day he issued the safe conducts he ordered Philip de Ulecotes to raze Eustace de Vesci's castle of Alnwick.[173] On July 19, the king directed his officials to give Robert and Eustace possession of their lands.[174] On the twentieth two of Robert's men were freed from the king's prison.[175] The next day they both received advance payments on the damages due them—Eustace £100 and Robert 100 marks.[176] In November the men who were estimating the damages suffered by the church were directed to inquire about those of Robert fitz Walter as

---

[170] " Praestito roll 12 John," *Rot. liberate,* pp. 181, 196, 223; *Rot. claus.,* I, 82, 120.
[171] Migne, *Patrologia,* ccxvi, 772-775.
[172] *Rot. pat.,* p. 99.
[173] *Ibid.*
[174] *Ibid.,* p. 101.
[175] *Ibid.*
[176] *Rot. claus.,* I, 146.

well.[177] But these two barons remained John's bitter foes and were to be the leaders of the great revolt.

During the early months of 1213 while King John was still actively hunting down men whom he suspected of being involved in the conspiracy of Robert fitz Walter, he took some steps to appease at least part of his baronage.[178] On February 25 he addressed letters patent to his subjects in Yorkshire and Lincolnshire. He was deeply moved by complaints that sheriffs and other royal officials had been extorting money from them that never found its way to the exchequer. He was sending Robert de Ros, William de Albini, Simon de Kyme, and Thomas de Moulton to investigate. The people of the shires were to inform these commissioners what sums the royal officials had taken since the king left England on his way to Ireland in 1210 and what pretexts had been used for taking them. They were also to report by how much the revenues of the hundreds, wapentakes, and tithings had been increased. The king also wanted to know whether any of his officers had been hearing pleas of the crown. Finally John asked for a complete report of all landed property held by Jews.[179] This is an extremely interesting document. The king was moved by the complaints of his subjects—but he seems to have been chiefly disturbed by the fact that he was not getting the money that was extorted. Thus while the letters start out as if their chief purpose was appeasement of discontent, the inquest they provided for was calculated to serve the interests of the king more than those of his subjects. All four of the commissioners named in the letters were to be either among the rebels mustered at Stamford in the spring of 1215 or among the twenty-five barons chosen to enforce Magna Carta. While there is no indication on the patent roll that similar letters were sent to other shires, the *Annals of Dunstaple* speak of an inquest into the behavior of sheriffs as if it were general.[180] Walter of Coventry mentions such an inquest, but places it after the making of peace with the church.[181] I am inclined to think that the inquest was restricted to these two shires and that

[177] *Ibid.*, p. 154.
[178] *Rot. pat.*, p. 98.
[179] *Ibid.*, p. 97.
[180] *Annals of Dunstaple*, p. 35.
[181] Coventry, II, 214.

the chroniclers were thinking about the rather vague general measures proposed in August.

Three changes in the holders of English shrievalties made during these same early months of 1213 may well have been connected with this campaign of appeasement. On January 30 Robert de Ros succeeded Hugh de Neville as sheriff of Cumberland.[182] Then on the same day that he despatched his letters ordering the inquest in Yorkshire and Lincolnshire John removed the sheriffs of these two counties. In Yorkshire Gilbert fitz Renfrew was replaced by Robert de Percy while Alexander de Pointon relieved Hubert de Burgh as sheriff of Lincolnshire.[183] Gilbert fitz Renfrew had paid extremely large profits into the exchequer and may well have enriched himself on the side.[184] As Hubert de Burgh had been in Poitou for some time, it was really his under-sheriff who was removed.[185] John's efforts to appease Lincolnshire and Yorkshire seem to indicate that he considered the barons of those shires the most seriously disaffected of his vassals.

While the political situation in England during the first four months of 1213 was essentially a continuation of that of the previous four years, that year as a whole saw extremely vital changes. The most significant of these were the result of the peace with the papacy. When King John came to an agreement with Innocent III, he cut one of the bonds that had bound his discontented barons to him. The basic issue in John's quarrel with the pope was the royal rights of patronage, and the question as to what privileges should be enjoyed by patrons was fully as important to the barons as to the king. The significance of this point is made clear by a letter addressed by Stephen Langton to the barons and knights of England in 1210.[186] He assured them that the pope had no intention of attacking their powers as patrons. But it must have been fairly easy for the king to convince his vassals that if he could not defend his rights, they had but little chance of

---

[182] *Rot. pat.*, p. 96.
[183] *Ibid.*, p. 97.
[184] Pipe rolls 12 and 13 John, Public Record Office.
[185] *Rot. pat.*, p. 97.
[186] Gervase of Canterbury, II, lxxviii.

doing so. While the king's eventual defeat cannot have served to lessen their fears, it destroyed his position as the fearless defender of lay privileges.

Then the peace reinstated in power in England three leaders of the disaffected barons—Eustace de Vesci, Robert fitz Walter, and Giles de Briouse, bishop of Hereford. While the part played by Bishop Giles in the baronial revolt is extremely obscure, he served as a link between the earlier and later risings. Through him the bitter hatred of the Briouses toward King John was passed on to other baronial elements. The existence in the minds of the barons of a strong memory of the Briouse affair seems the only reasonable explanation of the condemnation of Gerard de Athies and his relatives in Magna Carta. They had been John's chief agents in the crushing of the Briouses, but none of the rebels of 1215 except possibly Henry de Bohun had had any contact with them. As for Eustace de Vesci and Robert fitz Walter it seems clear that neither they nor the king ever pretended that the past had been forgotten or forgiven. John continued to hate these two barons, and they took their former place at the head of the disaffected.

The most important result of the agreement with Rome was the establishment in a dominant position in English politics of a truly great man—Stephen Langton, archbishop of Canterbury. Stephen was highly intelligent and had received the best education known in his day. He was the master of theology and canon law both in theory and practice. He was a man of strong character and personality, one inclined to be intransigent and with no love of compromise. Moreover Stephen was both a high ecclesiastic and a member of the English feudal class. Although he had spent his adult years in the service of the church, he had a deep interest in the internal policy of his native land. Therein lay the roots of his later difficulties with the papacy. Throughout the years when he was seeking admission to England as her primate, he fought John both as a foe of the church and as an unworthy king. In short he desired the full application in England of the canon law as interpreted by the papal court and also the proper observance of English secular law and custom by the royal government. Before he absolved John from excommunication Stephen obliged the king to promise to restore the good laws of his ancestors and invalidate all bad laws.[187] The king also swore to give all men justice according to the judgment of his court. In Stephen's mind John's peace with the church involved a promise to observe both canon and secular law.

Stephen Langton was trained to think of law, rights, and privileges in general terms. He was not primarily interested in who should hold a castle but rather in the law governing the possession of castles. He sought to have England governed by an orderly regime based on generally accepted legal principles. Now it is obvious that most English barons must have been fully capable of comprehending this idea. The feudal system was based on the assumption that every fief would have its customs formed by the lord's court. The law molded by the court of the English king was the common law of England. The idea of obliging the king to define this law and promise to observe it was not new—Henry I, Stephen, and Henry II had issued charters of liberties. But there is no evidence that before the return of Stephen Langton the opposition to King John had any general program of reform. We hear of individual grievances and of personal desires and ambitions rather than of basic principles. While it seems highly improbable that the English barons did not know about the charter of Henry I until it was shown to them by Langton, Wendover's tale may well contain an essential truth—that it was Stephen who led them to seek a general statement of legal principles instead of various benefits for individuals. In this connection it is interesting to notice that Robert fitz Walter who became the accepted leader of the baronial party had spent some time in France where Stephen was in exile. Is it too much to believe that Stephen had sold his program to Robert? But whether or not Stephen was responsible for the innovation of the line of thought that led to Magna Carta, he was clearly its doughty supporter and adherent. From the time of his consecration in 1207 to his suspension in 1215 he worked steadily to bring about a regime of established law in England.

---

[187] Wendover, II, 81.

It seems likely that his ideas were expressed in their earliest form in the so-called unknown charter by October 1213.

While John's submission to the papacy strengthened the baronial opposition by removing a strong reason for adherence to the king and by supplying it with more effective leadership, it also improved the king's own position. The Welsh had used John's excommunication as an excuse for their continual attacks on the Marches. After John's submission Pandulf and Langton persuaded them to make a series of truces.[188] But of far greater importance was the fact that the king obtained the pope's support against his barons. As long as John defied the papacy, Innocent III was glad to use against him any weapon that came to hand, and he had no objections to Langton's attacks on John as an unjust king. But the pope had no real interest in the internal polity of England. Innocent's chief aim was to increase the power, prestige, and dignity of the church and its head. By making his submission and becoming a papal vassal John had greatly furthered these ends to which Innocent was devoted. It immediately became to the pope's interest to show the value of papal support to a secular monarch. Moreover any movement against John became indirectly an attack on his overlord, the pope. We shall find Innocent piously exhorting John to deal justly with his barons, but he had little interest in the matter. What he cared about was the political and economic status of his vassal—the king. When Langton's fierce struggle for the principles of Magna Carta led him close to the baronial camp, he was suspended by the pope. Thus John by his submission obtained full papal support for his internal policy.

During this same year two events that had no connection with the conclusion of peace with Rome served to strengthen John's position. One was the restoration of William Marshal to the royal favor and to his former position in England. By this John gained the active aid of a wise and experienced counselor and administrator and a highly effective captain. Moreover the death of William de Brouse had left William Marshal the undisputed leader of the barons of the southern Marches of Wales. In July Walter de Lacy came to terms with the king and received possession of his lands

[188] *Rot. pat.*, pp. 100, 103.

in England and the Marches.[189] The return to favor of William Marshal and Walter de Lacy made the adherence of the lesser lords of the region fairly certain. And it was Walter de Lacy, Hugh de Mortimer, John de Monmouth, and Walter and Roger de Clifford who supplied through their knightly vassals and Welsh mercenaries a large part of the military force that John relied on during the baronial revolt. This group of Marcher lords was the only compact body of barons that remained consistently loyal.

Another event that probably strengthened John's position more than it weakened it was the death in October 1213 of Geoffrey fitz Peter. There seems to be no doubt that Geoffrey was steadfastly loyal to his master, but his last years must have been most unhappy. According to the *Histoire des ducs de Normandie* he had a bitter quarrel with John in 1212.[190] It certainly must have deeply embarrassed the aged justiciar to see the father-in-law of his two sons flee England under the stigma of treason. In short by 1212 Geoffrey was unable to keep his relatives and associates in order and was himself the victim of John's jealousy—perhaps even of his suspicion. It seems doubtful that had he lived he could have done anything to avoid the baronial revolt. While his death placed the great Mandeville barony in the possession of an enemy of the king, young Geoffrey de Mandeville, it also enabled John to appoint as justiciar a man who was completely his creature and in whom he had full confidence, Peter des Roches.[191]

King John hoped that as soon as he made peace with the church and was absolved from excommunication, he could launch his long-planned expedition to the continent. He summoned his host to muster at Portsmouth in late July.[192] It was a thoroughly foolish proceeding. The season was too far advanced to begin so ambitious a campaign and the king's vassals had already served in the host earlier in the year—in the army mustered to repel the threatened French invasion. The feudal levy had been called out in each of the last four years. To then summon it twice in a year was decidedly overdoing it. This was one of the objections voiced

---

[189] *Rot. claus.*, I, 147.
[190] *Histoire des ducs de Normandie*, p. 116.
[191] *Rot. pat.*, p. 110.
[192] Wendover II, 82.

The Seeds of Revolt

by the barons, but apparently they could think of others as well.[193] The realm was still under interdict.[194] Then according to Walter of Coventry they tried the old argument that they owed no service outside the realm. This last excuse is credited to the "northerners."[195] John wrote to the count of Toulouse that a great wind prevented him from setting forth.[196] It seems clear that whatever their reasons were the barons refused to go. The king was enraged and mustered what troops he had available to punish those he considered the chiefs of the opposition—the northerners. Langton went to him to remind him that when he was absolved he had promised to rule justly and that he had no right to attack a vassal without a judgment by his court. John told him to stay out of lay affairs, but apparently did not actually attack his foes.[197] Such is the story given by the chroniclers and there seems no reason for doubting it, even though there is no corroborative evidence.

While John was attempting to get his expedition under way in early August, Geoffrey fitz Peter and Peter des Roches presided over a council at St. Albans. Its chief purpose seems to have been to lay plans for inquiring about the damages suffered by the church, but it seems also to have made a gesture at reform in the government. The laws of Henry I were to be observed and the king's officers were not to commit extortions.[198] This sounds as if Langton had insisted on doing something to implement John's pre-absolution promises and had gotten the usual vague statements. King John had no objection to pleasant references to the good old days, and he disliked extortion that did not profit his exchequer. He was obviously seeking to keep the barons contented so that he could make his expedition to Poitou.

When Nicholas of Tusculum arrived in England in October 1213, he offered himself as a mediator between King John and the "northerners." Ralph of Coggeshall simply states that the two parties were reconciled.[199] But it seems likely that this was the agreement that is recorded in the so-called Unknown Charter

---

[193] *Ibid.*
[194] *Ibid.*, p. 80.
[195] Coventry, II, 217.
[196] Rymer, *Foedera*, I, 114.
[197] Coggeshall, p. 167; Wendover, II, 83.
[198] *Ibid.*, pp. 82-83.
[199] Coggeshall, p. 167.

of Liberties.[200] This document will be discussed at length among the antecedents of Magna Carta. It is apparently a set of rough notes on an agreement between John and his barons. The first item deals with the question that had arisen between Langton and the king when John sought to punish the "northerners" for refusing to sail for Poitou—the king agreed that he would not take a man without judgment. Another clause looks like a compromise in the actual dispute between king and barons. John granted that his men should not go in the host outside England except to Normandy or Brittany.

On February 9, 1214, King John set sail for Poitou.[201] With him went at least twelve of the barons who were to appear in the rebellious group that gathered at Stamford in the spring of 1215 —John de Lacy, constable of Chester, Richard de Montfichet, William de Mandeville, William de Beauchamp of Bedford, William de Huntingfield, William Malet, William de Lanvalay, Fulk fitz Warin, Maurice de Ghent, John fitz Robert, Nicholas de Stutville, and Thomas de Moulton.[202] Saher de Quency, earl of Winchester, Roger Bigod, earl of Norfolk, and Robert de Ros sent sons in their places.[203] But John's most bitter foes, the leaders of the disaffected vassals, Robert fitz Walter, Eustace de Vesci, William de Mowbray, Richard de Clare, earl of Hertford, Henry de Bohun, earl of Hereford, and Geoffrey de Mandeville, earl of Essex stayed in England. Thus while a fair number of the future rebels followed John to Poitou, the larger part including the leaders remained at home. On July 9 the king sent letters patent to England promising forgiveness of old grievances toward anyone who should cross to join him.[204] There is no evidence that any baron took advantage of this offer. Previously, on May 26, John had directed the justiciar, Peter des Roches, to levy a scutage at

---

[200] *Layettes du trésor des chartes,* I, 34-35, 423; William Sharp McKechnie, *Magna carta* (Glasgow, 1914), pp. 485-486.

[201] Wendover, II, 98; Coggeshall, p. 168.

[202] The first nine were present when the truce was concluded with Philip Augustus. *Layettes du trésor des chartes,* I, 405-406. The others received loans on the campaign. Pipe roll 16 John, Public Record Office.

[203] *Ibid.*

[204] *Rot. pat.,* p. 118.

the high rate of three marks per fee on all who did not have letters of quittance.[205]

There is ample evidence that while he was campaigning on the continent John was greatly disturbed over the situation in England. He had left the royal administration in the care of Peter des Roches and William Brewer. While it seems unlikely that he suspected their fidelity, he may well have had doubts about their discretion. The fact that the justiciar chose that summer to press attacks on the franchises claimed by two powerful and loyal barons, William de Vernon, earl of Devon, and Aubrey de Vere, earl of Oxford, indicates that such fears on the king's part were justified.[206] At any rate John twice sent special emissaries to England. On May 22 Peter des Roches and William Brewer were informed that the king was sending Richard Marsh to join them. They were to consult him on all the king's business.[207] On August 16 Thomas de Eardington was despatched to England to give secret instructions to a long list of royal officials.[208] Apparently William Marshal was entrusted with a special function—the making of all the necessary arrangements for the relaxation of the interdict.[209] It seems likely that he was also expected to serve as a check on the activities of the disaffected barons. On June 28 the earl of Pembroke went to St. Edmunds in an effort to prevent the election of the candidate for the abbacy who was supported by Earl Roger Bigod and Robert fitz Walter.[210]

John was fully aware that the barons were plotting against him during his absence. He complained to the pope about the activities of Eustace de Vesci and directed the justiciar to make certain that the sister of Robert fitz Walter was not elected abbess of Barking.[211] In October he requested the legate to act against the conspirators.[212] He also took steps to build up the strength of the

[205] *Rot. claus.*, I, 166.
[206] *Curia regis rolls*, VII, 158-159, 184.
[207] *Rot. pat.*, p. 139.
[208] *Rot. claus.*, I, 202.
[209] Rymer, *Foedera*, I, 118.
[210] "Electio Hugonis," pp. 76-77.
[211] *Rot. claus.*, I, 202; Rymer, *Feodera*, I, 126.
[212] *Ibid.*, p. 175.

royal party by giving important baronies to men on whom he could rely. In April Peter de Maulay was given Isabella, daughter of Robert de Turnham, with her barony.[213] In July the king's bastard son Richard was given Rohese of Dover and her barony of Chilham.[214] Another royal favorite, Richard de Rivers, received the heiress of the barony of Ongar with her lands.[215] Finally Ralph de Lusignan, count of Eu, was placed in possession of the great fiefs of Hastings and Tickhill.[216] Ralph's wife, Alice, countess of Eu, was the undoubted lady of Hastings and had a good claim to Tickhill. As Ralph was soon bought by Philip Augustus, this maneuver was of little actual value, but it was a sound idea. Ralph was a hardy warrior and might have been able to hold the honor of Tickhill against its chief mesne tenants who were mostly in the rebellious party. This was not, of course, John's chief purpose in placating Ralph de Lusignan—he needed his aid in Poitou —but it may well have been in his mind.

By far the most interesting feature of King John's domestic policy during the year 1214 was his relations with Geoffrey de Mandeville, eldest son of Geoffrey fitz Peter. As we have seen the *Histoire des ducs de Normandie* asserts that it was a quarrel between John and Geoffrey de Mandeville that led to the flight of Robert fitz Walter. When Geoffrey fitz Peter died, the king promptly accepted the homage of Geoffrey for the great Mandeville barony, but other possessions of the late justiciar were kept in the hands of the crown.[217] The king's German favorite, Terric Teutonicus, was given custody of the castle and honor of Berkhamsted and Geoffrey de Buckland was given charge of the manor of Ailsbury.[218] While this may have annoyed Geoffrey de Mandeville, it was an essentially proper proceeding. Berkhamsted and Ailsbury had been granted to Geoffrey fitz Peter and his heirs by his second wife, Aveline, whose eldest son, John fitz Geoffrey, was

---

[213] *Rot. pat.*, p. 113.
[214] *Ibid.*, p. 118; *Rot. claus.*, I, 168.
[215] *Rot. oblatis*, pp. 517-518.
[216] *Rot. pat.*, p. 116.
[217] *Rot. oblatis*, pp. 502-503.
[218] *Rot. pat.*, p. 105; *Rot. claus.*, I, 154.

under age.[219] Then Geoffrey was ordered to surrender the Tower of London to William de Cornhill, archdeacon of Huntingdon.[220] The Mandevilles had since the eleventh century claimed to be hereditary custodians of the Tower, but no strong king had ever acknowledged their right. This important stronghold was usually entrusted to the justiciar of England, and Geoffrey fitz Peter had held it in that capacity. John seems to have withheld only one thing to which Geoffrey de Mandeville had a clear right—the sword of the earldom of Essex and the third penny of the shire. While the chronicles accord Geoffrey the title earl of Essex, and I have followed their practice, he was not formally girt with the sword of the earldom and did not have the third penny.[221]

On January 26, 1214, King John gave his former wife, Isabella of Gloucester, to Geoffrey de Mandeville with the major part of the vast honor of Gloucester. The king retained the town and castle of Bristol. He also insisted that the men to whom he had granted fiefs from the escheated lands of the honor should retain their holdings and that those to whom he had given custodies pertaining to the honor should remain in possession.[222] Gilbert de Clare, son of Isabella's sister, shared two demesne manors of the honor with the widow of Amauri de Montfort and held some thirty of its knights' fees.[223] But Geoffrey received the palatine shire of Glamorgan, ten demesne manors in England, and some 270 knights' fees.[224] For this he offered the enormous sum of 20,000 marks to be paid within a year.[225] As the gross annual revenue of the lands of Geoffrey received cannot have been more than £550, it is hard to see how he could hope to meet these terms.[226] As a matter of fact he failed to make the first payment.[227]

[219] *Rot. chart.*, pp. 127-128, 151.
[220] *Rot. pat.*, p. 105; *Rot. claus.*, I, 154.
[221] *Curia regis rolls*, VII, 110-111.
[222] *Rot. pat.*, p. 109; *Rot. claus.*, I, 162, 209.
[223] *Ibid.*, p. 155; *Red book of the exchequer*, I, 156.
[224] *Ibid. Rot. pat.*, p. 109; *Rot. claus.*, I, 209.
[225] *Rot. oblatis*, pp. 520-521.
[226] Like most such figures this is largely a guess. The English manors assigned to Geoffrey yielded about £330 in 1205. *Pipe roll 7 John*, pp. 102-104. Glamorgan was farmed for £100 in 1208. *Pipe roll 10 John*, p. 24. An allowance of £100 for miscellaneous revenues seems ample.
[227] *Rot. claus.*, I, 163.

This grant has been interpreted as an effort on John's part to win over Geoffrey de Mandeville from the party of Robert fitz Walter. It seems to me equally likely that it was an attempt to get Geoffrey completely in the king's power. A baron who did not meet his payments at the exchequer could be imprisoned at the king's will and the lands for which the payments were due could be seized. The basic question is—was 20,000 marks anything like a reasonable fine for what Geoffrey obtained? It was twenty-four times the normal gross revenue of the entire honor without Bristol. We could judge the reasonableness of this ratio more adequately if we knew the age of Isabella. As she married John in 1189, she could not have been much under forty in 1214. She died in 1215, but she need not have been aged at that time. While it seems clear that she was most unlikely to produce an heir, Geoffrey may have hoped to enjoy her lands for a decade or more. Still the fine was extremely large and the terms of payment onerous. I cannot believe that John expected Geoffrey to be able to meet them.

While Geoffrey was trying to find the money for his first payments, John made another move. On July 11 he informed the justiciar that Geoffrey de Say had offered a fine of 15,000 marks for the Mandeville barony.[228] Peter was to consult with Richard Marsh and William Brewer about the matter. The result was a suit in the *curia regis* where Geoffrey de Say's claim was dismissed on a technicality—he had sued for the barony as held by Earl William de Mandeville when he died in 1189 and Geoffrey de Mandeville did not possess the barony in its entirety.[229] One cannot but wonder whether John toyed for a moment with the idea of giving Geoffrey de Mandeville the honor of Gloucester and Geoffrey de Say the honor of Mandeville, collecting 35,000 marks in fines, and having two grateful barons—or two who were at his mercy because they could not pay their fines. In all this weird series of maneuvers only one thing seems certain. If John was trying to win over Geoffrey de Mandeville, he was doing it very clumsily. Both Geoffrey de Mandeville and Geoffrey de Say remained stanch adherents of the baronial party.

[228] *Ibid.*, p. 166.   [229] *Curia regis rolls*, VII, 110-111.

Chapter VIII

MAGNA CARTA

ON OCTOBER 13, 1214, a defeated and sadly disappointed king landed at Dartmouth.[1] The campaign to which he had devoted years of preparation and enormous sums of money and which he had hoped would make him the undisputed master of western Europe had been a complete fiasco. His nephew Otto now had little chance of maintaining his position against Frederick of Hohenstaufen. The two most powerful of John's French allies, the counts of Flanders and Boulogne, and his bastard brother Earl William of Salisbury were prisoners of King Philip. John had strengthened his position in Poitou, but he well knew how temporary any gain was likely to be in that turbulent region. He had also captured a cousin of King Philip—Robert, eldest son and heir of Robert II, count of Dreux. Even if one accepts John's argument that the cousin of a king was a far more important capture than the illegitimate son of a king, his total accomplishment remains far from impressive.[2] Philip Augustus had decisively won his life-long contest with the Plantagenets.

John found his baronial foes bolder if not more numerous than before his departure for Poitou. There had been opposition to the collection of the scutage. The close rolls show that various sheriffs had distrained Eustace de Vesci, Roger de Montbegon, and Robert de Gresley, three of the northern barons.[3] Sometime during the early autumn either John or Peter des Roches had complained to the pope that Eustace de Vesci was defying the king's officers.[4] Mr. Mitchell has pointed out that no scutage was paid in Lancashire, Essex, and Hertfordshire and very little in Norfolk and Suffolk. No account was rendered at Michaelmas 1214 for the scutage due from Yorkshire. While some of the dissident lords such as Geoffrey de Mandeville and Gilbert de Ghent had paid part of their scutage, the greater number seem to have refused.[5]

[1] "Electio Hugonis," p. 92.
[2] *Rot. pat.*, p. 140.
[3] *Rot. claus.*, I, 213.
[4] Rymer, *Foedera*, I, 126.
[5] Mitchell, *Studies in taxation*, pp. 112-113 and note 84.

Shortly after the king's arrival in England, his enemies met at the abbey of Bury St. Edmunds. Under the guise of a pious pilgrimage they discussed their grievances. The charter of liberties of Henry I was accepted as a statement of the rights of the king's vassals. The barons assembled in the church and swore that if the king failed to grant them their just claims they would defy him and wage war against him.[6]

Obviously the composition of the baronial party that was to oblige John to issue Magna Carta is of major interest, but unfortunately our chief sources of information on this subject do not inspire one with unbounded confidence. The *Histoire des ducs de Normandie* gives us a brief list of barons who attended the meeting at St. Edmunds.[7] While this chronicle is in general a reliable one, the meeting took place at a time when the chronicler was not in England, and he probably had no direct knowledge of who was there. At any rate the list is too short to be of great value. Then Roger of Wendover supplies a much longer roll of those who gathered at Stamford in the following spring.[8] Wendover's roll includes forty-two names and gives us our fullest picture of the baronial party. But one hesitates to take Wendover's lists too seriously. A few pages further on he makes a statement so glaringly wrong that one is forced to question his knowledge of the subject. He says that after the barons had occupied London, they sent threatening letters to all who had not joined them and gives twenty-two names as a partial list of those to whom the letters were addressed. He then states that the majority of these men promptly joined the barons.[9] Now seventeen of these men certainly did not join the barons before the granting of Magna Carta, and eleven of these stood by John throughout the civil war. This seems to justify a certain lack of confidence in Wendover's lists. Finally Matthew Paris gives the names of the twenty-five barons chosen to enforce Magna Carta.[10] Paris was not a contemporary,

---

[6] Wendover, II, 111-112; Coventry, II, 217-218; *Histoire des ducs de Normandie*, pp. 145-146.
[7] *Ibid.*, p. 145.
[8] Wendover, II, 114-115.
[9] *Ibid.*, p. 117.
[10] Matthew Paris, *Chronica maiora*, II, 604-605.

and we have no knowledge of where he got his list. While the fact that thirteen of his names can be confirmed from a documentary source suggests that his list is on the whole correct, it should not be accepted as above criticism.

The close and patent rolls supply us with the names of fifteen men of importance who were in rebellion before the issuance of Magna Carta. In the middle of May John ordered the seizure of lands belonging to Geoffrey de Mandeville, earl of Gloucester, William de Mandeville, his brother, Robert fitz Walter, Robert de Vere, earl of Oxford, Henry de Bohun, earl of Hereford, Giles de Briouse, bishop of Hereford, William de Huntingfield, Henry de Braybrook, and Simon de Pattishall.[11] Various documents show clearly that Roger de Cressi, William de Montaigu, William Malet, and Robert fitz Paien were in arms as rebels.[12] A letter addressed to Roger Bigod, earl of Norfolk, in January seems to indicate that he was in the baronial group.[13] While it seems clear that Saher de Quency, earl of Winchester, was not in revolt when the above letter was addressed to Earl Roger, he had joined the barons by May 25.[14]

Thus we have the names of fifteen rebels supplied by the patent and close rolls, twenty-five by Matthew Paris, and forty-two by Roger of Wendover. Hence our knowledge of the secondary leaders of the opposition comes from the weakest source. On the whole it seems likely that this particular list of Wendover's is essentially accurate and can be accepted as a general picture of the baronial party. But the mere presence of a man's name on Wendover's roll should not be taken as conclusive evidence that he was a rebel at the time of the meeting at Stamford. It seems highly probable, for instance, that Wendover is mistaken in placing John de Lacy, constable of Chester, and his cousin John fitz Robert in this assembly. John de Lacy was clearly high in the royal favor on March 5 when all his extensive debts to the crown were forgiven.[15] The king also regarded him as loyal as late as May 31.[16] While John de Lacy was to show throughout the civil war a remarkable in-

---

[11] *Rot. claus.*, I, 200, 213.
[12] *Rot. pat.*, pp. 135, 138, 141.
[13] *Ibid.*, p. 126.
[14] *Ibid.*, p. 138.
[15] *Ibid.*, p. 129.
[16] *Ibid.*, pp. 134-142.

ability to make up his mind as to which side he wanted to support, it seems unlikely that he was at Stamford in mid-April. John fitz Robert was sheriff of Norfolk and Suffolk at the time the charter was granted. While the shires seem to have been in the actual control of John's half-brother, Roger de Cressi, one of the king's bitterest foes, John retained the custody of Norwich castle and his master's confidence.[17] When on May 15 the king ordered the bailiffs of Hubert de Burgh to seize the son of Roger de Cressi, he directed them to deliver their prisoner to John fitz Robert.[18] It seems most unlikely that John fitz Robert was at Stamford.

Using the names supplied by the close and patent rolls, Roger of Wendover, and Matthew Paris I have drawn up two lists to serve as bases for a discussion of the baronial party prior to the granting of Magna Carta. The first of these lists contains forty-five names and includes all those who by any stretch of the imagination could be described as barons. The second list of twenty-six includes those who seem to have been leaders of the party. As the chief purpose of the second list was to study the family connections of the rebel chiefs, the sons and younger brothers of rebellious lords were excluded. The following general remarks will be based on these lists.

Let us first glance at the geographical distribution of the leaders of the revolt. The contemporary chronicles emphasize the importance of the "northerners" and they were indeed a significant group. Twelve of the forty-five had the major portion of their lands in Yorkshire, Northumberland, Lancashire, and Cumberland. While this group could not boast of an English earl, it included the count of Aumale, two great barons, John de Lacy and William de Mowbray, and the king's bitter foe Eustace de Vesci. The barons of secondary rank were represented by Peter de Bruce, Richard de Percy, Robert de Ros, and Nicholas de Stutville. If one considers Lincolnshire a northern shire, as the contemporary writers probably did, six more names are added. One of these was the great lord Gilbert de Ghent whose claim to the title of earl of

---

[17] H. G. Richardson, "The morrow of the great charter," *Bulletin of the John Rylands Library*, XXVIII (1944), 441-442; *Rot. pat.*, pp. 136, 141.
[18] *Ibid.*, p. 141.

Lincoln was to be recognized by Louis of France. But this Lincolnshire group is less distinct than that in the far north. While William de Albini had extensive lands in Lincolnshire, his castle of Belvoir and much of his property was in Leicestershire. William de Huntingfield and Oliver de Vaux probably had their possessions about equally divided between Lincolnshire and East Anglia. Finally John fitz Robert was geographically a link between the northerners and the rebels of East Anglia and Essex. While his castles and baronies lay in Northumberland, he had important possessions in the east. Accepting Lincolnshire as a northern shire and including the borderline cases the northerners numbered twenty of the forty-five.

The next most important group consisted of twelve men whose lands lay in the easternmost shires—Norfolk, Suffolk, Essex, Middlesex, and Kent. This group included in addition to the elected leader of the party, Robert fitz Walter, Roger Bigod, earl of Norfolk, Richard de Clare, earl of Hertford, Geoffrey de Mandeville who styled himself earl of Gloucester and Essex, and Robert de Vere, earl of Oxford. While the titles of the last two lords suggest possessions outside this region, it seems unlikely that Geoffrey de Mandeville ever obtained effective possession of the honor of Gloucester, and Robert de Vere's lands lay almost entirely in Essex and Cambridgeshire. Below these great lords were two secondary barons, Geoffrey de Say and Richard de Montfichet.

A third somewhat less clearly defined group had its seat in the west of England—Shropshire, Herefordshire, Gloucestershire, and Somersetshire. Its most important members were Henry de Bohun, earl of Hereford, Giles de Briouse, bishop of Hereford, and the younger William Marshal. It included King John's old enemy Fulk fitz Warin, a cadet of the great house of Fitz Alan, Robert de Berkeley, William Malet, William de Montaigu, and Robert fitz Paien. Maurice de Ghent's lands were about equally divided between Gloucestershire and Somersetshire and Yorkshire. In all, this western group numbered ten.

Outside of these three groups there were only two men of any importance—Saher de Quency, earl of Winchester, and William de Beauchamp. Saher's ancestral possessions were insignificant and lay in Northamptonshire and Cambridge. He owed his power to his possession of half of the great honor of Leicester. William de Beauchamp's large barony was almost entirely in Bedfordshire.

While the location of the lands and castles of the rebellious barons was important from a military point of view, it seems unlikely that it can cast much light on the forces that created the baronial party. I can see no reason connected with geography that would make the lords of Essex and East Anglia more rebellious than those of Nottingham and Derbyshire. It looks as if the dominant factor was the attitude of the great barons. In Essex, East Anglia, Lincolnshire, Yorkshire, Lancashire, and Northumberland the most powerful barons were, with some few exceptions, the king's foes. In these regions there was a natural tendency for the lesser lords to join the baronial party. This was intensified with the beginning of actual hostilities as it then became actually dangerous to differ with one's more powerful neighbors. There were few rebels in the shires where the great barons stayed loyal. Thus the great feudal power of Ranulf of Chester, William de Ferrers, and Earl Henry of Warwick discouraged rebellion in Staffordshire, Nottinghamshire, Derbyshire, Warwickshire, and Leicestershire. The same was true of the earls of Arundel and Warren in Sussex and Surrey and Earl William of Salisbury in Wiltshire. Cornwall and Devon were kept in order by Earl William de Redvers, Henry fitz Count, Henry de Pomeroy, Robert de Cardinan, and Robert de Courtenay. In only one region does it seem probable that true geographic factors played a part in drawing the line between the king's friends and foes. As the Welsh were the king's enemies, the Marcher lords were strongly inclined to the royal party.

A number of scholars have suggested the possibility that ties of blood led many men into the baronial party. There is ample evidence that the family played an important part in thirteenth-century politics, but we know little of how family was defined in the minds of the men of the time. Did a man feel that he had family obligations toward his second cousin? The fact that landed property descended by inheritance was enough to make the barons of England expert genealogists. The most obscure relationships seem to have been well known from this practical point of view. An examination of the list of rebellious barons indicates that fairly distant blood relationship may have played a part in forming the baronial party. The list of rebel barons contains the names of thirteen descendants of the first Richard fitz Gilbert de Clare—all except his son Gilbert second cousins of Earl Richard de Clare. If, as seems likely, William de Mowbray's mother was a Clare, the roll of the clan comes to fourteen.[19] Six of these were descendants of the marriage between Aubrey de Vere, the chamberlain, and Adeliza de Clare. With the exception of John de Monmouth and William de Percy who was a minor every descendant of Richard fitz Gilbert who was of baronial rank was among the enemies of King John in 1215. This correlation between the blood of the house of Clare and opposition to John seems too close to be mere coincidence.[20]

While the importance of distant blood relationship may be open to some doubt, the closer ones, especially those of the family in the narrow sense, were clearly taken extremely seriously in the thirteenth century. When Roger de Lacy, constable of Chester, was taken in Chateau Gaillard, his uncle, Robert fitz Roger, was given the task of raising his ransom and became his pledge for a loan of £1,000 obtained from King John.[21] After Robert fitz Walter's capture in Vaudreuil, his first cousin, William de Albini, was authorized to mortgage Robert's lands to obtain money for his ransom.[22] When William de Briouse was in trouble with John, it was his nephew Earl William de Ferrers who tried to mediate between him and the king.[23] Perhaps the best evidence for the closeness of the relationship between uncle and nephew is the fact

---

[19] A monastic writer calls her daughter of Edmond, earl of Clare. Dugdale, *Monasticon*, VI, 320. No such person had ever existed. Banstead, Surrey, once a Clare manor, was part of her marriage portion. *Curia regis rolls*, V, 205.
[20] For the basic genealogy of the house of Clare see Round, *Feudal England*, p. 472. For that of Vere see his *Geoffrey de Mandeville*, p. 392.
[21] *Rot. liberate*, p. 103.
[22] *Rot. pat.*, p. 37.
[23] Rymer, *Foedera*, I, 107-108.

that a nephew was frequently accepted as a hostage for his uncle. Naturally the ties between brothers and half-brothers were still more binding. Moreover the men of the time were very generous in according the term brother. Thus one finds King John calling Geoffrey de Buckland the brother of Geoffrey fitz Peter.[24] Actually Geoffrey de Buckland was the brother of Geoffrey fitz Peter's brother-in-law. There is no need to labor the point further. Mediæval literature abounds in examples of the importance placed on kinship.

We have seen that William de Albini of Belvoir was the first cousin of Robert fitz Walter. He had the same relationship to Roger Bigod, earl of Norfolk, and to Gilbert de Ghent. It is possible that Saher de Quency was his nephew. Robert de Vere, earl of Oxford, Roger Bigod, earl of Norfolk, Simon, father of William de Beauchamp of Bedford, Robert fitz Roger, father of John fitz Robert, and Alice, grandmother of John de Lacy, had all been first cousins. Geoffrey de Say had married Earl Robert's sister. Peter de Bruce and William de Fortibus, count of Aumale, were first cousins, as were Geoffrey de Say and Earl Geoffrey de Mandeville, William de Mowbray and Gilbert de Ghent, Richard de Montfichet and Robert fitz Walter, and Eustace de Vesci and John de Lacy. In the relationship of uncle and nephew stood Gilbert de Ghent and Maurice de Ghent, William de Beauchamp and William de Lanvalay, and William de Albini and Robert de Ros. William de Lanvalay had married Robert fitz Walter's niece. Young William Marshal was married to the half-sister of the count of Aumale and two of his sisters were married to Hugh Bigod and Gilbert de Clare. The count of Aumale's wife was the sister of Richard de Montfichet. Eustace de Vesci and Robert de Ros had both married illegitimate daughters of King William of Scotland. Earl Henry de Bohun's wife was the sister of Geoffrey and William de Mandeville who were in turn sons-in-laws of Robert fitz Walter. Nicholas de Stutville was the stepfather of Gilbert de Ghent. John fitz Robert and Roger de Cressi were half-brothers.[25] In short it is clear that blood relationship may well have played an important part in forming the baronial party.

[24] *Rot. claus.*, I, 139.
[25] This is not quite certain. They may have been stepbrothers

It is important to remember that our knowledge of the genealogy of the English baronage is extremely limited. While connections in the male line are usually fairly obvious, those based on marriage are frequently obscure. I suspect that William de Mowbray's mother was a Clare, probably a sister of Earl Richard, but I can find no conclusive proof of this relationship. No one knows who was the wife of Roger de Lacy, constable of Chester. Geoffrey fitz Peter was the most important baron in England during John's reign. Yet the identity of his second wife is shown clearly only by a pair of obscure charters hidden deep in the *Calendar of ancient deeds*.[26] There seems little doubt that if our information were fuller, we should see many more blood relationships and marriage connections among the rebellious barons.

While in mediæval society as a whole feudal ties were almost as strong as those of close relationship by blood, it is difficult to estimate their significance in forming the baronial party. With one or two possible exceptions all the forty-five baronial leaders on my list were tenants-in-chief of the crown and hence definitely owed their service primarily to King John. Yet the part played by William Marshal in the quarrel between William de Briouse and the king seems to show that mutual feudal obligations among tenants-in-chief were of some importance even when the crown was directly involved. William Marshal refused to surrender William de Briouse to the justiciar of Ireland. While the *Histoire de Guillaume le Maréchal* suggests that he would have done so on a direct royal command, if King John's official account of the affair is correct, he ignored royal letters directing him to surrender his guest. Then King John's attitude toward two of William Marshal's knights, John de Erley and Henry fitz Gerold, who were tenants-in-chief of the crown when they remained in Ireland in open defiance of the king's command indicates that he himself regarded men whom he had, as he said, "loaned" to a great baron as being in a special category in respect to their obligations to him.[27] Perhaps one may say that the custom of the time allowed a tenant-in-chief of the crown to go somewhat further in supporting

[26] *Calendar of ancient deeds*, II, 91.   [27] *Rot. claus.*, I, 103, 106.

against the king a man to whom he owed feudal obligations than one to whom he had no such relationship.

It seems quite possible that among the "northerners" feudal relations played a part of some importance. As we have seen William de Mowbray had good reason to hate King John. Peter de Bruce, Nicholas de Stutville, and Eustace de Vesci were vassals of William de Mowbray.[28] Robert de Ros was an important vassal of William de Fortibus, count of Aumale, who was in turn a vassal of Earl Roger Bigod.[29] Outside the northern group feudal relationships were scattered, but may well have had some significance. While the blood relationship between Robert fitz Walter and Saher de Quency is highly speculative, there is no doubt that Saher was Robert's vassal.[30] Nicholas de Stutville held several fees of the barony of Belvoir from William de Albini.[31] Oliver de Vaux had married Petronilla, daughter and heiress of Guy de Craon, and held her barony of some twenty-two fees, but his ancestral lands consisted of a fief of thirty fees held from Earl Roger Bigod.[32] Thomas de Moulton was a vassal of the Craon barony.[33] While the bulk of William de Huntingfield's lands were held of honors in the king's hands, his castle of Frampton belonged to the Craon barony, and he was probably a distant relative of Petronilla.[34] Again the major part of the lands of Simon de Kyme were fees of the earldom of Chester, but there is some reason for thinking that he considered his closest feudal relationship to be with Gilbert de Ghent of whom he held three fees.[35] If one takes seriously Geoffrey de Mandeville's possession of the honor of Gloucester, Fulk fitz Warin and Simon de Kyme must be listed among his vassals.[36]

[28] *Red book of the exchequer*, I, 418-420; William Farrer, *Early Yorkshire charters* (Edinburgh, 1914), II, 12; *Kirkby's inquest* (The Surtees society, XLIX [1866]), pp. 24, 79-80.

[29] *Ibid.*, p. 243; *Red book of the exchequer*, I, 397.

[30] *Ibid.*, I, 349.

[31] *Pipe roll society*, XX, 99-100.

[32] Pipe roll 13 John, Public Record Office; *Red book of the exchequer*, I, 395; *Calendar of inquisitions post mortem* (Rolls series), II, no. 653.

[33] *Book of fees*, I, 193.

[34] *Ibid.*, pp. 183, 195, II, 1006; *Calendar of inquisitions post mortem*, I, 107.

[35] *Red book of the exchequer*, I, 383.   [36] *Ibid.*, II, 607, 610.

Obviously there must have existed among the barons purely personal relationships based on simple friendship, but these we can rarely learn about. There are few sources like the *Histoire de Guillaume le Maréchal*. We know that William Marshal was a close friend of Baldwin de Bethune, count of Aumale.[37] There is strong reason for believing that he cordially hated Saher de Quency.[38] But in general such personal likes and dislikes are unknown to us.

A contemporary chronicler makes a generalization about the baronial party that has to some extent been accepted by modern scholars—that it was essentially a group of young men.[39] Now we rarely have any information as to the date of a baron's birth. As a rule one can merely say when he succeeded to his inheritance and whether he was over twenty-one at the time. When what information we possess is applied to an examination of the list of forty-five rebel lords, the result does not seem to justify the generalization. It is possible to guess rather closely the ages of three young men. William Marshal the younger was about twenty-five, William de Fortibus about twenty, and Maurice de Ghent about twenty-eight.[40] There are eight others who may well have been in their twenties. While Hugh Bigod and Gilbert de Clare had not yet succeeded to their lands, their fathers had held their earldoms for thirty-eight and forty-two years respectively. Neither Hugh nor Gilbert can have been very young. Robert de Vere and Geoffrey de Say had succeeded to the family lands in 1214, but they too were middle-aged. Robert's brother, Earl Aubrey, had held the earldom for twenty years. Geoffrey de Say's father had clearly

---

[37] *Histoire de Guillaume le Maréchal*, lines 5879-5905, 6193-6236, 10130-10148.

[38] In speaking of William's foes at young Henry's court the author of the *Histoire* says he dares not name all for fear of men of their line. Saher was one of the few members of the household who was important later. Then when William reproached Philip Augustus for dealing with traitors, he clearly meant Saher and Robert fitz Walter. *Ibid.*, lines 5141-5162, 12688-12700.

[39] Coventry, II, 220; Powicke, *Stephen Langton*, pp. 211-212.

[40] William Marshal's parents were married in 1189 and those of William de Fortibus in 1195. Maurice de Ghent came of age in 1208. *Rot. oblatis*, p. 427.

lived to a ripe age—his elder brother had died in 1177 and his two cousins, Earl Geoffrey and Earl William de Mandeville, in 1166 and 1189 respectively. Gilbert de Ghent was about thirty-five. Henry de Bohun was forty, Robert de Ros forty-three, and Eustace de Vesci forty-four.[41] Robert de Berkeley, Peter de Bruce, William Malet, Simon de Kyme, Roger de Montbegon, William de Mowbray, and Richard de Percy, were all at least forty as they had held their fiefs for twenty to twenty-five years. Robert fitz Walter and Saher de Quency were over sixty-five.[42] The earls of Norfolk and Hertford may well have been older. William de Albini had been holding his barony of Belvoir for forty-eight years. On the whole it seems impossible to say that youth was a distinguishing mark of the baronial party. The chronicler who made the comment was clearly thinking of a few well-known cases. The presence of William Marshal the younger in the rebel ranks while his father was a stanch supporter of John must have attracted wide attention. In the autumn of 1215 young William de Lancaster served in the rebel garrison of Rochester and embarrassed his father Gilbert fitz Renfrew.

Another extremely interesting question is the size of the baronial party in relation to the whole English baronage. In an earlier chapter I used a list of one hundred ninety-seven English baronies as representing essentially all that existed. The holders of thirty-nine of these baronies are known to have been among the rebels prior to the issuing of Magna Carta. Then I used another list of the twenty-eight most powerful barons of England in 1199. By 1215 the major part of the honor of Richmond and one-half the honor of Leicester were in the king's hand. The original twenty-eight had been reduced to twenty-seven. Thirteen of these were rebels in 1215. The thirteen rebels held approximately 1,475 knights' fees against the 1,580 of those who were not in revolt. Unfortunately the figures for the baronage as a whole are not very

---

[41] *Rotuli de dominibus et pueris et puellis* (ed. J. H. Round, Pipe roll society, xxxv), pp. 1, 9, 84.

[42] Saher was a member of Henry the young king's mesne in 1173. Benedict of Peterborough, I, 45-47. Robert fitz Walter was at a tournament in France in 1180. *Histoire de Guillaume le Maréchal,* lines 4615-4617.

reliable. While only thirty-nine baronies are known to have been in the hands of rebels, one can only establish the loyalty of about as many others. In short the position of the majority of the baronage in this period before the issuing of Magna Carta is unknown. One might well argue that the true proportion among the barons as a whole probably followed that found among the great lords and that the baronage was essentially equally divided between the two parties. But at least the figures seem sufficient to destroy the old notion of a united baronage rising against King John.

Actually I suspect the true answer is more complicated. I am inclined to believe that there was a comparatively small group of rebels—say some forty-five men holding the thirty-nine baronies. Then there was another group, probably even smaller, who were ready to stand by John in arms. The great mass of the English baronage stayed out of the affair altogether. If one can judge by later events, most of the neutrals sympathized with the barons. By the time of John's death the holders of ninety-seven baronies were in rebellion as against the holders of thirty-six who remained loyal. Only eight of the twenty-seven great barons were still on John's side when he died. But even these figures are deceiving because they deal with technical allegiance. The earls of Arundel, Warren, Warwick, and Devon were loyal to John at the time of Magna Carta and remained so when the civil war broke out in the autumn of 1215, but they seem to have done nothing but protect their own estates. In 1216 the earls of Arundel and Warren transferred their allegiance to Louis of France and apparently ignored him as completely as they had John. Clearly all four of these earls were primarily interested in being left alone in their vast fiefs and followed whatever policy seemed best suited to attain that end. Actually it was the earl of Pembroke who sat on the fence most effectively. He himself was a stanch supporter of John while his eldest son and heir was a prominent rebel. The house of Marshal was safe whatever happened. Once the eventual defeat of the rebels was certain, the younger William Marshal rejoined the loyal camp in time to profit handsomely at the expense of some of his fellow rebels who had moved more slowly.

It is impossible to say much about the members of the rebellious party who were not of baronial rank. Our only source of information about the lesser foes of King John is the writs by which they were reinstated in their lands when they made their peace with the royal government. If all such writs were entered on the close roll, we have a complete list of all free-holders who participated in the revolt. As only one or two of the rebels of baronial status are missing from this list, it seems safe to assume that it is reasonably complete. It contains about 1,380 names. Thirty-five per cent of the barons who eventually joined the rebels were in revolt before the granting of Magna Carta. If this same ratio is applied to the free-holders as a whole, we have 480 in rebellion in this period. The geographical concentration of the rebels is more marked when all the free-holders are taken into account than when the barons alone are considered. A sample of 1,173 writs issued to individual sheriffs shows 20 per cent addressed to the north—Lincolnshire, Yorkshire, Lancashire, Northumberland, Cumberland, and Westmoreland—and 40 per cent to the east—Norfolk, Suffolk, Essex, Hertfordshire, Cambridgeshire and Kent. By adding the writs addressed to the sheriffs of Northamptonshire, Buckinghamshire, Bedfordshire, and Oxfordshire, 73 per cent of the total is accounted for. The same general result is obtained by examining a list of 724 rebels with lands in only one shire. The counties classified above as northern yield 27 per cent of the names and those considered as eastern 33 per cent. In contrast the counties of Shropshire, Staffordshire, Herefordshire, Gloucestershire, Cornwall, Devon, Dorsetshire, and Somersetshire furnish but 9 per cent of the names.

While I am convinced that the 1,380 free-holders who took part in the revolt against John were a very small part of the men of that status in England, I can produce no good evidence to prove my point. We have no way of determining the number of free-holders in the country. The most pertinent figure is that of existing knights' fees—some 6,500. But many of the men in question held in demesne far less than a knight's fee and some held more. Thus although I feel sure that the revolt was largely baronial and that only a small proportion of the lesser free-tenants took part, my conclusion must remain based largely on speculation.

It would be extremely interesting to know how many of the minor rebels were vassals who had followed their lords. In theory an English mesne tenant was under no obligation to follow his lord in rebellion—in fact his first duty was fidelity to the crown. At the same time it seems clear that a vassal who followed his lord into revolt was considered to have committed a less serious offense than a man who rebelled without such a feudal connection.[43] Unfortunately it is impossible to determine the feudal affiliations of the vast majority of the lesser rebels. The fact that the percentage of rebel barons from the various shires was roughly the same as that of the free-holders as a whole might indicate that vassals tended to follow their lords. But it may also mean simply that it was unwise to remain loyal to the crown in a region where the rebels were dominant.

While the barons who had sworn alliance at St. Edmunds postponed until January the presentation of their demands to the king and apparently hoped to keep their action a secret in the interval, it seems clear that John soon learned of the conspiracy. He despatched one of his favorite clerks, Walter Mauclerk, to Rome to seek the pope's support and to combat the efforts of any baronial emissaries who might journey there.[44] He also summoned to England a force of Poitevins under the command of the redoubtable Savaric de Mauleon.[45] This was an extremely shrewd move. King John was appealing to the pope against the barons and in such circumstances wanted to have his own conduct beyond reproach. To have brought in additional mercenary captains would have weakened his position before the papacy and aggravated the discontent of his vassals. Savaric de Mauleon was an experienced soldier, a skilful if not too scrupulous politician, a poet of considerable distinction, and one of the great nobles of Poitou. The barons of England might dislike him as a foreigner, but he was their fellow vassal and social and political peer.

[43] See Painter, *Feudal barony*, pp. 128-129.
[44] Rymer, *Foedera*, I, 120.
[45] *Rot. claus.*, I, 185, 187.

During the second week of January 1215 a group of barons met John in London. They demanded that he carry out the oath he had taken when he was absolved. He was to abolish his own innovations and those made by his father and brother and restore the customs that had existed under Henry I—or more properly the customs that Henry I had so blithely promised to observe in his charter of liberties. The chroniclers are too vague to permit one to make out just what the barons wanted John to do. They demanded that he issue a charter of liberties, but whether this meant simply a re-issue of the charter of Henry I or a more extensive document cannot be determined. If the barons presented to John some definite schedule like the Articles of the Barons, the chroniclers give no indication of it. John told the barons that what they asked was very grave and postponed giving his answer until Easter-tide. The archbishop of Canterbury, the bishop of Ely, and William Marshal swore that the king would then give them satisfaction.[46] The bishops of London, Winchester, Ely, Hereford, Bath, and Lincoln, the bishops elect of Coventry and Chichester, the earls of Surrey, Pembroke, Winchester, and Arundel, and Robert de Ros, Peter fitz Herbert, and William de Albini guaranteed the baronial delegation a safe journey home.[47]

On February 10 John learned that Savaric de Mauleon had landed in Ireland.[48] That same day saw royal agents sent into many of the shires " to explain our business." [49] Unfortunately we do not know what the business was. Perhaps their mission was to spread the royal version of John's dispute with his barons, but it is just as likely that their task was to prepare the king's fortresses for defense in case of civil war. About this same time King John ordered the seneschals of Gascony and Poitou to send him more mercenary troops. Then on March 4 the king made a truly masterly move—he assumed the cross of a crusader.[50] While it is difficult to define the privileges of a crusader in precise terms, in

[46] Wendover, II, 113-114; Coventry, II, 218; Rymer, *Foedera,* I, 120.
[47] *Rot. pat.,* p. 126.
[48] *Rot. claus.,* I, 187.
[49] *Rot. pat.,* p. 128.
[50] *Annals of Tewkesbury,* p. 61; *Annals of Osney,* p. 58.

general he was entitled to be protected by the papacy and secured in the possession of all that he had when he took the vow until after his return from the Crusade. Barons who demanded concessions from a crusader monarch were in a very dubious position. If they rose in revolt, they were definitely defying the papacy. There seems no reason whatever for believing that John had the slightest intention of journeying to the Holy Land. His assumption of the cross was simply a clever maneuver.

Apparently King John's next step was to have William Marshal and Earl William de Warren call the attention of the barons to the fact that he was a crusader as well as a vassal of the pope. He then asked Stephen Langton to compel the barons to perform the service they owed—presumably the payment of the scutage of Poitou. Stephen, according to John's letter to the pope, agreed to act if the king would send home his foreign troops.[51] On March 13 John informed his most recent Poitevin auxiliaries that the business for which he had needed them was finished and they were to go home.[52] There is, however, no evidence that Langton did anything to discourage the barons.

On April 13 there was a fruitless conference at Oxford between the king and at least some of his disaffected barons.[53] This may well have been the occasion when the barons hoped to receive the "satisfaction" promised them in London in January. Their failure to receive what they wanted led them to their first overt act of rebellion—they assembled in arms at Stamford.[54] John then sent Stephen Langton and William Marshal to ask the barons to say exactly what reforms they wanted. The two emissaries found the barons at Brackley and received a schedule of demands that they bore to the king. After hearing the barons' requests John indignantly refused to grant them.[55]

When Stephen Langton and William Marshal informed the barons that their demands had been rejected, the rebellious lords

---

[51] Rymer, *Foedera*, I, 129.
[52] *Rot. pat.*, p. 130.
[53] "Electio Hugonis," p. 124.
[54] Wendover, II, 114-115; Coventry, II, 219.
[55] Wendover, II, 115.

formally defied the king and chose Robert fitz Walter as their leader under the pretentious and essentially irrelevant title of Marshal of the host of God and Holy Church.[56] They then marched to Northampton and laid siege to its castle, one of the great royal fortresses of England. As they had no siege engines, they cannot have hoped to take the castle if it was vigorously defended, but they probably expected it to surrender.[57] While it is not certain that Henry de Braybrook, sheriff of Northamptonshire, was actually in the baronial host, it is clear that he was one of those who sympathized with the rebels.[58] Early in April John had learned that Henry was unreliable and had sent Richard Marsh to Northampton with power to make what dispositions seemed best for the safety for the castle.[59] As a result Geoffrey de Martini, a mercenary captain, was made constable of the castle. But as Henry de Braybrook was still sheriff and probably at least nominally Geoffrey's superior, the barons may well have hoped that he would arrange the surrender of the castle.[60] Fortunately Geoffrey made an energetic defense and after a futile siege of two weeks the barons moved on in search of easier conquests. They did not have to look very far. Bedford castle was a royal fortress, but William de Beauchamp was its hereditary constable. As soon as his fellow rebels appeared, he admitted them to the castle.[61] Bedford, however, was not a satisfactory substitute for Northampton. It was a second-grade fortress and far from a satisfactory refuge if the king moved against his foes with a large force.

At first glance King John's policy during the early months of 1215 seems hopelessly feeble and vacillating. At one moment he would be negotiating with his barons—at the next sending for foreign troops. Then he would reopen negotiations and send the troops home. At times he would summon his loyal barons to a rendezvous and then make no use of them. Actually, however, when one considers John's character and the general political and

---

[56] *Ibid.*, p. 116.
[57] *Ibid.* Coventry, II, 219; *Histoire des ducs de Normandie*, p. 147; *Annals of Dunstaple*, p. 43.
[58] *Rot. claus.*, I, 200; *Rot. pat.*, p. 136.
[59] *Ibid.*, p. 131.
[60] *Rot. claus.*, I, 193, 195.
[61] Wendover, II, 116.

military situation, his policy becomes comprehensible and reasonable even if far from admirable. King John had one definite purpose—the preservation at its fullest extent of the authority of the royal government. He was determined not to weaken in any way the power of the English crown. He had no intention of making any permanent concession to the demands of his barons. John never had any scruples as to the means he used to attain his ends, and he rather preferred devious to direct methods. If one accepts these assumptions about John's intentions and character, his policy fits well into the circumstances he faced.

The chief feature of the political situation in England in 1215 was the fact that the disaffected barons under the guidance of Stephen Langton had adopted a program that appealed to the feudal class as a whole. The leaders of the baronial party were the king's personal enemies. Their chief object, I believe, was to avenge old injuries real or fancied and to secure their private rights—lands, castles, and privileges that they felt John or his predecessors had deprived them of. But they had sufficient good sense and political acumen to accept Langton's broader ideas. First this new program had been little more than vague remarks about the charter of Henry I and the laws of King Edward. Then, probably in October 1213, they formulated the demands mentioned in the unknown charter. By April 27, 1215 they had a more elaborate list of what one can call constitutional demands. This put them in a strong political position. Many barons who had little interest in their private wrongs would sympathize with their general program. While I am by no means as sure as I once was that William Marshal actually had a hand in putting Magna Carta in its final form, I feel sure that he was in favor of its provisions. It was difficult for any feudal personage not to approve of a program that would strengthen him and his fellows against the crown.

King John on his side had few devoted servants on whom he could rely absolutely and only one of them could be classed as a great baron. Peter des Roches as bishop of Winchester was the lord of some eighty knights' fees and four strong castles. Peter de Maulay by his marriage to the daughter of Robert de Turnham was a baron of secondary rank as was John's bastard son, Richard, lord of Chilham. William Brewer, as we have seen in an earlier chapter, had built up a moderate sized barony. Robert de Vieuxpont was a powerful figure on the Scots border. But most of John's creatures were men of no feudal position. Thomas de Eardington, Philip de Ulecotes, Geoffrey de Neville, and Brian de Lisle were able administrators and captains, but the king had to supply the resources with which they served him. The same was true of the foreign captains—Fawkes de Bréauté, Philip Marc, Engelard de Cigogné and their lesser colleagues. In short the men whom John could rely on to follow him without question whatever he might do were few in number and comparatively unimportant in the feudal world.

There was a small group of Englishmen who held a dominant position in the realm. Stephen Langton's high reputation for ability and integrity, the prestige and spiritual power conferred on him by his exalted office, and the financial and military resources of the great archepiscopal barony made him the chief of these men. But close behind him came the earl of Pembroke. William Marshal's reputation for integrity, for the chivalric virtue of loyalty, was fully as high as that held by Stephen Langton. He had also the enormous prestige that was conferred by wide fame for knightly prowess. If one takes into account his fiefs in England, Wales, and Ireland, he held well over two hundred knights' fees, and his money incomes was probably far in excess of that enjoyed by any other English magnate. Moreover he was surrounded by a devoted group of friends and clients and was the leader of a powerful baronial group. As the greatest lord of South Wales and its marches and a well-known friend of the once great house of Briouse, he was the natural leader of the barons of that region. Two of King John's ablest and most trusted captains, John Marshal and Thomas de Sanford, were almost completely under the great earl's influence. In short William Marshal had everything that contributed to high position in mediæval society—advanced age, fame as a knight, and vast resources in men and money. Somewhat ahead of William Marshal in feudal power but well behind him in personal prestige was Earl Ranulf of Chester. The absolute master of his palatine shire of Cheshire and the greatest land-holder in Yorkshire and Lincolnshire Earl Ranulf was an immensely powerful baron. With his brother-in-law and close ally Earl William de Ferrers he dominated the counties of Staffordshire, Nottinghamshire, and Derbyshire. With these three men must be placed the earls of Arundel and Surrey. We know little of their personal qualities, but both had immense resources in men, money, and castles.

None of these men had any reason to love King John. Stephen Langton, William Marshal, and Ranulf of Chester had all suffered from his hostility. The king had seduced the sister of Earl William de Warren—who was incidentally his first cousin. If these great magnates stayed faithful to John, it would be because they felt that their duty or their interest demanded such a course. In the cases of Stephen Langton and William Marshal there seems to be little doubt that duty was the predominant consideration. Hence it was extremely important for John to keep his position technically correct according to generally accepted feudal custom. He dared not place himself manifestly in the wrong lest he lose his few powerful supporters. As the mass of lesser barons who sympathized with the program advanced by the rebels but hesitated to join a revolt would almost certainly follow the lead of these great lords, the king's whole position, his possession of the crown, depended on keeping their allegiance.

King John had one other mighty resource—the support of his overlord the pope. But here too he had to move with great care. Stephen Langton, the pope's friend and officer, was a firm advocate if not the creator of the baronial program. While Langton's concept of a realm governed by accepted law was of no great interest to Innocent III, and he was inclined to favor the man who had made him suzerain of England, the pope could not and would not support injustice against justice. He was inclined to listen to the arguments of John's agents rather than to those of the barons, but the arguments had to be reasonably good. Hence this was another reason why John's position had to be technically correct. The pope would aid him, but he had to appear to be worthy of aid.

A few days before he examined the schedule of baronial demands John sent his justiciar, Peter des Roches, to see to the state of affairs in the north. Letters were despatched to the king's chief agents in the region, Gilbert fitz Renfrew, John de Lacy, Robert de Vieuxpont, Geoffrey de Neville, Philip de Ulecotes, and Brian de Lisle, directing them to obey the bishop's orders.[62] At about the same time the lords of the southern marches of Wales were summoned to muster at Gloucester and then ordered to advance to Cirencester.[63] Clearly John wanted troops available if he felt it desirable to use them. The levies of the Marcher lords combined with the Poitevins of Savaric de Mauleon who were in the same region probably made a fairly formidable force. While we do not know the purpose of Bishop Peter's northern excursion, it seems likely that John wanted the lands of the northern rebels attacked if he decided to resort to force. It would appear that in the last days of April the king was planning to march against the baronial muster if his enemies committed an overt act. But when the barons laid siege to Northampton castle and thus placed themselves in open revolt, John did nothing very decisive. On May 5 the earls of Surrey, Salisbury, and Pembroke were sent out to perambulate the countryside with bodies of troops, probably to secure the royal castles near Northampton, but a few days later John was once again negotiating with his foes.[64]

Apparently a group of rebel barons that included Geoffrey de Mandeville and Giles de Briouse met John at Reading on May 10, and the king made a peace offer. He issued letters patent stating that he had promised the rebel lords that he would not arrest them or their men or seize their lands otherwise than by the law of the realm or the judgment of their peers until *"consideracio facta fuit"* by four men chosen by each party. The decisions of the four arbitrators would be subject to review by the pope. The bishops of London, Worcester, Coventry, and Rochester and Earl William de Warren would guarantee John's good faith.[65] Thus the king agreed not to use force against the rebels until some question had been considered by arbitrators and the decision reviewed by the pope. While this document does not state what was to be considered, a letter sent by John to Innocent III indicates that it was

---

[62] *Rot. pat.*, p. 134.
[63] *Ibid.*; *Rot. claus.*, I, 197.
[64] *Rot. pat.*, p. 135.
[65] *Ibid.*, p. 141.

the whole schedule of baronial demands.⁶⁶ Although no reference is made to any conditions that had to be accepted by the barons if this offer was to take effect, it must have been assumed that they would cease overt acts of revolt. Separate letters issued the same day promised Geoffrey de Mandeville and Giles de Briouse the judgment of the king's court in regard to the heavy fines that placed them in debt to the crown.⁶⁷ Once more John had strengthened his moral position—he had offered to submit to arbitration. Actually he was probably gambling on the advantages of delay and on his ability to sway the mind of Innocent III.

This attempt to make peace had no result. Either the barons rejected the offer or simply ignored it by continuing their siege of Northampton castle. On May 11 the king continued his military preparations. Fawkes de Bréauté and William de Harcourt were sent out to see to the defenses of the royal castles, and Winchester castle was turned over to Savaric de Mauleon to house his Poitevin troops.⁶⁸ Then on May 12 John took a decisive step. He ordered the sheriffs of England to seize the lands of the rebels and sell their chattels for the king's use.⁶⁹ Two days later special orders directed the seizure of the lands of Robert fitz Walter, Robert de Vere, Henry de Bohun, Giles de Briouse, William de Mandeville, William de Huntingfield, Henry de Braybrook, and Simon de Pattishall.⁷⁰ On May 15 the bailiffs of Hubert de Burgh were ordered to arrest the son of Roger de Cressi, but John with a characteristic chivalrous gesture forbade them to bother Roger's wife.⁷¹

During this second week of May disturbing reports and rumors reached King John. William de Montaigu, William Malet, and Robert fitz Paien were leading a rising in the southwest. On May 13 Henry de Pomeroy and John de Erley were appointed joint sheriffs of Devonshire and sent to suppress the revolt.⁷² The knights of the county were summoned to muster whenever Henry might direct and to obey his orders.⁷³ But John was still moving

⁶⁶ Rymer, *Foedera*, I, 129.
⁶⁷ *Rot. pat.*, p. 141.
⁶⁸ *Ibid.*, p. 135.
⁶⁹ *Rot. claus.*, I, 204.
⁷⁰ *Ibid.*, p. 200.
⁷¹ *Rot. pat.*, p. 141.
⁷² *Ibid.*, p. 135.
⁷³ *Ibid.*, p. 136.

cautiously. Peter de Maulay, constable of Corfe, was ordered to release William de Montaigu in bail if he had captured him.[74] Meanwhile the main baronial army had given up the siege of Northampton castle and had been received in Bedford by William de Beauchamp. The king heard rumors that the rebels were negotiating with the citizens of London for possession of that city. On May 16 John sent Earl William of Salisbury to London to try to prevent its surrender and the next day he despatched William de Cornhill, bishop of Coventry, and Hubert de Burgh to reinforce the earl.[75] As a member of the greatest of the London merchant families who had served for years at the exchequer in Westminster William de Cornhill had great influence with the Londoners. Hubert de Burgh had just returned from Poitou— presumably with a force of mercenary troops.

It seems unlikely that any of these emissaries actually reached London for the negotiations between the barons and the citizens and come to a fruitful conclusion. On the evening of Sunday, May 17, the citizens went to church leaving their gates unguarded so that the rebels could enter without difficulty. The barons occupied the city, plundered the dwellings of the king's partisans and the Jews, and tore down the latter's houses to obtain materials for repairing the city walls. The small but determined royal garrison in the Tower refused to surrender, but the rest of the city was in the hands of the king's foes.[76] On May 20 John ordered all his followers to do what harm they could to the traitorous citizens.[77]

The capture of London by the barons vitally changed the military situation. Before May 17 John could have crushed the rebels whenever he considered it politically feasible to do so. He had refrained from attacking them not because he lacked the force but in order to satisfy the pope and the rest of the baronage of the correctness of his conduct. As long as the rebel host lay in the open country, a rapid concentration of royal garrisons would have

[74] *Ibid.,* p. 135.
[75] *Ibid.,* pp. 136, 137.
[76] Wendover, II, 116-117; *Histoire des ducs de Normandie,* p. 147; Coventry, II, 220; *Annals of Waverley,* p. 282; *Annals of Dunstaple,* p. 43.
[77] *Rot. pat.,* p. 137.

been able to destroy it. Few in number and for the most part inexperienced in warfare the rebel barons could not have withstood John's hardy mercenary troops. If the mercenaries had been supported as they almost certainly would have been by the war-hardened knights of the marcher lords, the rebels' position would have been hopeless. But once sheltered behind the walls of London in alliance with its citizens the barons could defy a large army for a considerable time. Clearly John had waited too long. When the barons definitely put themselves in the wrong by besieging Northampton castle, the king should have massed his available forces and crushed them. It is, however, easy to explain John's delay. His Flemish auxiliaries, by far the best of his mercenary troops, arrived in England just before the fall of London.[78] With them on hand John could have destroyed the rebel army in the open field without endangering the safety of his castles by withdrawing too large a part of their garrisons for his field army.

The barons were prompt to exploit their victory. As soon as they were established in London, they addressed letters to all their fellow barons demanding their support. If they refused, the rebels would treat them as public enemies and ravage their lands.[79] It is unlikely that these threats had any great effect. The fact that the barons held London might move men already strongly inclined to their party like the count of Aumale, William de Albini, and John de Lacy to take the final step and join the revolt. But the baronial army cooped up in London could do little to protect the lands of its partisans. Scattered over England were something like a hundred castles held by royal garrisons, to a large extent mercenaries. These garrisons were already plundering the lands of the king's foes. The bulk of the English baronage waited quietly to see what was going to happen.

John, as usual, had difficulty in making up his mind. When his Flemish knights under the command of Robert and William de Bethune joined him at Freemantle soon after the fall of London, he sent them with Earl William of Salisbury to put down the rising in the west. When Earl William and his allies reached Sherborne,

---

[78] *Histoire des ducs de Normandie*, p. 147; *Rot. pat.*, p. 138.
[79] Wendover, II, 117.

they heard that the enemy was much more numerous than they were. To the great annoyance of the Flemings the earl retired to Winchester where the king was staying. John immediately sent them back to carry out their commission. This time the royal forces advanced against the rebels who fled without giving battle.[80] It is impossible to discover who these western rebels were. William de Montaigu, William Malet, and Robert fitz Paien were rebels at this time, but the chronicles call the force against which the Flemish were sent "northerners."[81] Perhaps "northerner" was simply used as a synonym for rebel. On the other hand it is quite possible that Maurice de Ghent whose lands lay both in the north and the west was involved in this rising. Then it may be that Giles de Briouse had stirred into revolt the tenants of the honors of Barnstaple and Totnes.

By the last days of May King John had decided on his course of action. He would make a temporary peace with his barons relying on the pope to invalidate any concessions he might have to make to obtain it. Then he could muster his power and crush his foes when the time was ripe. On May 27 the king asked Stephen Langton to arrange a truce and ordered his officers to observe it.[82] On June 15 John met his rebellious barons at Runnymede to begin the negotiations leading to the granting of Magna Carta.

While he was reopening negotiations with his barons, the king was paving the way for his future appeal to the pope. John's agent, Walter Mauclerk, had arrived in Rome on February 19. Ten days later Eustace de Vesci appeared to plead the baronial cause. He was commissioned to ask the pope to compel John to grant the barons' demands.[83] Apparently Walter won the argument. On March 19 Innocent wrote to Stephen Langton and his suffragans. He was greatly disturbed to hear of the dissensions between the king and some of his barons. He was particularly shocked at the report that Stephen and the bishops were involved and were said

---

[80] *Histoire des ducs de Normandie*, pp. 147-149.
[81] *Histoire des ducs de Normandie*, pp. 147-149; *Rot. pat.*, pp. 135, 138.
[82] *Ibid.*, p. 142.
[83] Rymer, *Foedera*, I, 120.

to favor the barons. The pope had no patience with armed conspiracies. The prelates were to work for peace, to declare the sworn alliances among the barons invalid, and to excommunicate any obdurate conspirators. They were to urge the barons to perform the service they owed the king and to placate him in every possible way. Then they might reverently ask him to grant their demands. The pope himself was asking John to grant his vassals' "just petitions." Similar letters were addressed to the barons.[84] A separate mandate to the barons directed them to pay the scutage of Poitou. As the barons of England had always paid scutage, to refuse to do so was to deprive the king of his rights.[85] On May 29 John despatched letters to the pope. He thanked Innocent for his letters to the prelates and barons, but regretted that they had been ignored by the recipients. John told his barons that England was part of the patrimony of St. Peter and that he was a crusader. He offered to abolish all the bad customs established by himself and Richard. When he asked the archbishop to force the barons to respect his rights as a crusader, Stephen agreed to do so if John sent home his mercenaries. But when the king kept his part of the agreement, the archbishop still did nothing. Finally John had offered to submit the disputes to arbitration, but this too had been rejected by the barons.[86] John had spent several months placing himself in an impregnable position. In his letter he laid that position before Innocent III. It gave him a base to build on when he asked the pope to invalidate Magna Carta.

While it is fairly easy to present a general account of the negotiations between King John and his disaffected barons prior to the issuing of Magna Carta, we have no precise knowledge of the issues that were under discussion at the various conferences. Three relevant documents have come down to us—the so-called Unknown Charter of Liberties, the Articles of the Barons, and Magna Carta itself.[87] The Unknown Charter is by now extremely familiar to all students of Magna Carta, but no one has found any real evidence that would serve to show its place in the negotiations. Then

[84] *Ibid.*, p. 127.   [85] *Ibid.*, p. 128.   [86] *Ibid.*, p. 129.
[87] For convenient editions of the first two documents see McKechnie, *Magna Carta,* pp. 485-493.

there is no evidence as to how long the Articles of the Barons had been in existence when it was presented to John at Runnymede. I have discovered no new evidence, but it seems worth while to make a few comments with the distinct reservation that they are no more valuable than those made by my predecessors.

The Unknown Charter is a comparatively brief document. Mr. McKechnie has divided it into twelve short chapters and for the sake of convenience I shall follow his numbering in my comments. It is not actually a charter. The first chapter begins " King John concedes." The second chapter and the rest of the document is in the first person singular—" If it happens that my baron . . . . I should . . . ." A formal charter would have been in the first person plural throughout. The document clearly represents someone's informal notes. Nothing is known of its history except that it came into the possession of a king of France, presumably Philip Augustus, and now rests in the National Archives in Paris. It is appended to a copy of the Charter of Liberties of Henry I. Between the charter of Henry I and the Unknown Charter is the note " This is the charter of King Henry through which the barons sought their liberties and the following King John concedes." [88] The argument has been advanced that as most of the document is in the first person, it must have been dictated by King John. It is, however, perfectly conceivable that a man taking notes on oral promises made by the king or even one drawing up a list of suggestions for oral promises would adopt this form.

The substance of chapters 1, 2, 3, 4, 5, 6, 9, 11 of the Unknown Charter is found in the Articles of the Barons and in Magna Carta. The substance of chapters 10 and 12 is found in the Charter of the Forest and presumably these questions were among those postponed in 1215. But these chapters of the Unknown Charter have interesting peculiarities. The first chapter reads " King John concedes that he will not take a man without judgment nor accept anything for justice, nor do injustice." Thus these extremely important concessions that were relegated to the 29th and 30th chapters of the Articles of the Barons and the 39th and 40th chap-

[88] *Layettes du trésor des chartes*, I, 34-35, 423.

ters of Magna Carta are here in first place. Then the Unknown Charter provides that the lands of a minor should be in custody of four knights of the fief and a royal officer. The Articles of the Barons makes no such suggestion, but Magna Carta provides that in case a royal custodian is removed for wasting the fief he should be replaced by two vassals of the young lord. Then two of these chapters of the Unknown Charter are more radical than those in the Articles of the Barons. Chapter 5 provides that when a royal vassal died, his chattels should be divided in accord with his will. The parallel chapter of the Articles of the Barons gives precedence to debts owed the Crown. Then chapter 9 of the Unknown Charter provides for the deforesting of all forests created by Henry II, Richard, and John. The Articles of the Barons speak only of lands afforested by John, but lands afforested by his father and brother appear among the subjects reserved for later discussion in Magna Carta.

Chapters 7 and 8 of the Unknown Charter are quite different from those of the Articles of the Barons that deal with the same subjects. Chapter 7 reads "I concede to my men that they shall not go in the host outside England except in Normandy and Brittany and that decently and that if anyone owes the service of ten knights it will be alleviated by the advice of my barons." Chapter 8 states "And if scutage happens in the land, one mark of silver will be taken from a knight's fee; and if the gravity of the host necessitates it, more shall be taken by the counsel of the barons of the realm." The Articles of the Barons make no reference to foreign service. The barons probably felt that the provision that scutage could be taken only with the counsel of the king's vassals protected them adequately against all abuses connected with the host. Nor is there any mention in the Articles or in Magna Carta of the alleviation of military service. Yet we know that in practice this alleviation was taking place during the reigns of Richard and John and was to become definitely recognized under Henry III.[89]

There is no external evidence to indicate the place occupied by the Unknown Charter in the negotiations between John and his

[89] Painter, *Feudal barony*, pp. 38-39.

barons. I shall confine myself to advancing some very tentative conclusions based on internal evidence. First I shall glance at certain suggestions that have been made that seem to me to be clearly untenable.[90] There are no grounds for calling this document "a forged charter." If anyone wanted to forge a charter, he would have made a better job of it. No literate man of the day could mistake this document for a regular charter. If Philip Augustus wanted a copy of a charter of liberties issued by John, he could certainly have obtained a summary if not an actual copy of Magna Carta. Nor does it seem possible that the Unknown Charter represents an intermediate stage between the Articles of the Barons and Magna Carta. It is more primitive in form than the Articles and contains matter not in either the Articles or Magna Carta. At that stage of the negotiations John would hardly have offered anything not asked for in the Articles.

To my mind the internal evidence indicates that the Unknown Charter is either a set of notes made on an actual charter granted by John in 1213, notes made from oral promises given by the king at that time, or proposals for such a charter. It could well represent promises made by King John when he came to terms with the northern barons through the mediation of Langton and Nicholas of Tusculum.[91] The provision that the barons owed no military service outside the realm except in Normandy and Brittany seems to me to make sense only if an expedition somewhere else was being contemplated at the time. The barons had refused to serve in Poitou—John agreed that they were not obliged to. The prominence given to the promise not to take anyone without a judgment also fits in well with this period. When John had sought to punish the northern lords for their refusal to go to Poitou, this right to a judgment was the argument advanced by Langton to halt the king's vengeful expedition.[92] And it was Stephen Langton, Eustace de Vesci, and Robert fitz Walter who would feel most keenly the need for such a promise, for their relatives and friends had recently suffered from the king's anger. While I am still inclined to believe that it was Stephen Langton who saw that this

---

[90] For a brief summary see McKechnie, *Magna Carta*, pp. 172-175.
[91] Coggeshall, p. 167.   [92] Wendover, II, 83.

right of a free man to a judgment was the most fundamental of all the baronial demands and who placed it first on this list, there is no proof whatever for this hypothesis.[93] I simply feel that it took a more than feudal mind to place this provision ahead of those that were purely feudal in scope.

Finally the presence of this document in the French archives seems to fit in with the theory that it represents promises made in 1213. King Philip had plenty of friends in England at that time. Stephen Langton, his fellow bishops, a number of lesser clergy, and Robert fitz Walter and Eustace de Vesci had just left his protection. While it seems unlikely that Langton's sense of propriety would have allowed him to send valuable information to King Philip, there is no reason for believing that Eustace or Robert would have had any such scruples. And the document did contain immensely valuable information—that John had agreed that his vassals did not owe him actual military service in Poitou. One cannot but wonder if John's desire to use Nantes as a base of operations in the summer of 1214 had some connection with his promise to his barons not to demand foreign service except in Normandy or Brittany.[94]

The Articles of the Barons was certainly presented to King John at Runnymede and the royal seal was attached to it by his command—probably on June 15. While I am inclined to believe that the Articles differed little if at all from the schedule shown John on April 27, my reasons are far from conclusive. Between the meeting at St. Edmunds in the autumn of 1214 and April 27, 1215, the barons had plenty of time and leisure to work out their demands in detail. After April 27 they must have been kept well occupied with their armed revolt and as a result had little opportunity to add to or modify their schedule. Then Roger of Wendover states that when John had heard the baronial demands as contained in the schedule he said that he would never concede them such liberties as it would make him a slave.[95] Now as applied to

[93] Sidney Painter, " Magna Carta," *American historical review,* LIII (1947), 48.
[94] Sidney Painter, *The scourge of the clergy, Peter of Dreux, duke of Brittany* (Baltimore, 1937), pp. 11-12.
[95] Wendover II, 115.

the specific demands in the Articles this was a highly exaggerated statement, but it is reasonable if it referred to the *forma securitatis* —the provision for the twenty-five barons to enforce the charter. In the Articles of the Barons as in Magna Carta they were a body set above the king. As John was a man of violence in expression as well as in action and Wendover is not over accurate, this argument has not very much weight. I simply offer it for what it is worth.

By and large Magna Carta as issued by King John was the Articles of the Barons carefully worked over by highly intelligent men with a thorough knowledge of the English government. In the first place certain vagaries of arrangement were corrected. The Articles discuss in chapter 4 the right of a widow to have her dower and marriage portion without paying a fine and to remain in her husband's house until she receives them. Then chapter 17 provides for the remarrying of widows. These two sections become chapters 7 and 8 in Magna Carta. The Articles insert the important section dealing with men who have been disseised of lands or rights by the crown between the chapter on the writ *praecipe* and that on inquisitions of life or members. In the great charter it is placed with similar provisions. Even more striking is the case of the last part of chapter 35 of the Articles that has little to do with the rest of the chapter but clearly belongs in chapter 3. It is put in its correct place in the great charter. Magna Carta in its final form was far from being a model of logical arrangement, but it was a great improvement in this respect over the Articles.

Then throughout the men who drafted the great charter added precision and exact definition. Thus chapter 1 of the Articles says simply—" after the death of their ancestors heirs of full age shall have . . . ." Magna Carta puts in place of " ancestors " " any earl, baron, or other tenant-in-chief by military service." This sort of improvement carried through the whole document turned the essentially vague and sloppy Articles into the clear and precise form for which Magna Carta is justly famous. In two cases this process was carried so far as to seem to change the meaning of the original provisions. Chapter 13 of the Articles states " assizes of nouvel disseisin and of mort d'ancestor shall be abbreviated and similarly of other assizes." I am not sure what this meant and apparently the men reworking the charter were puzzled. Perhaps they asked the barons what they meant. At any rate the result was clearly chapter 19 of Magna Carta—"and if on the day of the shire court they cannot take the assizes, as many knights and free tenants shall remain of those who were present as shall be sufficient to be able to make judgment . . . ." It looks as if the barons told the drafters that too much time of too many men was wasted taking assizes and chapter 19 was an attempt to solve the need. Then chapter 14 of the Articles provides that no sheriff shall interfere with pleas of the crown without the coroners. Chapter 24 of Magna Carta forbids sheriffs, constables, coroners, or other royal bailiffs to hear pleas of the crown. How these two chapters serve the same purpose is beyond me, but they were clearly intended to. Mr. McKechnie has shown that this process of giving greater precision to Magna Carta went on even after the first formal copies had been drawn up.[96]

Magna Carta contains two types of additions to the Articles of the Barons. Here and there clauses were added to make the provisions more workable. Thus the Articles provide that a custodian who abused his office should be removed, but made no provision for his replacement. Magna Carta corrects this defect by using an idea found in the Unknown Charter. Chapter 8 of the Articles directs the king to send justices to take assizes in the shires—Magna Carta adds "or the chief justice if we are outside the realm." Chapter 31 of the Articles provides for the free entry of merchants into the realm—Magna Carta makes an exception of merchants from enemy lands in time of war. The last section of chapter 48 providing that the king or the justiciar be notified of the voidance of evil customs of the forest was added after at least one of the formal copies was completed. It seems unlikely that these additions required much negotiation. They may well have been made by the drafters on their own authority.

The men who drew up the Articles of the Barons foresaw that

[96] McKechnie, *Magna Carta*, p. 166 and note 1.

John might claim the privileges of a crusader. Apparently the decision as to this was left to Langton and his suffragans, and they seem to have decided in John's favor. The restoration of lands and rights unjustly taken by Henry II and Richard was to await the king's return from the crusade. Finally there are a few real additions to the Articles of the Barons. Two of these are of little importance and hard to explain. Chapter 21 of Magna Carta provides that earls and barons had to be amerced by their peers and according to the nature of their offenses. Chapter 54 forbids anyone to be taken or imprisoned on the appeal of a woman unless the charge was the slaying of her husband. Throughout John's reign barons seem to have been accorded the privilege of being amerced by their peers. The second chapter would seem to be intended to make rape less hazardous, but that can hardly have been its chief purpose. A more important addition gives the king leave to postpone certain questions until his return from the crusade. Two of these do not appear in the Articles—the deforesting of lands afforested by Henry II and Richard and prerogative wardship. It looks as if the barons had an afterthought and asked that these be added. As John had no slightest intention of going on a crusade, he could cheerfully promise to consider them when he got back.

By far the most important addition to the Articles of the Barons found in Magna Carta is the chapter that establishes the procedure to be followed in obtaining the *commune consilium regni* for the levying of a scutage or gracious aid. It provides that the king should send individual writs of summons to the archbishops, bishops, abbots, earls, and "major barons." Then general writs were to be sent to the sheriffs summoning all other tenants-in-chief. The writs were to set a definite place of meeting, name a day at least forty days in the future, and tell the reason for the summons. On the appointed day those who were present were to proceed to do business even if all who had been summoned were not there.

The wording of this chapter leaves two interesting questions. What was a "major baron"? Was this term intended to describe the king's tenants by barony as against other tenants-in-chief or did it simply mean the important barons? As I have indicated elsewhere, I prefer the second of these alternatives.[97] It seems probable that "major barons" meant just that and that the petty tenants by barony were to be included in the general summons. Obviously this would leave the royal government some discretion as to who were to be summoned by individual writs. Then there is the question whether "all those who hold of us in chief" was intended to include the mesne tenants of baronies in the king's hands—the tenants-in-chief *de honore*. As a number of rather important rebel leaders belonged in this category, it seems likely that they were meant to be included.

Some writers have assumed that the assembly provided for in this chapter was the traditional great *curia regis* of the English kings. This would be in accord with feudal theory—a lord's *curia* consisted of all his vassals. But there is no evidence that any such body had ever been summoned to serve as a council. Moreover the mere fact that the proposed assembly is described in such detail in Magna Carta indicates that it was an innovation. If the *commune consilium regni* was to be obtained from the great *curia regis* as it had previously existed, it would have been sufficient to say just that. While this innovation was sound in feudal theory, it was probably utterly impracticable. According to my calculations the king's tenants-in-chief numbered about twelve hundred and included men who held only tiny fractions of a knight's fee. An assembly of that size would have been extremely unwieldy and the smaller tenants-in-chief would have found attendance an unbearable burden. As this chapter was dropped when the charter was reissued along with the one it was meant to implement, it seems improbable that its provisions were ever put to the test of actual use.

As we do not know at whose behest this chapter was inserted in Magna Carta, it is hard to speculate effectively on the reasons for its inclusion. The barons may have wanted to deprive the royal government of any discretion in issuing summonses by basing eligibility on tenure. As no tenurial classification other than the very broad one adopted would have included all the rebel leaders, they

---

[97] Painter, *Feudal barony*, pp. 50-51.

felt obliged to insist on it. But if this chapter was drafted at the request of the barons, it was an afterthought on their part. It was not in the Articles they presented to the king. It seems almost as likely that this assembly was John's idea. He may well have hoped to play off against the great lords the mass of lesser tenants-in-chief whom he believed to be more amenable to his control. The domination of such an assembly by the king would be particularly easy if, as seemed likely, few of the minor tenants-in-chief answered the summons. Then the council would consist of the great lords and the king's servants. While comparatively few of the military and civil officials of the royal government were barons by tenure, practically all of them were tenants-in-chief of the crown. Finally one cannot neglect the possibility that this chapter was concocted by a neutral political theorist—perhaps by Stephen Langton himself. If a logical legal mind imbued with feudal custom set about providing for the assembly that could properly give the counsel of the realm on the subject of imposts to be levied on a feudal basis, it would undoubtedly have arrived at this result—an assembly of all tenants-in-chief of the crown.

One more divergence between Magna Carta and the Articles of the Barons deserves mention. The Articles state that aids and tallages could be taken from London and other cities only by the *commune consilium regni*. Magna Carta speaks only of London and makes no reference to tallages. This change may well have been the result of a bitter debate. As we have seen the whole military position of the rebel barons depended on their possession of London and they had to keep the good will of the citizens. But tallage was a seignorial rather than a feudal right. John could have insisted with sound reason that it was none of his vassals' business how often or how heavily he tallaged his royal demesne. Moreover despite their desire to please the townsmen the barons would not be enthusiastic about pressing this question. Any limitation of a lord's power to tallage his demesne would have been a serious blow to their own revenues.

The provisions of Magna Carta as issued by King John fall naturally into four groups. The first dealing with the relations between the crown and the church consists only of the first part of chapter 1. It guarantees the English church all its rights including freedom of election. As this guarantee is couched in the traditional vague phraseology, it seems of little practical importance. No English king, not even John, would have admitted that he meant to deprive the church of her rights—he would simply disagree with the clergy as to what those rights were. Again other kings of England had promised free episcopal elections but had never allowed their promises to interfere with their practices. Freedom of election could only be secured by outlawing the methods by which the crown exerted its influence on the chapters. But apparently it seemed worth while to Langton and his fellow prelates to have ancient assurances renewed.

Then fifteen chapters deal with the feudal relations between the king and his vassals. Chapters 2 and 3 cover relief, 4 and 5 the right of custody, 6, 7, and 8 the right of marriage, and 12 and 14 the exaction of scutages and aids from tenants-in-chief. Chapter 15 states that the king will not "concede to anyone that he take an aid from his free men" except on the three recognized occasions. This does not mean that the king will not allow his vassals to take special aids from their men. It simply means that the king will not order his sheriffs to force the vassal's tenants to pay. While this provision may have been intended to please the mesne tenants, it seems more likely that it was aimed at one of John's fiscal devices. When a tenant-in-chief owed the crown a large sum, John was inclined to force him to ask an aid from his vassals to discharge the debt. The case of William de Mowbrays' debt to the crown and the aid exacted from his vassals was undoubtedly fresh in the minds of several of the rebel barons. Chapter 16 forbids a lord to demand more service than a fief owes. Chapter 29 forbids the king to demand money payments in commutation of castle-guard service if the vassal prefers to perform his service. Chapter 37 exempts certain serjeantries from prerogative wardship. Chapter 43 promises that tenants *de honore* will not be obliged to perform greater services to the crown than their fiefs had owed to the lords of the honors. Chapter 46 guarantees the barons their rights of patronage over the abbeys founded by their ancestors.

Thirty-two chapters deal with the procedures and policies of the royal administration. Ten of these have to do primarily with fiscal procedure. Chapter 9 requires the king's officers to take a debtor's chattels before they seize his land and to take all the property of a debtor before they distrain his pledges. Chapters 10 and 11 safeguard widows and children from usury. Chapter 25 promises that shires and hundreds will be farmed at the old farms without increments. This was an obvious blow at John's efforts to increase the royal revenue from these sources. Chapters 26 and 27 deal with the king's interests in the chattels of men who have died. Chapters 28, 30, and 31 limit the right of the king's officers to requisition supplies, horses, carts, and wood for the king's use. Chapter 32 guarantees that the crown shall enjoy the lands of a convicted felon for no longer than the customary year and a day.

Another twelve chapters are concerned with the administration of justice. Chapter 17 provides that common pleas, cases between subjects in which the crown had no direct interest, should not follow the king's court but should be heard in a certain place—presumably at Westminster. For a number of years it had been John's practice to have the major part of the judicial business of the realm performed by the justices that followed him from place to place. If his purpose was to keep personal control of the decisions rendered, this practice may well have annoyed the barons for that reason alone. But attendance at a migratory court must always have been both costly and inconvenient. Chapter 18 requires that the possessory assizes should be heard in the shires only and that royal justices should visit each county for this purpose four times a year. While it was undoubtedly desirable that these cases be settled promptly and it was a grave burden on all concerned to have to carry them to Westminster, this provision was entirely impracticable. To send two justices into each shire four times a year would have required a large increase in the number of justices and no shire really wanted these powerful royal agents to come so frequently. The issue of 1217 provided for one visit a year. Chapters 20, 21, and 22 regulated amercements. Chapter 24 forbade sheriffs, constables, and coroners to hear pleas of the crown. Chapter 34 forbade the use of the writ *praecipe* to remove a case from a feudal court. This provision should probably be classed as feudal rather than judicial in its purpose. It was an attempt to preserve some of the importance of the baronial *curiae*.[98] Chapters 36 and 40 prohibit the sale of justice. Chapter 39 is the famous section that protects all free-men from punishment without due process of law. As we have seen this was the first chapter in the Unknown Charter. It was extremely close to the heart of all John's foes both lay and clerical. But in attempting to safeguard themselves, their relatives, and their friends John's enemies devised a most effective shield against governmental tyranny. It seems likely that Stephen Langton at least realized that this chapter expressed a principle that was fundamental to any reign of law.

Four chapters of the charter are concerned with the administration of the king's hunting privileges—with the forests and river banks. Chapter 23 promises that only where it is customary shall men be forced to build bridges over streams to facilitate the royal hawking. Chapter 44 frees men not living in the forest from attendance at its courts unless they have business there. Chapter 47 provides for the deforestation of lands afforested by John and the removal of restrictions placed by him on hawking meadows. Chapter 48 directs that twelve knights shall be chosen in every shire court to inquire into evil, that is new, forest customs and to survey the conduct of the king's officers including the sheriffs. If they found evil customs and these were not corrected in forty days, the knights could correct them after notifying the king or the justiciar.

Finally five chapters dealing with the practices of the government fall into the class of general legislation. Chapter 33 forbids weirs in streams—a delightfully optimistic attempt to improve navigation. It was probably a pleasant and totally ineffective gesture to please the Londoners. Chapter 35 decrees that common measures shall be used in all the realm—a worthy idea that can have met with little opposition from either crown or baronage. Chapter 41 seeks to protect foreign merchants. Chapter 42 provides free entrance to and exit from England for all travellers in

---

[98] For a full discussion of this clause see Naomi Day Hurnard, " Magna carta, clause 34 " in *Studies in mediaeval history presented to Frederick Maurice Powicke* (Oxford, 1948), pp. 157-179.

time of peace. Chapter 45 promises that the king will appoint as officials only men who know the laws of the realm and mean to observe them. This may well have been aimed at the appointment of foreigners—or in fact at the appointment of anyone not pleasing to the barons.

These three groups of provisions have one general characteristic—they are aimed at what the barons considered abuses in the policy of the crown and the royal administration. Although a few of the forbidden practices were innovations made by John, most of them were long standing. These provisions would on the whole have been just as reasonable and pertinent if they had been made under Henry II or Richard. The fourth group was directly concerned with the immediate situation and with certain of John's practices. John had taken hostages from the barons whose loyalty he doubted and had obliged them to make out charters promising fidelity to him. Chapter 49 provides that both hostages and charters shall be returned. Chapter 50 directs the removal from office of Gerard de Athies, Engelard de Cigogné, Andrew, Peter, and Guy de Chancelis, Guy de Cigogné, Geoffrey de Martini and his brothers, and Philip Marc and his brothers and nephew. These men were all Angevins who had followed John to England. They were able soldiers and efficient if heavy-handed administrators. Gerard de Athies had led the royal attacks on William de Briouse. Geoffrey de Martini had held Northampton castle against the rebel host. It is easy to see why these men were hated—the puzzle is to understand why the list is not longer. When Roger of Wendover came to insert the charter in his history, he seems to have felt that the list could stand improvement. He added Fawkes de Bréauté and "all the Flemings."[99] In chapter 51 John promises to send home all his foreign troops. Chapters 52 and 55 contain the provisions that were of greatest interest to the barons as individuals. In chapter 52 John promised to restore all lands, castles, or rights taken by him without a judgment by his court. If a debate arose on any such question, it was to be settled by the twenty-five barons. Chapter 55 provides that all

[99] Wendover, II, 134.

illegal fines or amercements made by him shall be forgiven or settled by the twenty-five. Then chapters 56-59 give the Welsh and Scots allies of the barons what they themselves are promised. They are to receive anything taken from them, and their hostages are to be returned.

The barons had no confidence in King John's promises. They felt sure that he would try to persuade the pope to declare the charter invalid. Even if he failed in that, they expected him to ignore its provisions. Hence they tried to devise a scheme for guaranteeing its execution. The barons, presumably the rebels, were to choose twenty-five of their number to act as a committee to enforce the charter. If John or one of his officers violated a provision of the charter, the offense was to be reported to four barons of the twenty-five. They would ask the king or his justiciar to correct the matter. If no action were taken within forty days, the case would be put before the full committee. Then the twenty-five *cum communa totius terrae* would wage war on the king until he complied with the request. Any Englishman who wished could swear to obey the orders of the twenty-five in enforcing the charter. In fact the king would command all men to swear to support the committee. If a vacancy occurred in the twenty-five, the others would choose a man to fill it. In case of disagreement in the committee, the issue would be decided by majority vote. Finally John promised not to seek the invalidation of the charter.

This plan has been criticized on the ground that it established revolt and civil war as the means of enforcing the charter. But the final sanction behind all contracts is force, and rebellion or the threat of rebellion was the only means by which the barons could hope to control the king. The deficiencies of the plan lay in the barons' motives or lack of imagination—perhaps in both. In issuing Magna Carta John recognized formally the existence of a system of law that bound him as well as his people. The barons were unwilling to allow the royal government to interpret and administer that law. How could they expect the king to be willing to allow them to perform that function? The intelligent solution would have been some form of a tribunal that had the appearance at least of neutrality. A body composed of men like Stephen Langton and William Marshal might well have enforced the charter successfully. But the committee of baronial partisans could only lead to civil war. John could never trust his foes nor willingly submit to the humiliation of being ruled by them. Moreover the real interest of the barons, as they soon demonstrated, lay not in the general clauses of Magna Carta and their enforcement but in the recovery of the rights they claimed as individuals. The barons clearly thought of the committee of twenty-five primarily as a means of securing these private rights—lands, castles, and privileges. If one asks why the men who had sufficient imagination to devise the assembly of tenants-in-chief to give counsel in levying aids did not think of the possibility of having the committee to enforce the charter elected by such a body, the answer probably is that they did not want a neutral group. They wanted to secure their claims and they were fully aware that many of these claims rested on extremely tenuous legal foundations.

Magna Carta has often been described as a "feudal" document. This is both true and misleading. The basic idea underlying Magna Carta—that there was a system of law and custom that governed the relations between lord and vassals—was essentially feudal. It is not, however, very far removed from the church's conception of God's law. As I have suggested before, Langton may well have thought of this feudal law as a sort of subsidiary to divine law in the realm of secular politics. But John and his barons were undoubtedly thinking in the feudal terms of the environment in which they lived. Then, as we have seen, a number of chapters of Magna Carta dealt with purely feudal relationships—the lord's rights of relief, wardship, marriage, and the exaction of aids from his vassals. As the rebel barons were the king's vassals, these chapters were perhaps the ones that interested them most next to those designed to secure their individual claims against the crown. Certainly the chapters dealing with feudal relationships came first in the charter. But it is extremely important to remember that John was king as well as feudal lord of England and that this distinction was fully understood by the men of his day. The minute he learned of Richard's death John called himself *dominus Angliae*—that title was his by inheritance. But he was not king until he had been crowned with the assent of the barons of the realm. Now thirty-two of the sixty odd chapters of Magna Carta deal with the relations between the English king and his subjects. The charter defines these subjects who had rights that the king was bound to observe as *liberi homines,* free men. Thus the feudal concept of a system of law that governed the relations between lords and vassals was carried over into the realm of non-feudal political relationships. The rights of the freeman against the king were made as sacred as those of the vassal against his lord. Now this transference of a feudal concept into the field of non-feudal politics was not entirely new—it was implicit in certain chapters of the Charter of Liberties of Henry I. But the men who drafted Magna Carta consciously emphasized it. The last sentence of the first chapter states: "We grant to all the freemen of our realm, from us and our heirs forever, all the undermentioned liberties to have and to hold for them and their heirs from us and our heirs." The charter was not a grant to the tenants-in-chief of the crown but to all the freemen of England.

On June 19 King John issued letters patent formally notifying his officers that peace had been made "between us, our barons, and the freemen of our realm" and directing them to carry out the provisions of Magna Carta. The charter was to be read publicly in every shire—presumably in the shire court. Each sheriff was to see that the men of his shire took the required oath to the twenty-five barons. The twenty-five or a majority of them were to set a day and place for the men of the shire to take this oath before them or their duly appointed representatives. At the first meeting of the shire court twelve knights were to be elected to inquire into bad customs maintained by the sheriff or other royal officials. The king's servants were to see that all the provisions of the charter were observed.[100] While this writ implies that a copy of the charter was being sent with it, it seems doubtful that enough

[100] *Rot. pat.,* p. 180.

copies of the charter were ready by June 19.[101] Under the terms of the writ the sheriff would not actually need the text of the charter until the next meeting of his shire court.

Apparently these royal letters did not fully satisfy the barons. A week after they were issued, they were reinforced. Letters to the sheriffs and to the groups of knights elected to inquire into evil customs ordered the seizure of the lands and chattels of all men who refused to take the oath to the twenty-five barons. If anyone remained obdurate for two weeks more, his chattels were to be sold and the proceeds used for the crusade.[102] The fact that these letters were considered necessary indicates that the freemen of the realm were not showing unrestrained enthusiasm for taking the oath to the twenty-five. In fact the barons were still troubled over this matter in August.[103]

The conclusion of peace between John and his barons involved changes in the personnel of the royal government. Although no reference to the office of justiciar is made in the great charter, it is clear that the removal of Peter des Roches was one of the conditions of the peace. On the day agreement was reached, John appointed to this high office Hubert de Burgh.[104] This arrangement was obviously a compromise. Hubert had always been a loyal and, except for a brief period of estrangement, a trusted servant of John. Yet he was an Englishman and hence more acceptable to the barons than Peter. Moreover either because of ancient tenurial relations or because of relationship by marriage Hubert had the support of the powerful Earl Warren. Although he had had little experience as a judge and presumably no great knowledge of the law, he was an experienced administrator and a tried and able captain. He had been the king's chamberlain, the constable of Chinon, and the seneschal of Poitou.

John on his side was naturally disinclined to retain in office men who had been active partisans of the rebellious barons. On

---

[101] For an excellent discussion of the process of placing the charter in circulation see Richardson, " The morrow of the great charter," pp. 425-429.
[102] *Rot. pat.*, p. 145.
[103] Rymer, *Foedera*, I, 133.
[104] Matthew Paris, *Chronica maiora*, VI, 65.

June 25 Reginald de Cornhill and Henry de Braybrook were deprived of their shrievalties. Hubert de Burgh replaced Reginald de Cornhill in Kent and Surrey while William de Duston took the place of Henry de Braybrook as sheriff of Northamptonshire.[105] Four days later John Marshal was appointed sheriff of Norfolk and Suffolk in place of John fitz Robert.[106] Then Magna Carta provided for the removal from office of certain foreign mercenary captains. Here King John showed no great haste. It was not until July 8 and July 19 that Engelard de Cigogné was deprived of Gloucestershire and Herefordshire. In Gloucestershire he was replaced by Ralph Musard, a local baron, while Herefordshire was added to the group of shires in the hands of the new justiciar.[107] When Hubert de Burgh took over Norfolk and Suffolk from John Marshal on July 25, he was sheriff of four counties.[108] During July two foreigners mentioned in the charter were removed as constables of royal castles. Geoffrey de Martini was directed to surrender Northampton castle to the sheriff, Roger de Neville.[109] Peter de Cancellis, constable of Bristol, was replaced by Philip de Albini, a loyal servant of John's who was a relative of the lord of Belvoir.[110] But Philip Marc, sheriff of Nottingham and Derby, remained in office.

Undoubtedly the provisions of Magna Carta that were of greatest interest to the baronial leaders were those providing for the reduction of extortionate fines and amercements and the restoration of lands, castles, and privileges improperly held by the crown. King John was anxious to delay the execution of these provisions of the charter, but the barons insisted on immediate action. The reasons behind the baronial attitude are easy to comprehend—once they disbanded their forces and abandoned their stronghold, the city of London, any attempt to coerce the king would have to start all over again from the beginning. One cannot be so positive about John's motives. He may well have had grave doubts about the justice of many of the baronial claims and a sincere desire to examine them closely before acting. On the

[105] *Rot. pat.*, pp. 144-145.
[106] *Ibid.*, p. 144.
[107] *Ibid.*, pp. 148-149.
[108] *Ibid.*, p. 150.
[109] *Ibid.*, p. 146.
[110] *Ibid.*, p. 149.

other hand he may have already despatched messengers to Rome to persuade the pope to invalidate the charter. Certainly it was to his advantage to delay if he hoped to avoid making restoration.

The result was a series of compromises. Some claims, in general the most reasonable ones, were granted at once while the consideration of others was postponed. Letters close of June 19 addressed to Earl William of Salisbury make clear what was happening. John reminded his brother that he had promised to restore lands and castles that had been seized without proper legal action. He had asked Henry de Bohun, earl of Hereford, to allow him to postpone the restoration of the castle and barony of Trowbridge. Earl Henry had agreed that Earl William might hold the castle until June 28, but he had insisted on the immediate restoration of the "flat lands." The earl of Salisbury was directed to put Earl Henry's agents in possession of the barony.[111] As we have indicated above the rights of the controversy over the honor of Trowbridge are hard to determine. The fact that eventually Earl Henry ceded part of the barony to his rival might be taken as evidence that there was justice on both sides, but it could also mean simply that the earl of Hereford was too slow about submitting to the government at the close of the civil war.[112] Certainly the barony had been seized without final action in the *curia regis* and hence should have been restored under the terms of the charter. On August 1 Earl William received extensive grants from the royal demesne to compensate him for his loss of Trowbridge.[113]

During the last half of June, 1215, King John placed a number of estates in the possession of their baronial claimants. Count William of Aumale received the manor of Driffield in Yorkshire.[114] Henry I, Richard, and John had regarded this manor as part of the royal demesne, but count William's grandfather, William le Gros, had held it under Henry II.[115] As the highly inconstant count of Aumale shifted to the royal party during this period, the grant of Driffield may have been more of a bribe than a restora-

---

[111] *Rot. claus.*, I, 215.
[112] *Book of fees*, II, 720-723, 737, 741.
[113] *Rot. claus.*, I, 223-224.
[114] *Rot. pat.*, p. 154.
[115] *Pipe rolls 2, 3 and 4 Henry II*, pp. 26, 46, 86; *Pipe roll 22 Henry II*, p. 164.

tion.[116] Earl Richard de Clare was given the town of Buckingham to which his claim was absolutely sound at least as a custodian.[117] Earl Richard had given Buckingham, the *caput* of the honor of Giffard, to William de Briouse the younger in marriage with his daughter.[118] The earl had a good claim to the custody of the town until young John de Briouse came of age. Roger de Montbegon was given some land that John had granted him as count of Mortain but had seized during one of Roger's frequent periods of disgrace.[119] The manor of Ailsbury and the honor of Berkhamsted were given to William de Mandeville.[120] As these lands had been formally granted to Geoffrey fitz Peter, William's claim was good.[121] There is, however, some doubt as to whether he was actually given seisin.

The castle of Fotheringay which had been taken into the king's hands at the time of Robert fitz Walter's revolt in 1212 was restored to David, earl of Huntingdon.[122] Saher de Quency received the fortress of Mountsorrel that belonged to his half of the honor of Leicester.[123] The great castle of Richmond was restored to its hereditary constable, Ruald fitz Alan.[124] These grants represented the recognition of unquestionable rights. Robert fitz Walter received the custody of Hertford castle.[125] Robert's claim to the custody of this castle was not very strong. His wife's ancestor, Peter de Valognes, had been sheriff of Hertfordshire under William I and may well have had the custody of the chief castle of the shire.[126] There is no evidence that Peter or his successors held that office after the death of the Conqueror. A charter given to Peter's son Roger, by the Empress Matilda makes no reference to Hertford castle and Matilda gave the office of hereditary sheriff of Hertfordshire to Geoffrey de Mandeville.[127] It seems most unlikely that if Roger de Valognes claimed the hereditary custody of

[116] *Rot. pat.*, p. 152.
[117] *Ibid.*, p. 143.
[118] *Ibid.*
[119] *Rot. claus.*, I, 215.
[120] *Ibid.*, p. 217.
[121] *Rot. chart.*, pp. 127-128, 151.
[122] *Rot. pat.*, p. 144.
[123] *Ibid.*, p. 145.
[124] *Ibid.*, p. 143.
[125] *Ibid.*, p. 144.
[126] H. W. C. Davis, *Regesta regum Anglo-Normannorum*, 1066-1154 (Oxford, 1913), I, nos. 93, 235, 277.
[127] Round, *Geoffrey de Mandeville*, pp. 167, 286.

Hertford castle, it would not have been mentioned in one of these grants. In 1200 Robert fitz Walter was given a day to prove his claim in the *curia regis*. There is no record of any hearing, but in 1202 Robert was given the custody of the castle and held it until 1209.[128] As the letters patent appointing him constable make no reference to any hereditary right, it seems likely that John gave him the custody without deciding the question. William de Lanvalay was given custody of Colchester castle.[129] King Henry I had granted Colchester and its castle to Eudes his *dapifer*.[130] After Eudes' death the castle and town were in the custody of Hamo de St. Clare, a prominent vassal and perhaps a kinsman of Eudes.[131] In the reign of Henry II Colchester was in the custody of Richard de Lucy.[132] Apparently King Richard in the last few months of his reign placed this fortress in the care of William de Lanvalay's father who was a descendant of Hamo de St. Clare. In 1200 William the elder offered 200 marks for the custody of Colchester as Richard had granted it to him. He and his widow held it until 1209.[133] Hence William's claim to hold Colchester as his father's heir seems to have been sound. There is, however, no clear evidence that the crown had ever recognized Hamo de St. Clare or William de Lanvalay the elder as hereditary constables. William Mauduit was given the custody of Rockingham castle.[134] Williams' great-grandfather had married late in the reign of Henry I the daughter of Michael of Hanslope, hereditary constable of Rockingham.[135] In 1190 his grandfather offered King Richard £100 for the custody of the castle.[136] In 1195 William's father, Robert Mauduit, paid 100 marks for his relief and the custody of Rockingham "as long as the king pleases."[137] This seems to mean

[128] *Curia regis rolls*, I, 116; *Rot. pat.*, p. 17.
[129] *Ibid.*, p. 151.
[130] William Farrer, *An outline itinerary of King Henry the first*, p. 12.
[131] *Pipe roll 31 Henry I*, p. 138; Farrer, *Honours and knights' fees*, III, 291.
[132] *Pipe rolls 2, 3, 4 Henry II*, p. 135.
[133] *Pipe roll 1 John*, p. 87; *Rot. oblatis*, p. 89.
[134] *Rot. pat.*, p. 144.
[135] Farrer, *An outline itinerary of King Henry the first*, p. 141.
[136] *Pipe roll 2 Richard I*, p. 36.
[137] *Pipe roll 7 Richard I*, pp. 203-204.

that his claim to be hereditary custodian was not recognized by Richard. In 1199 Robert offered John £100 to have the custody of Rockingham " as he had it before." [138] But in 1205 the castle was in the custody of Hugh de Neville who held it either directly or through deputies until 1215.[139] In short while William had a good claim based on possession by his ancestors, it does not appear that either Richard or John had recognized it. Finally John ordered the constable of the castle of York to deliver it to William de Mowbray pending an inquisition as to whether or not he had a right to be its hereditary constable.[140] The only evidence I can find that connects the Mowbrays with the constableship of York is a grant to a monastery of the mill of York castle by William's great-grandfather Nigel de Albini.[141] There is no indication that Henry II, Richard, or John had ever recognized such a claim.

In addition to lands and castles John restored to his foes certain less tangible properties. Richard de Montfichet was made forester in fee of the forests of Essex.[142] This office had been held by Richard's grandfather and his father had fined for it with King John in 1200.[143] Orders were issued to the sheriffs of all the counties in which lay the lands of the honor of Gloucester that Geoffrey de Mandeville was to have the *regalia* of all religious houses founded by his wife's ancestors and all the franchises enjoyed by her father Earl William of Gloucester. Two of the chaces belonging to the honor were to be perambulated and given to him.[144] Robert de Vere, earl of Oxford, was given the third penny of the pleas of Oxfordshire.[145] Philip de Ulecotes was instructed to allow Eustace de Vesci to have his customary rights in respect to hunting dogs.[146]

While the close and patent rolls show us what baronial claims were granted by King John in the weeks after the issuing of

---

[138] *Rot. oblatis*, p. 9.
[139] *Pipe roll 7 John*, p. 256.
[140] *Rot. pat.*, p. 143. *Rot. claus.*, I, 215.
[141] *Early Yorkshire charters*, VI, 77.
[142] *Rot. pat.*, p. 144.
[143] William Farrer, *Feudal Cambridgeshire* (Cambridge, 1920), pp. 234-235; *Pipe roll 2 John*, p. 48.   [145] *Ibid*.
[144] *Rot. claus.*, I, 216.   [146] *Ibid*.

Magna Carta, we know little about those that were postponed for later consideration. In fact only two of these can be established with any certainty. According to Walter of Coventry Geoffrey de Mandeville claimed the hereditary constableship of the Tower of London on the ground that this fortress had been in the custody of his father, Geoffrey fitz Peter.[147] This statement is not quite fair to Geoffrey. King William II granted the custody of the Tower to William de Mandeville, and he apparently held it under Henry I. Both Stephen and Matilda granted Geoffrey de Mandeville, the first earl of Essex, the hereditary constableship.[148] During the reign of Henry II the Tower had been ordinarily in the custody of the justiciar, and it is likely that Geoffrey fitz Peter held it in that capacity. As the first earl of Essex had forfeited all his possessions under Stephen, a claim based on his charter had little validity, but it was probably no feebler than those being advanced by other barons. It was in all probability the extreme military importance of the Tower that caused John to insist on the postponement of the consideration of Geoffrey's claim. In the meantime the Tower was placed in the more or less neutral hands of Stephen Langton.

We know of another postponed claim through two interesting documents discovered by Mr. Richardson. In the first of these Geoffrey de Mandeville, Saher de Quency, and Richard de Clare informed Brian de Lisle, royal constable of Knaresborough, that the twenty-five barons had decided that Knaresborough castle belonged by right to Nicholas de Stutville. He was directed to keep the oath he had taken to obey the twenty-five barons and to deliver the castle to Nicholas.[149] In the second document the same three lords ordered Robert de Ros, "custodian" of Yorkshire to use all the force of the shire to aid Nicholas to obtain the castle. Both writs were witnessed by Robert de Vere, earl of Oxford.[150] They were issued on September 30 after the barons had broken off relations with John and attempted to set up their own government.

[147] Coventry, II, 221.
[148] Stenton, *English feudalism,* pp. 222-223; Round, *Geoffrey de Mandeville,* pp. 37-38, 89, 141.
[149] Richardson, "The morrow of the great charter," p. 443.
[150] *Ibid.*

We shall mention these documents again in connection with later events. For the moment our interest lies in the fact that they inform us about another postponed claim.

About the year 1175 King Henry II granted the castles of Knaresborough and Boroughbridge with the lands pertaining to them to William de Stutville for the service of three knights.[151] On December 7, 1189, this charter was confirmed by King Richard in return for a fine of £2,000.[152] In 1199 William offered John 3,000 marks to have his charters confirmed and for several other favors.[153] William de Stutville died in 1203 heavily in debt to the crown, and his son Robert apparently lacked the funds to pay the relief demanded by John. Although Robert was not yet a knight, he must have been of age for he gave his consent to the curious arrangement by which the king obtained his relief. Hubert Walter, archbishop of Canterbury, offered the king 4,000 marks to have custody of the Stutville lands for four years. Then Robert would come into possession—presumably without further payment. On July 9, 1203, King John issued two charters. One confirmed Robert de Stutville in the possession of all his father's lands while the other gave Hubert custody of them for four years.[154] But Robert died before Hubert Walter. In August 1205 his uncle, Nicholas de Stutville, the younger brother of William, offered the enormous sum of 10,000 marks for the family lands. The castles of Knaresborough and Boroughbridge were to be retained by the crown until the fine was paid.[155] Nicholas did not allow this obligation to disturb him unduly. In 1208 he owed 9,998½ marks of his fine and the same amount was still due from his son in 1230.[156] Thus under the terms of his agreement with John Nicholas had no right to the castles in 1215. But he could and probably did argue that the fine of 10,000 marks was extortionate. Nicholas' fine included 2,100 marks owed to the crown by his brother. Thus the actual relief is reduced to about 8,000

---

[151] *Ibid.*, pp. 442-443.
[152] *Ibid.; Pipe roll 2 Richard I*, p. 68.
[153] *Pipe roll 1 John*, p. 56; *Cartae antiqae rolls*, no. 102.
[154] *Rot. chart.*, p. 108.
[155] *Ibid.*, p. 166.
[156] *Pipe roll 10 John*, p. 148; *Pipe roll 14 Henry III*, p. 275.

marks. If one assumes that Hubert Walter was a good business man, the Stutville lands must have been worth something over 1,000 marks a year. But as Nicholas did not have the honor of Knaresborough, his income was probably about half this sum. In short it is easy to see how Nicholas could consider that he had been forced to offer an unreasonable fine. It is, however, possible to see why John should have felt otherwise. Clearly both Richard and John felt that William de Stutville had done extremely well at the expense of the royal demesne. Each of these monarchs had demanded £2,000 for the confirmation of Henry II's charters. John seems to have considered 4,000 marks a suitable relief for William's son, Robert. On this basis 8,000 marks was not an unreasonable relief to demand from an uncle succeeding his nephew —especially when an important part of the lands involved had never been held by their common ancestor. I have gone into this claim by Nicholas de Stutville at such length because Mr. Richardson seems to assume that it was well founded and that John was obviously in the wrong. It seems worth while to point out that the question was debatable.

In addition to removing his foreign favorites from office and restoring the lands, castles, and privileges illegally seized John had promised in Magna Carta to return to the barons the hostages whom he held for their good behavior and to send home his mercenary troops. As we have no list of the hostages in John's possession in June 1215 we cannot say positively that he released all of them, but he certainly freed a fair number.[157] In the case of the mercenary troops it seems likely that he sent home the most recent arrivals and kept those who had been in England for some time. The Flemish knights and serjeants who had arrived just as the barons captured London and had participated in crushing the rising in the west were sent home.[158] The mercenary captain Hugh de Boves was directed to dismiss the troops at Dover.[159] But the companies of Fawkes de Bréauté, Engelard de Cigogné, Philip Marc, and Savaric de Mauleon were clearly retained.

[157] *Rot. pat.*, p. 143.
[158] *Histoire des ducs de Normandie*, p. 151.
[159] Rymer, *Foedera*, I, 134.

Before the gathering at Runnymede broke up, the king and the barons arranged to hold a meeting at Oxford on July 16 to settle the issues still pending. Mr. Richardson has shown the importance of this conference.[160] On July 15 the king notified Langton and the barons that he could not be at Oxford on the day appointed and was sending in his place the archbishop of Dublin, the bishop of Winchester, Pandulf, the earls of Pembroke, Warren, and Arundel, and Hubert de Burgh.[161] John himself arrived at Oxford on July 17 and stayed there until July 23. He was apparently quite sick. While the story of the barons insisting that the king be carried out of his room to preside over his court may be apocryphal, it would hardly have arisen if the king were in good health.[162] Each side brought its grievances to discuss at this council. The barons complained that Engelard de Cigogné was still sheriff of Herefordshire and his kinsman Peter de Chancelis constable of Bristol. John satisfied this grievance by replacing Engelard with Hubert de Burgh and Peter with Philip de Albini.[163] At the same time the king pointed out that John fitz Robert was still acting as sheriff of Norfolk and Suffolk even though John Marshal had been appointed to succeed him. This was settled by giving the shrievalty to Hubert de Burgh who seems to have been one of the few men trusted by both sides.[164] The barons also agreed to allow Robert de Ros to be superseded as sheriff of Cumberland by Robert de Vaux, but as Robert de Ros was still holding the position in January 1216, the arrangement was of little value.[165] The grant of the custody of Colchester castle to William de Lanvalay seems to have been made at this conference.[166] Then apparently Earl Ranulf of Chester had heard that men were getting lands and castles to which they had rather vague claims. Although he was a loyal supporter of John, he saw no reason for not taking advantage of his opportunities. He

[160] Richardson, " Morrow of the great charter," pp. 426-429.
[161] *Rot. pat.*, p. 149.
[162] *Histoire des ducs de Normandie,* p. 151.
[163] *Rot. pat.*, p. 149.
[164] *Ibid.*, p. 150. Richardson, " Morrow of the great charter," pp. 441-442.
[165] *Rot. pat.*, pp. 150, 163.
[166] *Ibid.*, p. 151.

claimed and received the lands of his kinsman, Simon de Montfort, earl of Leicester.[167] Finally there was a debate as to how far the twelve knights elected in each shire could go in abolishing customs of the forest. The barons apparently insisted that the powers of these committees should not be limited, but the bishops sided with the king. The archbishops of Canterbury and Dublin and the bishops of London, Winchester, Bath, Lincoln, Worcester, and Coventry issued letters declaring that no customs necessary to the administration of the forests should be abolished.[168]

While these questions are interesting because of the light they cast on the policies of the two parties, they were comparatively minor matters. The real issues were the possession of London and the position of the barons in relation to the crown. At this council in Oxford John seems to have argued that it was time for the barons to give up the city and issue charters guaranteeing their loyalty to him. The barons replied that they were unwilling to do these things until all the men of England had taken the oath to the twenty-five and John had satisfied all their claims to lands, castles, and privileges. The barons knew that London was the key to their power and that the king was most anxious to get possession of it for that very reason. This is shown very clearly by a letter sent by Robert fitz Walter to William de Albini about the end of June. Apparently the barons had planned to hold a tournament at Stamford on July 6. Robert informed William that it had been postponed for a week and the place changed to a location near London. The reasons for this move were clearly stated. "You know well how great a convenience it is to you and us all to hold the city of London which is our refuge and how much damage it would be to us if by our neglect we should lose it." Robert went on to say that the barons had been warned that "certain persons" expected them to leave the city and were planning to seize it. William was to come to the tourney with horses and arms. Whoever performed best would receive a bear donated by a lady.[169]

[167] *Ibid.*, p. 150.
[168] Rymer, *Foedera*, I, 134.
[169] Wendover, II, 137-138.

As King John found it impossible to shake the determination of the barons, he finally granted them the delay they sought. An agreement was drawn up between the king and thirteen baronial leaders—Robert fitz Walter, the earls of Hertford, Essex, Norfolk, Winchester, Oxford, and Hereford, William Marshal the younger, Eustace de Vesci, William de Mowbray, John fitz Robert, Roger de Montbegon, and William de Lanvalay. The barons were to hold London until August 15 as the king's custodians paying him the revenues due from the city. The archbishop of Canterbury was to continue to hold the Tower. The king was not to introduce troops into either the city or the Tower. During this same period all men who had not taken the oath to the twenty-five barons were to do so and everyone who had claims for the restoration of castles, lands, or privileges were to present them to the king or the twenty-five. All property seized from the rebels during the civil war was to be returned. If the king failed to carry out this agreement, the barons were to continue to hold London.[170] King John had lost the debate, but he did gain one point—he obtained a formal announcement that the barons had failed to perform one of their promises. The archbishops of Canterbury and Dublin, the bishops of London, Winchester, Bath, Lincoln, Worcester, Coventry, and Chichester, and Pandulf issued letters declaring that when peace had been made, that is when the great charter was sealed, the barons had in their presence promised to give the king security for their good behavior in any form except by the surrender of castles or hostages. The king had demanded that each baron issue letters in a set form. "Know that we are bound by oaths and homage to our lord John, king of England, to faithfully conserve his life, members, and worldly honor against all men who can live and die and to guard and defend his rights, the rights of his heirs, and his realm." The barons had refused to issue such letters.[171] John had lost the battle of the council table, but he was preparing to bombard his foes with papal bulls and wanted to be in as strong a moral position as possible.

It is extremely difficult and probably utterly futile for an his-

---

[170] Rymer, *Foedera,* I, 133. [171] *Rot. pat.,* p. 181.

torian to attempt to pass judgment on either John or his foes. I am convinced that the king never had the slightest intention of observing Magna Carta to a greater extent than was absolutely necessary. But it is important to remember that this conviction is based on an interpretation of John's character and general policy rather than on his actions during the month after the charter was sealed. The writers who have chosen to test the king's sincerity by his behavior can make a strong case in his favor. John promptly issued the writs required to put Magna Carta into operation and reinforced them as seemed necessary. He removed his unpopular justiciar and most of his foreign sheriffs and constables. He sent home at least a fair part of his mercenary troops. Furthermore he granted a large number of claims for the restoration of lands, castles, and privileges. Apparently the only criticisms of his conduct that the barons could formulate on July 16-23 were that he had not compelled everyone to take the oath to the twenty-five and had not granted all the claims that had been made. In regard to the first of these questions John seems to have done all he could. He had ordered the sheriffs to seize the lands and chattels of all who refused to take the oath. But it must have been practically impossible to enforce such an order. As we have seen, the rebellious barons represented only a part, probably a minor part, of the feudality of the realm. To persuade men to take an oath to obey the mandates of a group for which they had no particular sympathy and which may have included personal enemies must have been extremely difficult. The fact that practically all the restorations made were to the benefit of members of the committee of twenty-five must have raised doubts about this group's disinterested concern for the "community of the realm." In regard to the question of the restoration of lands, castles, and privileges there is an important point to bear in mind. There were few royal demesnes, castles, or rights that some baron could not claim on grounds fully as sound as those on which some of the claims that were granted rested. If the king granted all the claims that his barons could concoct, the royal power would be reduced to a mere shadow. In short it can be argued with plausability that John's actions between June 19 and July 24, 1215, were those of a man who sincerely intended to carry out his promises. There is but one possible flaw in this argument. The letters of Innocent III annulling Magna Carta were issued on August 25. If John despatched his emissaries to request this action before the meeting at Oxford, the argument that he sincerely intended to observe the charter cannot stand. If these emissaries were sent after that meeting, John's case has strength. He had done his best to carry out his promises yet his barons refused to give up London and to issue charters guaranteeing their loyalty to the royal house. As the journey from London to Rome took about thirty days, it is conceivable that John's envoys did not leave until after the council at Oxford.[172]

There seems to be only one justification for the attitude of the barons—they hated and distrusted the king. They were convinced that he had no intention of keeping his promises if he could possibly avoid doing so. As I believe they were right, I cannot but sympathize with them. But if one judges them by their actions, their position becomes indefensible. They demanded that the king restore what he had taken during the civil war yet they stubbornly held on to London. They insisted that all men take the oath to the twenty-five; but they refused to seal the letters guaranteeing their loyalty to John. The twenty-five barons saw to it that their claims received attention first. It is interesting to notice that Nicholas de Stutville whose claim was still unsatisfied in late September was not one of the twenty-five. Moreover if we are to believe the contemporary chroniclers the barons conducted themselves in a highhanded manner throughout the realm. They insulted the king at Oxford and they defied and mistreated his officials in the shires.[173] John's unwillingness to have his realm ruled by the twenty-five barons seems to have been justified by the committee's behavior.

Either during or just after the meeting at Oxford new papal letters arrived in England, but, as Professor Powicke has pointed out, they were of little use to the king.[174] They were apparently

---

[172] Charles Bémont, *Chartes des libertés Anglaises* (Paris, 1892), pp. 41-44; Landon, *Itinerary*, p. 186.
[173] *Histoire des ducs de Normandie,* p. 151; Coventry, II, 222.
[174] F. M. Powicke, " The bull ' Miramus plurimum ' and a letter to Arch-

written as soon as Innocent learned of the baronial muster at Stamford. The pope recalled his earlier letters in which he had commanded the barons to perform the service they owed the king and to present their claims to him humbly and in which he had asked John to grant his vassals' just requests. King John had offered his barons justice, but they had taken up arms against him. They were not even deterred from this by the fact that John was a crusader. It was both criminal and absurd for men who had supported John when he was quarreling with the church to rebel against him when he had given satisfaction to Rome. Moreover they had violated their oaths of homage and fidelity. The pope wished and felt obliged to protect his vassal—especially as this vassal was also a crusader. Hence he had ordered the archbishop of Canterbury and his suffragans to excommunicate the rebels and place their lands under interdict unless within eight days they made peace with the king. These letters were dated June 18.[175] As the sole copy preserved lacks the beginning, we do not know to whom they were addressed, but it is clear that similar letters were sent to Langton and his fellow bishops. It is easy to understand why Stephen Langton ignored these letters. While it can hardly be said that the barons had sought their rights humbly, they had made peace with the king.

A fortnight or so after he sent this letter of June 18, Pope Innocent received John's letter of May 29. As we have seen the burden of this letter was the archbishop's refusal to carry out the orders contained in the pope's letter of March 19 and the barons' failure to accept any of the offers made by the king and to respect his status as a crusader. While John's letter did not ask for the appointment of a papal commission friendly to the king, his envoys may well have made such a suggestion orally.[176] At any rate on July 7 the pope addressed a letter to the bishop of Winchester, the

bishop Stephen Langton, 5 September 1215," *English historical review*, XLIV (1929), p. 89.

[175] G. B. Adams, " Innocent III and the great charter," *Magna Carta commemoration essays* (ed. H. E. Malden, Royal historical society), pp. 43-45.

[176] See H. G. Richardson, " The morrow of the great charter—an addendum," *Bulletin of the John Rylands library*, XXIX (1945), 191.

abbot of Reading, and Pandulf. Innocent expressed his astonishment at the attitude of Stephen Langton and his suffragans. Their failure to aid John actively endangered not only the English realm but also the success of the crusade. Hence the pope himself felt obliged to act. He declared the disturbers of the English realm and all their accomplices excommunicate and placed their lands under interdict. The archbishop and his suffragans were directed to proclaim this excommunication in proper form. If the prelates neglected to obey this mandate, they were to be suspended from office. The three commissioners or any two of them had full power to enforce these commands.[177]

The agreement made between John and the barons at Oxford implied that the latter would surrender London and the Tower to the king on August 15 unless John violated its terms. On August 20 the bishops and barons of the realm assembled again at Oxford and apparently requested the king's presence. John neither attended in person nor sent representatives of sufficient rank to negotiate in his name. He simply despatched a Hospitaller, a Templar, and Ralph de Normanville to carry a message to the assembly.[178] According to Walter of Coventry the purport of this message was just what one would expect—the king had carried out his promises and the next move was up to the barons.[179] A week later the bishops and barons held another conference at Stanes, but this seems to have been entirely ignored by John though it is possible that the bishop of Winchester and Pandulf were there. There is a suggestion in the chronicles that the existence of the papal letters of July 7 was announced at this meeting. I fully agree with Mr. Richardson that the story of Langton's semi-farcical attempt to pervert the pope's purpose by proclaiming an excommunication in ambiguous terms is completely unacceptable.[180]

It seems likely that it took John and his advisers several days to decide what to do with their fine new mandate. It was far more

[177] Powicke, "Miramus plurimum," p. 91.
[178] *Rot. pat.*, p. 153.
[179] Coventry, II, 223.
[180] *Ibid.*, p. 224. Richardson, "Morrow of the great charter—addendum," p. 195.

useful than the letter of June 18. Innocent had himself pronounced the excommunication of the rebels, and Langton was directed to proclaim the sentence. But the archbishop could obviously answer that this letter like the previous one envisaged a situation that no longer existed. The country was not, in theory at least, in a state of civil war. Peace had been made and papal letters written in ignorance of that fact should not be taken too seriously. The king's counsellors were fully aware of these possible objections and concocted an argument that they hoped would answer them.

On September 5 the three commissioners addressed a long letter to Stephen Langton and his suffragans. After quoting in full the papal letters of July 7, they launched into their own argument. The commissioners knew that the pope had sent the English prelates many letters directing them to aid John against the disturbers of his realm. It was notorious that Robert fitz Walter, the earls of Winchester, Clare, and Gloucester, Eustace de Vesci, Richard de Percy, John de Lacy, William de Albini, William de Mowbray and many others had conspired against the king and the peace of the realm that was part of the patrimony of St. Peter, had taken up arms, and had defied their lord against the "*triplicem formam pacis* that was honest and reasonable and worthy of acceptance by God-fearing men." Moreover they had by fraudulent machinations occupied the city of London, the *caput* of the realm, in contempt of the *forma pacis* which the pope had ordained in the presence of and by the consent of their accredited envoys. They had held the city against the king and severely mistreated the inhabitants who were faithful to him. Some of these men even though they sought it as crusaders could obtain no redress. Then in alliance with the citizens of London and other sworn foes of the king they had injured the royal dignity. They had granted lands, abolished approved customs of the realm and instituted new laws. They changed what had been ordained by their lord the king with the counsel of his magnates. They showed respect neither for the business of the Holy Cross, the pope's mandates, or their oaths of fidelity. Hence the commissioners declared the disturbers of the realm excommunicate, placed their lands under interdict, and enjoined Langton and his suffragans to proclaim the sentence. The commissioners went on to declare that all conspiracies against the king were dissolved. All constitutions or decrees and all enfeoffments or grants of land made by the barons without the king's consent either in the past or in the future were declared void. Anyone using grants by the barons was excommunicate. The city of London and its citizens were included in this sentence of excommunication and interdict. Finally the commissioners launched the same sentence against a group of clerks including Giles de Briouse, bishop of Hereford, William fitz Walter, archdeacon of Hereford, and John de Ferreby who had gone to Rome with Eustace de Vesci in the late autumn of 1214.[181]

This interesting document has, I believe, been generally misinterpreted. Both Professor Powicke and Mr. Richardson take the *triplicem formam pacis* to have been Magna Carta although they recognize the difficulties raised by this hypothesis.[182] It is hard to explain why Peter des Roches and Pandulf should call Magna Carta "honest and reasonable and worthy of acceptance of God-fearing men" when they must have known that John's envoys were at Rome asking the pope to declare it invalid. But this difficulty is removed by a close examination of the letter—the *triplicem formam pacis* cannot have been Magna Carta. Clearly the commissioners are describing events in chronological order. The barons conspired, took up arms, and defied the king against this *triplicem formam pacis*. Then they occupied London "in contempt of the *forma pacis* which the pope had ordained in the presence of and by the consent of their accredited envoys." Now the conspiracy, the taking up arms, the defiance of the king, and the occupation of London all took place before Magna Carta was issued and could hardly be called acts in contempt of it. As a matter of fact the earliest reference to this *forma pacis* is found in Innocent's letter of June 18. There the pope said "unless the said barons within eight days after the receipt of our letters . . . shall accept and carry-out the *formam* described above provided by us

[181] Powicke, "Miramus plurimum," pp. 92-93.
[182] *Ibid.*, pp. 87-88. Richardson, "Morrow of the great charter—addendum," p. 193.

in the presence of their messengers after long deliberation," they were to be excommunicated. Now the *forma* referred to here was clearly repeated from an earlier papal letter that has not survived —one sent before the barons had actually taken up arms. While this letter was much like the missive of March 19, it was not quite the same. The barons were to seek humbly and devoutly to placate the king and were to perform all the services they owed. The king was to grant their just petitions. If the two parties could not agree, the questions at issue were to be settled in the king's court by the barons' peers according to the laws and customs of the realm. This plan was probably presented to Eustace de Vesci and his fellow envoys in March. It was the *triplicem formam pacis* that was "worthy of acceptance by God-fearing men."

The existence of Magna Carta was what embarrassed the commissioners—what made this letter difficult to write. They may have intended to make no reference to it. They certainly gave no indication that the king had agreed to its terms and issued it as a solemn charter. The statement that the barons had "abolished approved customs of the realm and instituted new laws" may have been intended as a reference to Magna Carta, but it could equally well have been meant to describe the activities of the twenty-five barons. I am inclined to think that the plan of the commissioners was simply to ignore Magna Carta and make the activities of the twenty-five barons a continuation of the revolt against John. One thing is clear. If Magna Carta was mentioned in the letter, all who observed it were included in the sentence of excommunication. As I doubt that even Peter des Roches would declare excommunicate all those who observed a royal charter, however obtained, I am forced to the conclusion that there was no reference to it in the letter. The acts of the twenty-five were declared invalid and all who observed them were excommunicated. In short when Pope Innocent wrote the letter of July 7, he knew nothing of Magna Carta and envisaged an England torn by a baronial revolt. The three commissioners made their covering letter fit the conditions that were in the pope's mind.

Stephen Langton refused to obey the papal mandate. He argued that the pope had not understood the situation in England. In this he was clearly right. The very disingenuousness of the commissioners' letter would have been enough to disgust a man of the archbishop's temperament and character. The commissioners promptly suspended him from office, and he departed for Rome to attend the Lateran Council and to bear his story to the pope. Pandulf soon followed him for the same purpose.[183]

Stephen Langton had failed, but he had failed honorably. He had hoped to establish a reign of law in English secular politics. To that end he had persuaded a group of disaffected barons who hated the king and lusted for lands, castles, and privileges to formulate a general program of reform—one that would benefit not only the barons but all the freemen of England. But he could not overcome John's intransigence and the all-consuming greed of the barons. He could neither persuade John to accept the charter sincerely and try to make it work nor induce the barons to be reasonable in their demands for personal benefits. Above all he could not convince either side that the other could be trusted—a rather difficult task as neither side was trustworthy. I cannot feel that Stephen really disobeyed the pope's orders. He had been commanded to excommunicate the barons if they did not make peace with the king. They did make such a peace. The archbishop had left England before the arrival of the papal letters that declared this peace void. As we shall see later there was one respect in which Stephen's conduct was open to question—his delivery to the barons or at least his failure to deliver to the king the Tower of London and the castle of Rochester. As direct military aid to rebels this was unseemly conduct in the primate of all England.

Towards the end of September papal letters dated at Anagni on August 24, 1215, arrived in England. After an extended review of his previous letters to the king, prelates, and barons of England Innocent III solemnly annulled Magna Carta. John had been compelled by force to make an agreement that was not only vile and wicked but illicit and iniquitous. It had diminished and degraded both his rights and his honor. Hence Magna Carta was condemned. If John observed it or the barons sought to oblige

[183] Coventry, II, 225; Wendover, II, 155; Rymer, *Foedera*, I, 139.

him to, they were subject to excommunication.[184] Thus the charter and everything it provided for were condemned. John was absolved from his promises to observe it and the men of his realm from their oaths to obey the twenty-five barons.

Sometime before the arrival of the papal letters annulling Magna Carta open war had broken out once more between the king and the barons. On September 13 John despatched a group of envoys to Rome bearing letters informing Innocent III that his barons were in revolt and asking the pope's aid.[185] Four days later Henry fitz Count was ordered to seize the Cornish lands of Robert fitz Walter.[186] The civil war had begun in earnest.

---

[184] Bémont, *Chartes des libertés,* pp. 41-44.
[185] *Rot. pat.,* p. 182.
[186] *Rot. claus.,* I, 228.

CHAPTER IX

THE CIVIL WAR

THE fortunes of war are determined by three closely interrelated sets of forces—military, political, and economic. In the Middle Ages the materials of war were expensive, but except for one item, war-horses, they were practically indestructible. The making of swords, shields, lances, hauberks, cross-bows, and cross-bow bolts required many hours of skilled labor. When a war broke out, one either had enough arms and armor or one did not—there was little one could do to make up a deficiency. The procuring of war-horses was a serious problem for all mediæval armies and one rarely solved satisfactorily. A heavy loss of horses meant dismounted cavalry. In short expenditure for material while a war was in progress was usually very slight. The costs of war lay in feeding feudal troops and feeding and paying mercenary soldiers. The most valuable of all resources was a reserve of cash or highly negotiable goods such as jewels and silks. Next came the control of the produce of the land. In all these respects King John probably had a decided advantage over his enemies. While in theory every free-born Englishman had the military equipment suited to his station, it seems doubtful that all of them did. But there can be little doubt that John's mercenary troops were adequately armed. In the same way it is hard to believe that small English tenants who were expected to serve as mounted serjeants actually worried too much about always having a good war-horse. John's serjeants usually had two or three on hand at all times. Moreover the king's command of his duchy of Aquitaine opened to him the war-horse markets of southern Europe while his foes had no source of supply outside the realm. Then King John, despite the costs of his Poitevin campaign, still had large reserves of money in his treasuries with additional supplies of jewels and silk cloths. Moreover he controlled throughout the war the most profitable of English industries—the tin mines of Devon and Cornwall. Finally as we shall see he had an enormously valuable resource—strong castles in the midst of his foes' lands. It seems clear that a very large proportion of the revenues from the lands of the rebels was taken for the king's use.[1] The barons held London and must have drawn some profit from it, but it cannot have been a major item in the balance-sheet. The barons probably had another advantage. They certainly did not pay all their troops, and they may not have paid any of them. Nevertheless on balance the economic advantage must have been with King John.

The political forces involved in the war between John and his barons are extremely difficult to evaluate because we have only an inadequate idea of the political mores of the day. It is clear that the king was cordially hated by a fair number of his barons and regarded with dislike by most of the others. His opponents believed that he had violated his solemn promises stated in the great charter. Presumably most of the freemen of England had sworn to obey the twenty-five and to support them in war against the king if he failed to keep his agreements. Yet John was still the crowned and anointed king of England. The importance of this fact is difficult to estimate, but it must have been considerable. Robert de Ros was a rebel baron and one of the twenty-five. At the outbreak of the war between John and the barons in April he was sheriff of Cumberland and custodian of Carlisle castle. On July 24 he was replaced as sheriff by Robert de Vaux, but he kept the castle in his hands. Yet when the king wrote to him in January 1216 to point out that Carlisle had been entrusted to him while he was a loyal vassal, he promptly ordered his constable to deliver it at the king's order, and it was soon surrendered to Robert de Vieuxpont.[2] Thus a rebel lord refused to use against the king a royal castle entrusted to him as John's liege-man. One of Matthew Paris' stories tells how at the siege of Rochester William de Albini refused to allow a cross-bowman to take a shot at

---

[1] See references to *tenseriis* or special taxes taken by the constables of castles from the king's foes. *Rot. pat.*, pp. 166-169; *Rot. claus.*, I, 236, 244, 247, 250, 253. They were important enough to have the returns audited. *Rot. pat.*, p. 167.

[2] *Ibid.*, pp. 150, 163; *Rot. claus.*, I, 246.

the king.[3] The clause in Magna Carta allowing the barons to wage war against John contained the reservation "saving our person, the queen's and those of our children." Moreover every English free man had sworn fidelity to the king against all men. While many a man followed his immediate lord into revolt, the primary obligation was always there. A rebel who returned to his allegiance could never be charged with violation of feudal propriety. Then, as we shall see, John reinforced his position as king and feudal lord by obtaining steadily increasing support from the church. The barons attempted to counteract these influences by declaring Louis of France king of England. But in the face of the papal denunciations and in the absence of any formal coronation Louis' position cannot have been taken very seriously. I doubt very much that the group of great barons who changed sides shortly after Louis' arrival did so because they believed he was a rightful king—they simply misjudged the military situation.

The military situation in September 1215 was decidedly favorable to the king. In the thirteenth century the key to the military control of a country was the possession of its castles—especially the first-class ones. The art of fortification was far in advance of that of siegecraft and a strong castle that was adequately supplied and determinedly defended could hold out for months against a large army with the best siege engines. The garrison of a castle ruled the countryside about it. Only the presence of a field force stronger than the garrison could check its activities. Moreover the holder of a number of castles in a region could quickly create a field army out of their garrisons. In short while a strong army could march at will through a region dominated by hostile castles, only long, expensive, and difficult sieges could reduce them. Once the army had passed, the garrisons controlled the country once more. Moreover an army that had passed through a group of hostile castles always had a potential field army in its rear. This was what Louis of France forgot when he sent a part of his forces north in 1217—and the result was the crushing defeat that ended his hopes of becoming king of England.[4]

[3] Matthew Paris, *Chronica maiora*, II, 626-627.
[4] Painter, *William Marshal*, p. 213.

While it is impossible to make a completely accurate list of the English castles that were in a defensible state at any particular time, I have counted 209 that seem certainly to have been used during the civil war. Of these 72 were royal, 14 episcopal, and 123 baronial. With the exception of Bedford, Carlisle, Colchester, and Hertford, and possibly Rockingham and York all the royal castles were in September 1215 in the hands of men thoroughly loyal to John. Four of the episcopal castles belonged to Peter des Roches' see of Winchester and the three castles of the see of Durham were in the hands of Philip de Ulecotes. Hugh de Welles, bishop of Lincoln, had placed his three fortresses in the king's hands. Giles de Briouse's episcopal stronghold was probably in the hands of a royal custodian in September and certainly was after his death in November. Rochester was the only episcopal castle that was not in the possession of John's partisans. Fifty-one of the baronial castles belonged to barons loyal to the king and seven more belonging to men not in revolt were in John's hands. Twelve castles that belonged to rebel lords were held by royal constables. Only fifty-three baronial castles were in the possession of rebel barons. In short John and his men held 149 castles against 60 held by his foes.

The actual disparity between the two parties in respect to fortresses must have been much greater than these figures indicate. Some of the baronial castles were barely defensible and others were very weak. The castle of Anstey in Hertfordshire was simply the ancient *motte* of the counts of Boulogne refortified to some extent—probably by placing a new stockade on its summit.[5] Freiston in Lincolnshire and Whitwick in Leicestershire were usually called *domi* rather than castles and were probably little more than well-fortified manor houses.[6] Many, perhaps the majority, of the baronial castles had no stone fortifications. While it is impossible to judge with any certainty the condition of most castles in 1215, it seems likely that the rebel barons held no more than twenty formidable fortresses and that very few of these could

[5] *Rot. claus.*, I, 350.
[6] *Ibid.*, p. 13; *Select pleas of the crown* (ed. F. W. Maitland, Selden Society, I), p. 18.

compare in strength with the great royal strongholds. On the other hand some fifty of the royal castles seem to have been first-class fortresses, and the barons loyal to John held many as strong as the best of those in the possession of the rebels.

When one considers men instead of fortresses, the king's advantage appears even greater. During the reigns of Richard and John the greatest baron rarely led more than ten knights to a campaign.[7] Even if one were to assume that actual service was rotated among the baron's vassals, only a part of the knights of England would have had military experience. But it seems far more likely that the barons collected scutage from their vassals and hired knights to follow them to war and that the same men were hired for campaign after campaign. Then there were a fair number of barons who had actually served very few times. In short it is likely that the majority of English knights never got nearer to real fighting than paying their scutage. Among the barons themselves comparatively few had any extensive military experience. Robert fitz Walter, Saher de Quency, William de Mowbray, William de Albini, Roger de Cressi, and Robert de Ros were experienced captains, and they undoubtedly had some tried followers, but the total of trained men must have been small. And it is probable that most of these were in the host sheltered behind the walls of London. In general a baronial castle must have been garrisoned by collecting the free-holders from its lord's fiefs in the neighborhood.[8] On the king's side the picture was very different. His castles were garrisoned by professional soldiers under seasoned captains. He could procure and pay additional mercenary troops. The only group of barons with continuous and extensive military experience, the lords of the Welsh Marches, were loyal to him. Until Prince Louis arrived with his French troops, it was a war of professionals against amateurs.

The outbreak of civil war led quickly to the collapse of the normal local administration in the English shires. The king's government in the various counties was in the hands of the military leaders who might or might not hold the office of sheriff. In the

[7] Mitchell, *Studies in taxation*, pp. 97, 110, 111, 302-303.
[8] Stenton, *English feudalism*, p. 205.

regions where their chief strength lay the barons set up their own local officials. While the only list that we have of these baronial *custodes* probably belongs to the brief period of civil war before the granting of Magna Carta, it is clear that the same system was maintained later.[9] As the course of the war depended largely on the ability, loyalty, and resources of the local leaders of the two parties, it seems best to make a brief survey of England from this point of view.

The king's interests in the far north were in the care of three men—Philip de Ulecotes, Hugh de Balliol, and Robert de Vieuxpont. Although Philip was a creature of King John, he was an Englishman who had married the heiress of a royal serjeant who was apparently hereditary coroner of Northumberland.[10] Philip was an experienced captain of mercenary troops. In the fall of 1215 he was sheriff of Northumberland and custodian of the vacant see of Durham. In his hands were the great royal fortresses of Bamborough and Newcastle-on-Tyne and the episcopal strongholds of Durham and Norham.[11] Hugh de Balliol was the most powerful baron of Northumberland and Durham. He was a loyal supporter of John and acted as second in command to Philip de Ulecotes.[12] In September 1215 Robert de Vieuxpont held only his own barony and its castles—the northern two-thirds of the present county of Westmoreland. Robert was a member of a cadet branch of the Norman house of Vieuxpont. His father, William, had married a sister of the great northern baron Hugh de Moreville.[13] In short while Robert's lordship of Westmoreland dated only from John's grant in 1205, he had fairly deep roots in the region. He was an able and experienced captain and administrator. There is little evidence to indicate who led the rebel forces in the northern shires. Although Walter of Coventry's list

[9] Coventry, II, 224; Richardson, "Morrow of the great charter," pp. 431-432, 443.
[10] *Pipe roll 2 John*, p. 20; *Rot. chart.*, p. 76; *Book of fees*, I, 204, 250.
[11] The grant of the custody of Durham castle and the lands between the Tyne and Tees to Robert de Vieuxpont on August 13, 1215, seems never to have gone into effect. *Rot. claus.*, I, 225.
[12] *Rot. pat.*, p. 186.
[13] *Calendar of charter rolls*, I, 450-451.

of baronial *custodes* gives Robert de Ros as custodian of Northumberland, other evidence shows that in the fall of 1215 he was the custodian of Yorkshire.[14] As Eustace de Vesci was one of the chief baronial leaders and the center of his power lay in Northumberland, it seems likely that he was the rebel commander. His second in command may well have been John fitz Robert of Warkworth. In September 1215 Robert de Ros still held as custodian the royal castles of Cumberland, but it seems clear that he did so through his constables and was not himself resident in the shire. The chief rebel barons of the north-east were Robert de Vaux, titular sheriff of Cumberland, and Gilbert fitz Renfrew, lord of the barony of Kendal that comprised the southern part of modern Westmoreland. Despite the ability of his three captains the situation in the far north must have disturbed John seriously. Cumberland was pretty firmly in rebel hands and the majority of the barons of Northumberland were in revolt. When one remembers that King Alexander of Scotland was one of John's bitterest foes, the gravity of the situation becomes apparent.

In the region between the Tees and the Wash, eastern Yorkshire and Lincolnshire, there was no dominant royal commander. Although William de Harcourt bore the title of sheriff of Yorkshire, he was actually simply the constable of the great fortress of Scarborough and controlled the subsidiary castle of Pickering. Except for the vale of Pickering that was held by these two castles and the count of Aumale's lordship of Holderness with its castle of Skipsea all Yorkshire east of the Ouse seems to have been in rebel hands. The sheriff of Lincolnshire was Walter de Coventry, Earl Ranulf of Chester's seneschal of his barony of Bolingbroke, but as Walter held no castle, he can have been little more than a casual raider of rebel lands. Lincoln castle was held for the king by its hereditary constable, Nichola de la Haye. South of Lincoln was a triangle of fortresses under the command of Philip Marc, the mercenary captain who was sheriff of Nottinghamshire and Derbyshire. These consisted of the royal castle of Nottingham and two strongholds of the see of Lincoln, Newark and Sleaford.

---

[14] Coventry, II, 224; Richardson, " Morrow of the great charter," p. 443.

Still farther to the south the count of Aumale's castle of Bytham and Earl Warren's castle of Stamford strengthened the royal hold on southern Lincolnshire. Coventry names William de Albini whose castle of Belvoir lay in Leicestershire near the Lincolnshire border as baronial custodian of the latter shire, but it seems likely that Gilbert de Ghent whom Louis of France was to create earl of Lincoln was the baronial leader in the county. While Gilbert probably did what he could to fortify the old *motte* at his chief seat, Folkingham, he had no castle of any importance.[15]

West of the region that we have just discussed lay a line of castles commanded by Brian de Lisle. In Yorkshire he held Knaresborough and Boroughbridge, in Derbyshire Bolsover, the Peak and Horsley. Brian was also custodian of the archbishopric of York, but this cannot have been of much military importance. Brian's position must have been extremely uncomfortable. Knaresborough and Boroughbridge were isolated from other royal castles and lay in the midst of a countryside ruled by the rebels. There is reason for believing that they were subject to frequent attacks.[16] In Derbyshire Brian was not so much troubled by rebels as by Earl Ranulf of Chester. Earl Ranulf and his brother-in-law Earl William de Ferrers were masters of the open country in Staffordshire, Derbyshire, and Nottinghamshire and felt that they ought to control the royal castles of the region. In May 1215 John had granted Ranulf Newcastle under Lyme, the chief stronghold of Staffordshire, as a fief.[17] But while the two earls had no great trouble in persuading the king to grant them custody of Bolsover and the Peak, they apparently never persuaded Brian to obey the royal mandates.[18]

Of all the royal commanders north of the Trent Earl Ranulf of Chester was potentially by far the most important. Philip de Ulecotes, William de Harcourt, Philip Marc, and Brian de Lisle were essentially merely super-constables. They commanded groups

---

[15] *Royal and other historical letters illustrative of the reign of Henry II* (ed. W. W. Shirley, Rolls series), I, no. 52.
[16] Richardson, " Morrow of the great charter," p. 443.
[17] *Rot. chart.*, p. 216.
[18] *Rot. pat.*, pp. 153, 188, 192, 193.

of fortresses with their garrisons, but no one of them could muster a field army that was more than a raiding party. While the count of Aumale and Robert de Vieuxpont could undoubtedly draw some troops from their fiefs, they were not among the really great barons of the realm. But Ranulf of Chester could draw from his palatine shire a force of hardy Marcher knights with long experience in warfare to add to the English levies of himself and Earl William de Ferrers. While the other royal commanders could do little more than use their garrisons to plunder rebel lands, Earl Ranulf was in a position to take the offensive against the king's enemies. Moreover as such an offensive would be highly profitable to himself, he was almost certain to conduct it.

The royal castles of Shropshire were held by Thomas de Eardington, sheriff of Shropshire and Staffordshire. He apparently also still had in his hands the strongholds of the Fitz Alan baronies of Clun and Whitchurch that had come into his possession as custodian while William fitz Alan was a minor. Another tried servant of the crown, William de Cantilupe, the seneschal of the household, was sheriff of Warwickshire and Leicestershire, but his chief duty was to act as constable of Kenilworth castle. Leicestershire was largely dominated by rebel fortresses—John de Lacy's Castle Donington, Saher de Quency's castle of Mountsorrel, and the stronghold of Belvoir. The chief power in Warwickshire was its earl. Henry de Beaumont, earl of Warwick, and his father-in-law, Thomas Basset of Headington, held the castle and earldom of Warwick for John. Walter de Clifford, sheriff of Herefordshire, Walter de Beauchamp, sheriff of Worcestershire, and Ralph Musard, sheriff of Gloucestershire, were minor barons loyal to the king. But they too were little more than constables of the chief castles of their shires. The real ruler of these counties was William Marshal, earl of Pembroke. Earl William seems to have acted as a viceroy making grants of rebel lands and concluding treaties with the king's foes.[19] While most of the barons of the Welsh Marches had remained loyal to John, the king's commanders in the region had serious problems. Llywelyn

---

[19] Painter, *William Marshal*, pp. 184, 187.

and other Welsh princes were in alliance with the barons and constituted a continuous threat to the safety of the Marches. Then there were in the region some of John's bitterest foes. The vigorous and colorful Fulk fitz Warin was operating in the region at the head of an armed band. Moreover when the civil war commenced in September, Giles de Briouse was in the rebel party. He made peace with John in October, but died in November.[20] His successor as active head of the family was his younger brother Reginald. Reginald had recently married Llywelyn's daughter and the result was an alliance that was extremely dangerous to the safety of the Marches.[21] Fortunately Earl William Marshal had possession of the Briouse castles in the region after Giles' death and he and Reginald were on personally friendly terms.[22] William made a local treaty with Fulk fitz Warin and it seems likely that he and Reginald had a tacit agreement not to bother each other.[23]

On September 17, 1215, King John tried a bold experiment to secure the loyalty of Cornwall. Henry fitz Count was the illegitimate son of Earl Reginald of Cornwall. King Richard had given him two Devonshire manors that had belonged to his father. John had added several other estates and had granted Henry the escheated barony of Bradninch.[24] Henry fitz Count was an able and vigorous captain who served John well. It must have annoyed him continuously to think that only the bar sinister kept him from ruling the great palatine earldom of Cornwall. When he saw that civil war was inevitable, John appointed Henry sheriff of Cornwall with the promise that when peace was restored he would investigate his rights to the earldom. As Henry clearly had no rights, this promise had little real meaning, and it is fairly certain that John meant it simply as a means of keeping Henry loyal. Henry fitz Count was undoubtedly fully aware of this and

---

[20] *Rot. pat.*, pp. 157, 159.
[21] Painter, *William Marshal*, p. 251.
[22] *Rot. pat.*, p. 159. William's daughter, Eve, married Reginald's son before 1218. Painter, *William Marshal*, p. 281.
[23] *Rot. claus.*, I, 270.
[24] *Book of fees*, I, 97; *Pipe roll 4 John*, p. 250.

decided to have the advantage of possession before peace came. He demanded that the men of Cornwall do homage to him as their lord. Had Henry waited until the arrival of Louis of France made John's position really serious, he might have succeeded. As it was he was removed on November 16 and replaced by Robert de Cardinan, the most powerful of Cornish barons.[25] As he already had the custody of the great barony of Dunster, Henry was a powerful figure in the west throughout the war and remained loyal to the crown, but he never obtained the earldom of Cornwall.[26]

The security of Devonshire was fairly well assured by the loyalty of Henry fitz Count and the two dominant barons of the shire—William de Redvers, earl of Devon, and Robert de Courtenay, lord of Oakhampton. As William de Redvers was too old to take any active part in the war, the shrieval office and the defense of the shire fell to Robert. Dorsetshire and Somersetshire had as their sheriff John Marshal, nephew of Earl William, but the chief royal commander in the region was the constable of the great fortress of Corfe. Corfe was as nearly impregnable as a castle could be and was considered by John to be the safest place in his realm. There he kept his heir and the bulk of his treasure. In November 1215 he placed Corfe under the command of Peter de Maulay.[27] In Wiltshire the king's interests were represented by the sheriff, Earl William of Salisbury, but he had no control over the constables of the castles of Marlborough and Devizes, Hugh de Neville and Thomas de Sanford. While William Brewer was sheriff of Hampshire, the dominant lord in the shire was Peter des Roches and the royal troops were Poitevins under the command of Savaric de Mauleon. Surrey and Sussex were largely in the hands of Peter des Roches and the earls of Arundel and Warren. The sheriff of Berkshire held Wallingford castle, but his authority in the shire was shared by the constable of Windsor. In Kent there was one supreme royal commander—Hubert de Burgh, justiciar of England, sheriff of Kent, and constable of Dover Castle.

North of the River Thames and east of the River Welland lay the chief center of the rebellion. The king's authority was repre-

[25] *Rot. pat.,* pp. 155, 159.   [26] *Rot. claus.,* I, 137.   [27] *Ibid.,* p. 241.

sented by the constables of the scattered royal castles supported by the strongholds of loyal barons. In Northamptonshire the king had Northampton, in Cambridgeshire Cambridge and Wisbech, in East Anglia Norwich and Orford and in Hertfordshire Berkhamsted. In East Anglia he could rely on some assistance from Castle Rising and Buckenham that belonged to the earl of Arundel and from the Warren stronghold of Castle Acre. But these loyal fortresses were isolated. Around them lay the lands of rebel barons and between them were castles in rebel hands. A large part of this region was eventually to form the bailiwick of Fawkes de Bréauté, but in the fall of 1215 there was no general royal commander in the region, and the baronial custodians were far more powerful than the royal sheriffs.

Thus if one looks at England as a whole John's military dominance was secure except in three regions—Cumberland, Yorkshire, and the district north of the Thames and east of the Welland. While his castles in the two latter districts were firmly held, the garrisons were too weak and scattered to do more than plunder the baronial lands in the neighborhood. For offensive action against the enemy's castles they needed aid. In the west Ranulf of Chester and William Marshal could muster field armies strong enough for local offensive action, but they dared not lead their troops far from home. John's great lack was a field army with which to attack the rebellious barons. He had already taken some steps to secure such a force. As early as August 13 Richard Marsh had been despatched to Poitou to raise troops.[28] After the final break with the committee of twenty-five the king sent agents to Flanders and Brabant to enlist additional mercenaries.[29] By September 28 he was momentarily expecting the arrival of the mercenary captain Hugh de Boves with a strong force.[30] Meanwhile the king stayed on the Kentish coast awaiting the arrival of his army.

Early in October King John learned that baronial forces were laying siege to two of the royal castles that formed a cordon

---

[28] *Rot. pat.*, pp. 152-153.
[29] *Histoire des ducs de Normandie*, pp. 152-154.
[30] *Rot. claus.*, I, 229.

around the section of England controlled by the rebels—Oxford and Northampton.[31] At about the same time the king heard that a severe storm had caught at sea a fleet bearing his mercenary troops, and that Hugh de Boves and many of his men had been drowned.[32] On October 2 royal letters patent directed the constables of ten castles to release as many troops as they could spare for field service under Earl William of Salisbury. Two days later similar letters were issued for Fawkes de Bréauté.[33] While it is possible that two field forces were collected from these garrisons —one to relieve Oxford and Northampton and the other to reinforce John in Kent—it seems more likely that John changed his mind and sent Fawkes instead of Earl William on the first of these missions. At any rate it is clear that during the first ten days of October John had very few troops under his command in Kent.

Meanwhile the baronial leaders in London had decided to undertake a cautious offensive. About mid-way between London and Canterbury stood Archbishop Langton's castle of Rochester. Apparently Stephen had agreed to deliver this fortress to a royal custodian to be held until after his return from the Lateran Council in Rome. On August 9 John had directed the archbishop to surrender it to Peter des Roches.[34] But when Stephen left England in mid-September, Rochester was still under the command of Reginald de Cornhill. Although Reginald had originally received Rochester as John's representative while he was sheriff of Kent, he had continued to hold it as Stephen's constable after his loss of the shrievalty, and he was a strong partisan of the rebel barons. Robert fitz Walter decided to take advantage of this situation to seize and garrison Rochester. Although John had apparently been expecting a move of this sort and had been just south of Rochester from September 28 to October 5, the news that a baronial force had left London by the Dover road found him in Dover. The king immediately marched back to Canterbury. There word came to him that the barons had occupied Rochester and had pressed on

[31] Coventry, II, 226.
[32] *Rot. claus.*, I, 230; *Histoire des ducs de Normandie*, p. 157.
[33] *Rot. pat.*, p. 156.
[34] *Ibid.*, p. 181.

as far as Ospring. According to the *Histoire des ducs de Normandie* John then retired to Dover once more, but this seems to be an error. The king seems to have stayed in Canterbury from October 7 to October 9. The chronicler is, however, probably correct in his statement that when the barons learned that John was at Canterbury, they prudently withdrew to Rochester.[35]

During the two days that John spent at Canterbury his mercenary troops began to arrive. The Flemish knights and serjeants commanded by Robert de Bethune had sailed late enough to escape the storm that dispersed the fleet of Hugh de Boves.[36] With these reinforcements the king felt strong enough to begin a limited offensive while he was waiting for the rest of his auxiliaries. On October 9 he marched from Canterbury to Ospring and on the twelfth moved to Gillingham on the coast just east of Rochester. Meanwhile the barons had placed a formidable garrison in Rochester castle. The commander was William de Albini, lord of Belvoir, a close relative of Robert fitz Walter and perhaps the ablest and most experienced captain in the rebel party. With him were William de Lancaster, son and heir of Gilbert fitz Renfrew, Robert Arsic, a minor baron of Kent and Oxfordshire, William de Avranches, a Kentish baron, Thomas de Moulton and Alexander de Pointon, mesne tenants of the honor of Richmond who had won prominence as royal officials, Reginald de Cornhill, Robert de Loveland, hereditary custodian of the royal prison of the Fleet, and many lesser rebel lords. The chroniclers agree that there were about 100 knights in Rochester in addition to serjeants and crossbowmen.[37] As the baronial army was essentially a feudal one, it seems likely that it contained a high proportion of knights and was short of light troops.

From Gillingham John marched along the southern bank of the Medway to Rochester. He found Robert fitz Walter and a party of rebels holding the bridge that carried the London-Dover road over the Medway and a brief skirmish ensued. Apparently the king

---

[35] *Histoire des ducs de Normandie*, p. 157; Wendover, II, 146; Coggeshall, pp. 173-174.

[36] *Histoire des ducs de Normandie*, pp. 154, 158.

[37] *Ibid.*, p. 157; Wendover, II, 146, 151; Coggeshall, p. 176; Coventry, II, 226.

failed to capture the bridge and lost a few men, but he captured Oliver de Argentan. As Oliver's brother, Richard, could not afford to pay the ransom demanded by John, he sought and obtained from his fellow rebels permission to free his brother by joining the royal party.[38] Robert fitz Walter's successful defense of the bridge did not hamper the king in occupying Rochester and the rebel leader soon withdrew to London while John laid formal siege to Rochester castle.

Through the remainder of October and all of November King John and his army pressed their siege of Rochester castle. Although William de Albini had not had time to provision the fortress adequately, he and his men conducted a determined and vigorous defense. The walls were so high and strong that the king's siege engines made little impression and he was obliged to resort to the slow process of mining both the outer walls and the keep. The keep was located in the southeastern corner of the *enceinte*. Apparently John's miners dug a vast series of galleries under the angle of the outer walls and the southeastern corner of the keep. These galleries were shored with wooden beams. When everything was ready, a herd of pigs to which had been tied burning torches was released in the galleries to set fire to the shoring. Even after the corner of the keep had collapsed and admitted John's troops, William de Albini and his men continued to defend the rest of the keep, but eventually they were obliged to surrender. King John was enraged by the garrison's stubborn resistance and announced his intention of hanging every man in the castle, but Savaric de Mauleon persuaded him to change his mind. Savaric pointed out that the war was not over and that the barons might well capture him or some other loyal lord. Savaric had no desire to be hanged.[39] Actually it is hard to believe that John would have hanged the leaders of the garrison. Dead they would be of no use to him while alive they were worth large ransoms.[40]

---

[38] Coggeshall, p. 175.

[39] Wendover, II, 148-151; Coventry, II, 226-227; Coggeshall, pp. 175-176; *Histoire de ducs de Normandie*, p. 163; *Rot. claus.*, I, 231, 234, 238.

[40] Coventry states that John hanged one cross-bowman whom he had nourished from boyhood. Wendover says several cross-bowmen who had

When William de Albini and his companions had entered Rochester castle, the baronial leaders had sworn to relieve them if they were besieged by John. Unless the king and his army were so incredibly careless as to fail to keep watch on the bridge over the Medway, relief of Rochester from London along the Dover road was impossible. A relieving army would have to detour and approach Rochester from Maidstone. Yet on October 26 the baronial forces solemnly marched as far as Dartford along the Dover road. There they learned that the king was coming to meet them and decided that discretion was the better part of valor. They promptly retired to London and left the garrison of Rochester to its fate.[41] It is hard to believe that this march to Dartford was seriously intended as an attempt to relieve Rochester—it seems more likely to have been a mere gesture to relieve the consciences of the rebel chiefs. The only other effort made to save the Rochester garrison was an attempt at doing it by negotiation. On November 9 John issued letters of conduct for Earl Richard de Clare, Robert fitz Walter, Geoffrey de Say, and the mayor of London to hold a conference with Peter des Roches, Hubert de Burgh, and the earls of Arundel and Warren.[42] If this meeting actually took place, it had no result. If the barons made an offer, it may well have been to surrender Rochester castle if the garrison could go free.

During the siege of Rochester the civil war proceeded at a slow pace in the rest of England. King Alexander of Scotland unsuccessfully laid siege to the great border fortress of Norham.[43] Geoffrey de Neville, the chamberlain, and Fawkes de Bréauté roamed the region between Oxford and Lincoln with an armed band. On November 28 Fawkes captured the castle of Hanslope, seat of the Mauduit barony.[44] It seems likely that the royal castle of Rockingham of which William Mauduit was hereditary constable was taken by Geoffrey de Neville at this time.[45] Perhaps

inflicted heavy casualties on the besiegers were hanged. The *Histoire des ducs de Normandie* says no one was hanged. As the author was probably at the siege, this seems the best source.

[41] Coventry, II, 226; Wendover, II, 148-149.
[42] *Rot. pat.*, p. 158.
[43] *Chronica de Mailros*, p. 121.
[44] Wendover, II, 163.
[45] *Rot. pat.*, p. 168.

this same period saw the capture of Earl David of Huntingdon's stronghold of Fotheringay.[46] Fawkes also took Bedford castle from William de Beauchamp.[47]

Day by day as John lay before Rochester he received additional reinforcements of mercenary troops. The influx was on such a large scale that the king appointed a special agent, Brother Roger of the Temple, to pay the passage of the arriving soldiers.[48] By the time Rochester was taken, John had a formidable field army and was ready to move against his rebellious barons. There were obviously two alternative procedures. The king could lay siege to London in the hope of capturing the entire baronial host and thus ending the rebellion at one stroke. As we do not know the number of troops available to John, the size of the army in London or the strength of the city, it is impossible for us to judge whether or not this plan would have been feasible. Certainly in 1217 William Marshal showed no enthusiasm for an attack on London. As the advantages of a direct attack on London must have been as obvious to John as to us, one can only assume that he considered it hopeless. The other alternative was to leave a force to contain the baronial army while he himself reduced the rebels' castles and ravaged their lands. This was the course pursued by John. He left his brother Earl William of Salisbury, Savaric de Mauleon, Fawkes de Bréauté and a strong force of mercenaries to watch London while he himself marched to the north.[49] While the king took with him a body of mercenaries, he was probably relying on the support of such lords as Earl Ranulf of Chester and Robert de Vieuxpont once he reached the regions in which they were operating.

During the first months of the civil war both John and his foes had been active on the political front. On September 13 the king had written to Innocent III announcing that his barons were in open revolt and begging the pope's aid. With these letters he sent a strong group of emissaries—the archbishops of Bordeaux

[46] *Rot. claus.*, I, 247.
[47] Wendover, II, 163.
[48] *Rot. claus.*, I, 234, 236-238; *Rot. pat.*, pp. 158, 160.
[49] Wendover, II, 162-163.

and Dublin, Richard Marsh, his chancellor, the abbot of Beaulieu, three lesser clerics, and John Marshal and Geoffrey Luttrel.[50] Their task was to refute any statements that Stephen Langton or the barons' agents might make against the king and to win for John the full support of the papacy. In this they could undoubtedly rely on the active assistance of Pandulf who seems to have gone to Rome at about the same time. It must have been about a fortnight after the despatching of this embassy that the papal letters of August 25 arrived in England. In these letters Innocent declared Magna Carta void and threatened with excommunication anyone who observed it or sought to have it observed.[51] The effect of these letters on the barons seems to have been slight. They probably hoped that Stephen could persuade the pope of the justice of their cause. This was an idle dream. John's legates were completely successful in Rome. The suspension of Stephen was confirmed; Walter de Gray, one of John's most faithful servants, was elevated to the archbishopric of York; and the pope issued letters excommunicating many rebels by name and authorizing his commissioners to add other names to the list.[52] These last letters were issued on December 16 and must have arrived in England in mid-January. From then on no one could doubt that to be a rebel was to be excommunicate.

While King John was mustering the thunders of Rome, the barons were seeking more mundane aid. As we have seen the king's foes had been in communication with Philip Augustus since as early as 1209. In 1212 there had been rumors afloat that they planned to choose as king of England Philip's vassal and good friend Simon de Montfort. It seems likely that the French king encouraged the rebels in the spring of 1215 and he may well have had agents in England. It is only fair to point out that in following this policy he was only repaying John in his own coin—the English king throughout his reign had negotiated with every baron of France whom he believed might be disaffected. In August 1215 John tried to win over Peter of Dreux, duke of Brittany, by offer-

---

[50] *Rot. pat.*, p. 182.
[51] Bémont, *Chartes des libertés*, pp. 41-44.
[52] Wendover, II, 160-161, 167-171.

ing him the great honor of Richmond.[53] It is impossible to discover just when the negotiations between Philip and the rebel barons began to take definite form, but sometime in September or October they sent a delegation to Philip promising the English throne to the king's son, Louis, if he would come to their aid. While the chroniclers differ as to the composition of the embassy, it probably consisted of Saher de Quency, Geoffrey de Mandeville, and Henry de Bohun.[54] Wendover includes Robert fitz Walter, but it seems unlikely that the titular chief of the baronial party would leave his troops to go to France—or if he did that there would be any baronial army when he got back.[55]

John was fully aware that these negotiations were in progress. He attempted to please Philip by granting the merchants of his land full freedom to trade in England and also sent an embassy to Philip's court.[56] According to Ralph de Coggeshall his final effort was to send the French king forged letters by which the barons of England appeared to state that they had made peace with the king.[57] Such a maneuver would not have troubled John's conscience and he may well have sent the forged letters either to delay or to confuse the negotiations. Philip finally agreed to allow Louis to go to England if the barons would give hostages for their loyalty. Prince Louis immediately proceeded to collect a force of men to reinforce the barons until he himself could cross with his host. During December and January two bodies of French troops crossed the channel and joined the barons in London.[58] Fortunately for John the French knights had no more enthusiasm for fighting than did their English allies and they stayed peacefully in London complaining about the poorness of the wine supply. Nevertheless the arrival of these troops seemed to be a guarantee

---

[53] *Rot. pat.*, p. 152.

[54] *Histoire des ducs de Normandie*, p. 160; Coventry, II, 226; Coggeshall, p. 177; Anonyme de Bethune, *Chronique* (ed. Léopold Delisle in Recueil des historiens des Gaules et de la France, XXIV), p. 770.

[55] *Wendover*, II, 173.

[56] *Rot. pat.*, pp. 154-155; Coggeshall, p. 180.

[57] *Ibid.*, p. 177.

[58] On the preparations of Prince Louis and the first contingents of French knights see Ch. Petit-Dutaillis, *Etude sur la vie et le regne de Louis VIII* (Paris, 1894), pp. 70-96.

that Louis was serious in his intention to invade England and hence must have seriously disturbed King John. Not only would a rival king be of decided political advantage to the barons, but the French knights when vigorously led were excellent soldiers. Once Louis arrived, John would face a formidable field army commanded by the son of the feudal suzerain of many of his own mercenary troops.

King John with his division of the royal army left Rochester on December 6. He then spent ten days in Surrey, Berkshire, and Hampshire while he stowed away in his castles the prisoners taken in Rochester.[59] On December 17 he marched northwards reaching Northampton on the twenty-first, Rockingham on the twenty-third, and Nottingham on the twenty-fourth. The day after Christmas he left Nottingham to begin his campaign against the northern barons. From his manor of Langar he despatched messengers to summon the garrison of Belvoir to surrender. This important stronghold was commanded by one of William de Albini's sons and two of his knights. The king's messengers suggested that if the garrison refused to surrender, the constable of Corfe would forget to supply any food to their captive lord. Nicholas de Albini hastened to Langar and formally surrendered the castle to John. After placing two mercenary captains, the brothers Geoffrey and Oliver de Buteville, in Belvoir, the king turned north to Newark.[60] The capture of Belvoir was an important victory. With Nottingham, Newark, Sleaford, and Lincoln it formed a strong and closely-knit group of royal strongholds controlling a valuable region. From Newark John despatched orders to Roger de Clifford to attack Geoffrey de Mandeville's castle of Hanley in Worcestershire and to Thomas de Eardington to seize and raze Tamworth in Staffordshire.[61] In all probability these were the only baronial castles left to the west of the king's line of march with the possible exception of Mountsorrel.[62]

[59] *Rot. pat.*, p. 161; *Rot. claus.*, I, 241.
[60] Wendover, II, 164; *Histoire des ducs de Normandie*, p. 163.
[61] *Rot. pat.*, p. 162; *Rot. claus.*, I, 244.
[62] Mountsorrel's fate is puzzling. On January 1, William de Cantilupe was ordered to deliver it to a mercenary captain. *Rot. pat.*, p. 162. Later

The Civil War

From Newark John marched to Pontefract in Yorkshire. There he was met by its lord, John de Lacy, constable of Chester, who offered his submission. Earl Ranulf of Chester who had joined the royal host pleaded his constable's cause to such good effect that John forgave the repentant rebel. John de Lacy swore that he would always faithfully serve John and his heirs by Queen Isabel. He would not observe any oath he had made to the king's foes nor would he support any charter declared invalid by the pope. If he failed to remain loyal, he would be disinherited forever. Finally he gave his brother, Roger, as a hostage.[63] About the same time the king also accepted the submission of the most mercurial of all English barons, Roger de Montbegon.[64] As one of the chief purposes of John's campaign was to punish King Alexander of Scotland for his raids into Northumberland, he hastened through Yorkshire leaving its local problems to be settled later. He did, however, write to Robert de Ros commanding him to surrender Carlisle to Roger de Vieuxpont.[65] Ranulf of Chester made a slight detour on the northward march to seize Richmond castle.[66] In all probability Middleham castle was surrendered to the earl at about the same time.[67]

King Alexander had advanced deeply into England and had burned the town of Newcastle-on-Tyne, but on learning of John's approach he withdrew hastily into Scotland. The English king captured Berwick, plundered the Scots marches in the vicinity, burned Berwick and retired southward to Newcastle.[68] In his marches through the Northumbrian coastal region he captured the

reference is made to a man taken there. *Rot. claus.,* I, 249. Yet Wendover lists it as one of the two castles still in baronial hands when John returned from the north. Wendover, II, 167. It was certainly in possession of its lord, Saher de Quency, in 1217.

[63] *Histoire des ducs de Normandie,* p. 163; Rymer, *Foedera,* I, 137.
[64] *Rot. claus.,* I, 244-245.
[65] *Rot. pat.,* p. 163.
[66] *Ibid. Rot. claus.,* I, 245.
[67] Middleham is not mentioned until February 17 but its lord made submission on January 9 at the same time as the constable of Richmond. *Ibid.,* pp. 245, 248.
[68] *Histoire des ducs de Normandie,* pp. 163-164; Wendover, II, 166; Coventry, II, 229.

baronial castles of the district—Mitford, Morpeth, Wark, Alnwick and probably Warkworth.[69] Farther south Henry de Neville surrendered his castle of Brancepeth in Durham.[70] Moreover Gilbert fitz Renfrew came to John in Northumberland and made his submission in the same terms as John de Lacy. Gilbert gave ten hostages and surrendered his two castles.[71] About this same time the constable of Carlisle under orders from his lord, Robert de Ros, delivered that fortress to Robert de Vieuxpont. On January 31 Robert de Vieuxpont was given custody of the lands of Robert de Vaux.[72] Thus Robert de Vieuxpont had firm control of all Westmoreland and Cumberland. The only castle not in his hands was the count of Aumale's stronghold of Cockermouth. To further strengthen the royalist grip on the north Ranulf of Chester was appointed sheriff of Lancashire with the custody of its castles.[73]

On February 7 John arrived before Peter de Bruce's castle of Skelton. As he stayed there four days, it seems likely that the garrison put up some resistance, but it cannot have been very determined.[74] The king then moved on southwards through Yorkshire and Lincolnshire reaching Bedford on February 29. He left behind as sheriff of Yorkshire and custodian of the castles of Scarborough, Pickering, and York one of his ablest, most experienced, and most trusted servants, Geoffrey de Neville, the chamberlain.[75] The king's northern campaign had been highly successful. A contemporary chronicler states that the only rebel castle left in the north was Robert de Ros' stronghold of Helmsley, and there seems to be no reason for doubting this statement.[76] Moreover he had levied heavy penalties on those who had shown favor to the rebels. The citizens of York and Beverley paid a total of £2,000 for his forgiveness.[77] Finally he had plundered and ravaged the lands of his foes in a thoroughly ruthless and efficient manner.[78] Two of the twenty-five barons, John de Lacy and Roger

---

[69] *Rot. claus.*, I, 246; *Chronica de Mailros*, p. 122.
[70] *Rot. oblatis*, p. 572.
[71] *Rot. chart.*, p. 221; *Rot. claus.*, I, 246.
[72] *Ibid.*, pp. 246, 247.
[73] *Rot. pat.*, p. 164.
[74] *Ibid.*, p. 167.
[75] *Ibid.*, p. 165.
[76] Wendover, II, 167.
[77] *Rot. oblatis*, pp. 569, 570-572, 574.
[78] Wendover, II, 165-167.

de Montbegon had made their peace while a third, Robert de Ros, had made gestures in that direction.[79]

Earl William of Salisbury, Savaric de Mauleon, and Fawkes de Bréauté whom John had left to contain the baronial army in London soon came to the conclusion that their foes had no intention whatever of leaving the city walls. Hence they decided on a plundering expedition into Essex and East Anglia. They ravaged the lands of the king's foes from the suburbs of London to the Wash. The mercenary troops under command of Walter Buc seem to have been peculiarly effective in persuading the people of the countryside to give up their movable property through the use of ingenious tortures. Although Savaric laid siege to two castles, Pleshy and Colchester, he does not seem to have captured either of them.[80] But two of Earl William's captains, William Talbot and Robert de Burgate, went on a private expedition that eventually led them to Doncaster in southern Yorkshire.[81] On the way they captured the south Lincolnshire castles of Moulton and Frampton.[82] At the close of their trip they turned over to John 450 marks of *tenseriis* from the lands of his foes.[83]

Early in March John moved into the eastern shires to complete their subjugation. He took Framlingham, the chief castle of Earl Roger Bigod, Castle Hedingham, the seat of Earl Robert de Vere, and the royal castle of Colchester.[84] In the latter fortress he found a mixed French and English garrison as it had been reinforced from London at the time of Savaric de Mauleon's abortive siege. The French were allowed to return to London, but the English troops were held for ransom. When the French arrived in London, the barons charged them with betraying their English companions and threatened to hang them all, but they were finally persuaded to leave the affair to be settled by Prince Louis.[85] The relations be-

[79] *Rot. pat.*, p. 165.
[80] Wendover, II, 163, 171-172; Coggeshall, pp. 176-178.
[81] *Rolls of the justices in eyre for Yorkshire in 3 Henry III* (ed. D. M. Stenton, Selden Society, LVI), pp. 208-209.
[82] *Rot. pat.*, pp. 164, 167.
[83] *Ibid.*, p. 169.
[84] *Histoire des ducs de Normandie*, p. 163; Coventry, II, 229; Coggeshall, pp. 179-180.
[85] *Ibid.*, p. 180.

tween the French and English in London had already been strained early in the month when Geoffrey de Mandeville, earl of Gloucester and Essex, had been killed in a tournament by a French knight.[86] The Colchester affair aggravated the mutual ill-will. According to the *Histoire des ducs de Normandie* Earl Robert de Vere made submission to John during this campaign.[87] Certainly he, Earl Roger Bigod, and Earl Richard de Clare entered into negotiations with the king.[88]

At the beginning of April 1216 only the walls of London and the prospective arrival of Prince Louis stood between the baronial party and complete destruction. Except for a few isolated strongholds all the castles of England were either razed or occupied by royal garrisons. The lands of the rebels had been thoroughly ravaged by John's mercenary troops. Moreover the mercenary captains and the Englishmen loyal to the king had been given the custody of the estates of the rebellious lords and were collecting their revenues. Thus Savaric de Mauleon had the custody of the lands of Geoffrey de Mandeville while Robert de Bethune enjoyed those of Earl Richard de Clare.[89] If it had not been for Louis of France, John could simply have sat before London until his barons made their submission. But Prince Louis was a serious menace. He was considered an energetic and able captain. Under his command the knights of France could be expected to earn to some extent at least their reputation for being the best warriors of western Europe. Moreover many of John's mercenaries came from his lands, and it was doubtful whether they would fight against their natural lord. Faced with this situation King John made two moves. He tried to persuade his barons to make peace before Louis arrived, and he made what preparations he could to meet the threatened invasion. On April 14 at Reading John issued two sets of letters close. Letters to all the ports of the eastern and southern coasts between the Wash and Lands End directed that all available

---

[86] *Ibid.*, p. 179; Wendover, II, 176; *Histoire des ducs de Normandie*, p. 164.
[87] *Ibid.*, p. 165.
[88] *Rot. pat.*, pp. 169, 171, 172.
[89] *Ibid.*, p. 161. *Rot. claus.*, I, 251; *Histoire des ducs de Normandie*, pp. 163, 165.

ships be concentrated at the mouth of the Thames.[90] Other letters directed the sheriffs of England to proclaim safe-conducts for all rebels to make peace within a month after Easter. Those who failed to take advantage of this opportunity were to be disinherited.[91]

While King John was mustering his resources to repel Prince Louis, his ecclesiastical allies were not idle. On Easter day the pope's commissioners directed Geoffrey de Buckland, dean of St. Martin's, the chapters of St. Paul's and St. Martin's, and the convent of Holy Trinity to proclaim the excommunication of the rebel barons in London and of the French troops that had already arrived.[92] Moreover there arrived in France about this same time the Legate Gualo who had been despatched by the pope to prevent French interference in the English civil war. On April 24 Gualo met with Philip Augustus and his son at Melun to discuss the matter. It is useless to go into the involved and specious arguments advanced by Prince Louis to establish his claim to the English throne. As we have seen, the fact that just before his death Richard clearly considered John his heir is sufficient answer to the charge that the latter was disinherited by the judgment of his peers in his brother's court. And any condemnation of John by the court of Philip Augustus could have no effect on his right to the English throne. The only argument that had any force was that John had forfeited his throne by breaking the promises made to his barons and that was unlikely to impress the legate. As a matter of fact Louis' claim was hopelessly feeble. Even if John had been disinherited by Richard, Louis was not the latter's heir—he was simply the husband of a daughter of one of Richard's sisters. If John was not the rightful king, then the true queen of England was Eleanor of Brittany, sister of Arthur, who was wearing her life away in an English prison. Gualo refused to accept Louis' arguments and left Melun threatening to excommunicate him if he invaded England. Gualo himself departed for the island kingdom to lend his support to King John.[93]

[90] *Rot. claus.*, I, 270.   [91] *Ibid.*   [92] Wendover, II, 174-175.
[93] *Ibid.*, pp. 176-180; Rymer, *Foedera*, I, 140; *Coventry*, II, 229; Petit-Dutaillis, *Louis VIII*, pp. 72-95.

King John spent the last ten days of April and the first three weeks of May in Kent awaiting the invasion. He probably felt fairly confident that the great fleet he had massed in the Thames could destroy Prince Louis' squadron. But fortune was against him. On the evening of May 18 a storm arose that wrecked many of John's ships and entirely dispersed his fleet.[94] Louis took to his ships on May 20 and reached the English coast unopposed.[95] On May 22 King John marched to Sandwich in the apparent intention of resisting Louis' landing or at least fighting a battle once he was ashore. But the risk was too great. Many of John's mercenaries came from France and their pay was in arrears. If they went over to Louis, one battle might decide the fate of England. The king retired along the coast to Dover. There he heavily reinforced the garrison with some of his best mercenary troops. He himself then withdrew towards Winchester.[96]

Louis and his army advanced rapidly through Kent taking the castles of Canterbury and Rochester. While he was besieging the latter castle a group of English barons arrived from London to do him homage. On June 2 Louis reached London where he was enthusiastically received by the citizens, clergy, and soldiers. There he received the homage of the rest of the rebel lords. On June 6 he marched from London against Earl Warren's castle of Reigate which he found empty. He then moved on to take Guildford and Farnham. On June 14 the French prince captured the city of Winchester and laid siege to its castles. Meanwhile King John withdrew steadily westward. By the time the two castles in Winchester had surrendered, he was at his stronghold of Corfe. Louis on his side proceeded to capture the castles of Porchester and Odiham.[97]

The arrival of Prince Louis, John's retirement before him, and his victories had an immediate political effect. As Louis lay in Winchester, the earls of Salisbury, Arundel, and Warren and the

[94] *Histoire des ducs de Normandie,* p. 168.
[95] *Ibid.,* Wendover, II, 180; Coventry, II, 229.
[96] *Histoire des ducs de Normandie,* pp. 169-170; Wendover, II, 180; Coventry, II, 229.
[97] *Histoire des ducs de Normandie,* pp. 171-174; Coventry, II, 229-230; Wendover, II, 182; Coggeshall, pp. 181-182.

count of Aumale made their submission to him.[98] This must have been a stunning blow to King John. These four men controlled thirteen castles and had some four hundred and thirty knightly vassals. At about the same time Warin fitz Gerold, one of the chamberlains of the exchequer and lord of a castle and over a hundred knights' fees, joined the French prince.[99] The desertion by his half-brother, Earl William of Salisbury, whom he had always trusted and favored must have been peculiarly humiliating to the king. Then while Louis was besieging Odiham Hugh de Neville sent word that he was ready to surrender Marlborough to him. A party under the command of Robert of Dreux was promptly sent to Marlborough and Hugh delivered the stronghold to it.[100] Finally John fitz Hugh went over to Louis.[101] While the loss of the great earls was the more serious politically, the defection of these two trusted intimates must have been a severe personal blow to John.

After his capture of Odiham, Prince Louis returned to London. He apparently felt that it would be well to consolidate his hold on the southeastern shires before adventuring farther afield. He did, however, send young William Marshal to Worcester to take advantage of the defection of Walter de Beauchamp, sheriff of Worcestershire. William occupied the town of Worcester, but this impertinence was too much for his father. The earl of Pembroke ordered his son to move out, and the young Marshal retired just as a royalist force under Earl Ranulf of Chester reached the city.[102] William Marshal could view with equanimity a son in the rebel camp and might even consider it prudent to have the family well entrenched in both parties, but he would not have his son seizing towns in his own bailiwick. Soon Walter de Beauchamp had been brought to penitence by his Marcher neighbors and was back in the royal camp.[103] Meanwhile Louis had left London,

[98] *Histoire des ducs de Normandie*, p. 174.
[99] *Rot. claus.*, I, 277; *Rot. pat.*, p. 190.
[100] *Histoire des ducs de Normandie*, pp. 175-176.
[101] *Rot. claus.*, I, 277.
[102] *Annals of Worcester*, p. 406; Painter, *William Marshal*, pp. 187-188.
[103] *Rot. claus.*, I, 280.

marched into Kent, and laid siege to Dover. Another force under the count of Nevers was sent to invest Windsor.[104]

King John spent the months of July and August in the western part of his realm wandering from Corfe on the Dorset coast to Shrewsbury and back to Corfe again. Meanwhile the rebel barons attempted to shake the royalist hold on the English shires. Prince Louis created Gilbert de Ghent earl of Lincoln and sent him off to reduce the chief castle of his shire. Gilbert took the town without great difficulty, but the castle held out against him—in fact Gilbert was to spend the rest of the war besieging Lincoln castle until he was captured in the battle that ended the siege.[105] King Alexander of Scotland with a strong force marched all the way across England to meet Louis at Dover, but after he lost his brother-in-law and ally, Eustace de Vesci, in an attack on Barnard Castle, he left the royalist strongholds alone.[106] Except for the capture of the comparatively weak royal castle of Cambridge by a baronial force none of the fortresses held by John's partisans seem to have fallen.[107] The general statements of the chroniclers have to be looked at carefully. Thus Roger of Wendover states that Alexander of Scotland subjected the whole county of Northumberland except the castles held by Philip de Ulecotes and Hugh de Balliol.[108] As these two captains had all the castles in the shire, Alexander can have done little more than march through a respectful countryside.

Early in September King John at the head of an army collected from his garrisons moved eastward to commence a new offensive.[109] He seems to have at first intended to raise the siege of Windsor and approached as close as Reading, but his force was probably not very strong and he decided against an open battle with the count of Nevers and his army. Instead he made a rapid plundering expedition into Essex and Suffolk. But the count of Nevers and his followers were heartily tired of their fruitless siege. They decided to try to cut off John. As the attempt was made with little energy,

---

[104] *Histoire des ducs de Normandie,* p. 177; Wendover, II, 191-193; Coventry, II, 230.
[105] Wendover, II, 190.
[106] *Ibid.,* pp. 193-194.
[107] *Ibid.,* p. 192.
[108] *Ibid.,* p. 191.
[109] *Rot. pat.,* p. 194.

the king easily avoided his foes and marched north to drive Gilbert de Ghent away from Lincoln. Nevers marched to Dover to join Louis.[110] The chroniclers suggest that the count was bribed by John. While he was a nobleman of highly dubious reputation and may well have betrayed his lord, no such hypothesis is necessary to explain his actions. Windsor was a first-rate fortress commanded by an able captain, Engelard de Cigogné, and its reduction was probably beyond the power of the force commanded by the count. Moreover a large part of his army consisted of English barons who never showed any inclination for determined action.

John stayed in Lincolnshire until October 4 and then swept south once more into Norfolk. This too was a mere plundering raid and by October 11 he was headed north once more. He took sick at the abbey of Swineshead in southern Lincolnshire and on October 19 died in the bishop of Lincoln's fortress of Newark. With him were his old friend Peter des Roches, three Marcher lords, and John Marshal. Some days later he was buried in the cathedral church of St. Wulstan in Worcester.

On October 10 King John gave Margaret de Lacy, wife of Walter de Lacy and daughter of William de Briouse, permission to clear three carucates of land in the royal forest of Acornbury to found a religious house for the salvation of the souls of William de Briouse, Matilda his wife, and William his eldest son.

---

[110] Wendover, II, 193.

INDEX

Aaron, Joseph, 141.
Aaron of Lincoln, 29, 141.
Abergavenny, lordship of, 22, 41-43, 239.
Abingdon, abbot of, 134.
Acornbury, priory of, 377.
Adams, G. B., "Innocent III and the great charter," 342.
Aid, 16, 53, 215.
Ailsbury, manor of, 39, 282, 331.
Albini, Aveline de, sister of Earl William of Arundel, wife of William de Montchesney and Geoffrey fitz Peter, 35-36. *See also,* Essex, countess of.
Albini, Gunnora de, wife of Nicholas de Stutville, 257.
Albini, Nicholas de, son of William III of Belvoir, 368.
Albini, Nigel de, 333.
Albini, Philip de, 329, 337.
Albini, Ralph de, brother of William II of Belvoir, 257.
Albini, William III de of Belvoir, 48, 122, 142, 208, 242, 273, 289, 291-292, 294, 296, 300, 309, 338, 344, 350, 353, 356, 362, 364, 368.
Alburbury, manor of, 49.
Alençon, count of, Robert, 148.
Alnwick, castle of, 252, 272, 370.
Alpesia, damoiselle, 235.
Alveston, manor of, 49.
Amercements, 111, 121, 223.
Andres, William of, *Chronica,* 191.
Angers, bishop of, 154.
Angers, castle of, 9, 131.
Anjou, barons of, 3.
Anjou, county of, 1, 2, 8-10, 112, 115, 131, 159.
Anjou, law of succession in, 1-2.
Annales Cambriae, 245.
Annals of Burton, 186.
Annals of Dunstaple, 134.
Annals of Margam, 5.
Annals of Osney, 184.
Annals of St. Edmunds, 229.
Annals of Tewkesbury, 184.
Annals of Waverley, 131.
Annals of Winchester, 191.
Annals of Worcester, 185.
Anstey, castle of, 352.
Anstey, Hubert de, 34.
Aquitaine, duchess of, *see* England, queen of, Eleanor of Aquitaine.
Aquitaine, duchy of, 1-2.
Archives de missions scientifiques et littéraires, 253.
Arcy, Norman de, 220.
Argences, Richard de, 149.
Argentan, Oliver de, 363.
Argentan, Richard de, 363.
Arras, bishop of, 182.
Arsic, Robert, 220, 362.
Articles of the barons, 300, 311-318, 320.
Arundel, castle of, 21.
Arundel, earl of, William I de Albini, 111.
Arundel, earl of, William III de Albini, 20-21, 35, 178, 194, 213, 230, 290, 297, 305, 337, 359-360, 364, 374.
Ashbourne, manor of, 26.
Athies, Gerard de, 120, 123, 206, 243-245, 265, 275, 324.
Aumale, count of, Baldwin de Bethune, 24, 40-41, 130, 295.
Aumale, count of, William I de Fortibus, 41, 235.
Aumale, count of, William II de Fortibus, 235, 252, 288, 292, 294-295, 309, 330, 355-357, 370, 375.
Aumale, count of, William le Gros, 330.
Aumale, countess of, Hawise, 24, 40, 113, 219, 235.
Avranches, castle of, 27.
Avranches, William de, 362.
Axholme, isle of, 23.
Axminster, manor of, 77.

Bacon, Roger, 258.
Ballard, Adolphus, *Borough charters,* 124.
Balliol, Hugh de, 252, 354, 376.
Balon, John de, 220.
Bamborough, castle of, 265, 354.

Bampton, barony of, 71.
Bampton, Juliana de, wife of William Painel I of Bampton, 74.
Bardolf, Doun, 71.
Bardolf, Hugh, 10, 13, 45, 71-73, 92.
Barking, abbey of, 281.
Barnard Castle, castle of, 252, 376.
Barnstaple, barony of, 22, 38, 42-43, 45, 99, 309.
Baronial conspiracies, 33, 54, 190, 250, 253-255, 267-270.
Baronial custodians of shires, 334, 353, 355-356.
Baronial party, 1215-1216, 286-299.
Baronial revolt of 1173-1174, 11, 12, 14, 23, 32.
Barons: debts of to crown, 44, 73, 225, 258, 307; desires of, 13-14, 303; grievances of, 13-14, 203-204, 206, 217-218, 220, 229, 256, 258, 276; "northerners," 257, 280, 288, 294, 309, 314; program of, 276, 301, 303; resources of, 19; the twenty-five, 207, 213, 243, 273, 325, 338-339, 340, 341.
Basset, Ralph, 73.
Basset, Thomas, 7, 119, 357.
Bassingbourn, John de, 269.
Bath, bishop of, Jocelin de Welles, 175, 177-179, 182, 300, 338-339.
Bath, see of, 174.
Bayeux, city of, 159.
Bayford, manor of, 67.
Beauchamp, Simon de, of Bedford, 59, 292.
Beauchamp, Walter de, of Elmley, 357, 375.
Beauchamp, William de, of Bedford, 59, 220, 280, 289-290, 292, 302, 308, 365.
Beauchamp, William de, of Elmley, 44, 239.
Beauchamp of Somersetshire, barony of, 85.
Beaufort-en-Vallee, 9.
Beaulieu, abbey of, 54, 153.
Beaulieu, abbot of, Hugh, 168-169, 173, 176-178, 181-182, 189, 366.
Beaumont, Henry II de, see Warwick, earl of.
Beaumont, Isabel de, sister of Robert III, earl of Leicester, wife of Simon III de Montfort, 34.
Beaumont, Margaret de, sister of Robert III, earl of Leicester, wife of Saher II de Quency, 32.
Beaumont, Robert I de, see Leicester, earl of.
Beaumont, Robert II de, see Leicester. earl of.
Beaumont, Robert III de, see Leicester, earl of.
Beaumont, Roger de, brother of Robert III de, see St. Andrews, bishop of.
Beaumont, Waleran de, see Warwick, earl of.
Beaumont, William de, see Warwick, earl of.
Bedford, castle of, 59, 302, 308, 352, 365.
Belvoir, castle of, 48, 289, 356-357, 368.
Bémont, Charles, *Chartes des libertés*, 341.
Benington, castle of, 259, 269.
Berkeley, Robert de, 289, 296.
Berkhamsted, castle of, 39, 360.
Berkhamsted, honor of, 39, 282, 331.
Berwick, town of, 369.
Bethune, Alice de, daughter of Baldwin de, wife of William Marshal the younger, 41.
Bethune, Anonyme de, *Chronique*, 367.
Bethune, Baldwin de, son of Robert V de Bethune, advocate of Arras, see Aumale, count of.
Bethune, Robert de, 309, 362, 372.
Bethune, William de, 309.
Beverley, citizens of, 157, 370.
Bigod, Hugh, brother of Earl Roger, 21.
Bigod, Hugh, son of Earl Roger, 292, 295.
Bigod, Roger, see Norfolk, earl of.
Binham, priory of, 259, 260.
Biset, Henry, wife of, 234.
Blisworth, manor of, 73.
Bohun, Henry de, see Hereford, earl of.
Bohun, Humphrey I de, 40, 210, 263.
Bolebec, Walter de, 24.
Bolingbroke, barony of, 355.
Bolsover, castle of, 356.
Bonet, John, 119.

Book of fees, 13.
Bordeaux, archbishop of, 365.
Boroughbridge, castle of, 335, 356.
Botereaux, William de, 119.
Boulogne, count of, Reginald de Dammartin, 149, 188, 192, 194, 228, 265, 285.
Boulogne, honor of, 34, 75.
Bourn, barony of, 68.
Bouvines, battle of, 228.
Boves, Hugh de, 265, 268, 336, 360-362.
Bracton's note book, 40.
Bradninch, barony of, 38, 74, 358.
Brakelond, Jocelin de, 101.
Bramber, castle of, 41.
Bramber, rape of, 22, 41-42.
Brancepeth, castle of, 370.
Branchester, John de, 79-80.
Braybrook, Henry de, son of Robert de, 268, 287, 302, 307, 329.
Braybrook, Robert de, 122, 268.
Bréauté, Fawkes de, 87, 218, 241, 243, 265, 304, 307, 324, 336, 360-361, 364-365, 371.
Brecon, archdeacon of, *see* Giraldus Cambrensis.
Brecon, lordship of, 22, 41-44, 239.
Breton, Guillaume le: *Gesta Philippe Augusti*, 191; *Philippidos*, 191.
Brewer, Alice, 72, 78.
Brewer, Isabel, daughter of William the elder, wife of Baldwin Wac, 78.
Brewer, Richard, son of William the elder, 78.
Brewer, William, 10, 31, 35, 71-78, 80, 87, 92, 97, 107, 109, 119-120, 123, 178, 194, 197, 205-206, 228, 230, 233, 242, 260, 281, 284, 303, 359.
Brewer, William, the younger, 72, 78, 85.
Bridgewater, castle of, 77.
Bridgewater, manor of, 74, 77.
Brinklow, castle of, 23.
Brinklow, manor of, 30.
Briouse, Annora de, daughter of William III de, wife of Hugh de Mortimer, 239.
Briouse, Giles de, son of William III de, *see* Hereford, bishop of.
Briouse, John de, son of William III de, 45.

Briouse, John de, son of William IV de, 331.
Briouse, Margaret de, daughter of William III de, wife of Walter de Lacy, 45, 377.
Briouse, Matilda de, wife of William III de, 230, 236, 242-250, 377.
Briouse, Philip de, son of William I de, 41.
Briouse, Philip de, brother of William II de, 42.
Briouse, Reginald de, son of William III de, 43, 243, 247-249, 358.
Briouse, William I de, 41.
Briouse, William II de, son of Philip de, 41-42.
Briouse, William III de, son of William II de, 7, 22, 28, 37, 41-47, 55, 70-71, 85, 123, 155, 188, 205-206, 221, 225, 228, 238-250, 254, 258, 264, 277, 291, 293, 377.
Briouse, William IV de, son of William III de, 28, 46, 236, 243, 245, 247-250, 331, 377.
Bristol, castle of, 238, 283, 329.
Bristol, town of, 144, 215, 284.
Brito, Walter, 78.
Brittany, duchess of, Constance, 3-4, 8, 13, 20-21, 26-27.
Brittany, duchess of, Eleanor, 373.
Brittany, duchy of, 3-6.
Brittany, duchy of, barons of, 3-5.
Brittany, duke of, Arthur Plantagenet, 1-11, 17, 26-27, 44, 54, 85, 163, 229, 236-237, 249-250.
Brittany, duke of, Conan IV, 3.
Brittany, duke of, Geoffrey Plantagenet, 1, 3-4.
Brittany, duke of, Guy de Thouars, 26-27.
Brittany, duke of, Peter of Dreux, 366.
Bruce, Peter de, 221, 288, 292, 294, 296, 370.
Bruges, castellan of, Adam Keret, 265.
Brunswick, Otto of, *see* Emperor, Holy Roman.
Buc, Walter, 371.
Buckby, manor of, 32.
Buckenham, castle of, 21, 360.
Buckingham, town of, 331.
Buckland, Geoffrey de, 82, 282, 292, 373.

Buckland, William de, 82, 292.
Burdels, Hawise de, 234.
Burgate, Robert de, 247, 371.
Burgh, Geoffrey de, brother of Hubert de, 270-271.
Burgh, Hubert de, 25, 30-31, 44-45, 48, 62, 82, 84-86, 92, 107, 122-123, 229, 238, 249, 274, 288, 307-308, 328-329, 337, 359, 364.
Burgh, Thomas de, brother of Hubert de, 107.
Burgh, William de, brother of Hubert de, 44-45, 85.
Buron, barony of, 77.
Burton, manor of, 33.
Bury St. Edmunds, abbey of, 144, 285, 315.
Buteville, Geoffrey de, 368.
Buteville, Oliver de, 368.
Bytham, castle of, 356.

Cainhoe, barony of, 163.
Caldecot, castle of, 262.
Calendar of ancient deeds, 36.
Calendar of charter rolls, 35.
Calendar of documents relating to Ireland, 187.
Calendar of inquisitions post mortem, 294.
Calendar of liberate rolls, 232.
Cambridge, castle of, 360, 376.
Camera, Simon de, 79. *See also*, Chichester, bishop of.
Cammel, honor of, 25.
Canfield, castle of, 24.
Canterbury, archbishop of, Hubert Walter, 3, 10-12, 15, 39, 54-55, 60-64, 70, 79, 93-95, 97, 104, 144, 156-157, 161-164, 178, 184, 228, 335-336.
Canterbury, archbishop of, Stephen Langton, 171-174, 177-182, 185-186, 190-192, 194-196, 198-199, 230, 255, 274-277, 279, 280, 300-301, 303-305, 309, 311, 314-315, 318, 323, 326, 334, 337-339, 342-347, 361, 366.
Canterbury, archbishop of, Thomas Becket, 38.
Canterbury, castle of, 374.
Canterbury, province of, suffragans of, 164-166.
Canterbury, Gervase of: *Actus pontificum*, 64; *Gesta regum*, 47.

Cantilupe, Fulk de, 171-173.
Cantilupe, William de, 45, 84, 87, 119, 121, 231, 357, 368.
Canville, Gerard de, 56, 59, 81, 84, 174, 221.
Canville, Richard de, son of Gerard de, 150.
Cardigan, castle of, 37, 238, 241.
Cardinan, Robert de, 290, 359.
Carisbrooke, castle of, 22, 31.
Carlisle, castle of, 350, 352, 369-370.
Carrick, Duncan of, 248.
Cartae antiquae rolls, 26.
Cartae antiquae rolls, 15.
Cartulary of Oseney abbey, 64.
Carucage, 113, 125, 128-129, 156-157.
Castle Acre, castle of, 21, 360.
Castle Baynard, castle of, 269.
Castle Elmley, castle of, 44.
Castle Goodrich, castle of, 37, 238.
Castle Hedingham, castle of, 24, 371.
Castle Rising, castle of, 21, 360.
Castlecarrock, Robert de, 258.
Castles: baronial, 19, 352-353, 371-372; building and repair of, 26, 265; royal, 26, 108-109, 265, 350-357.
Causton, manor of, 85.
Cazel, Fred A., Jr., "The marriage of Isabelle of Angoulême," 48.
Chacombe, Hugh de, 121, 135.
Chamber, the king's, 67, 83-87, 103, 110; chief clerk of, 65, 86, 103. *See also*, Lucy, Philip de; Marsh, Richard; Cornhill, William de.
Chamberlain of the household, 84-87, 103. *See also*, Burgh, Hubert de; Neville, Geoffrey de.
Chamberlain of London, 88, 137. *See also*, Cornhill, Reginald de.
Chamberlains of the exchequer, 59, 67. *See also*, Fitz Gerold, Warin; Mauduit, Robert.
Champagne, countess of, Blanche of Navarre, 159.
Chancelis, Andrew de, 324.
Chancelis, Guy de, 324.
Chancelis, Peter de, 324, 329, 337.
Chancellor, of England, 62-65, 67. *See also*, Walter, Hubert; Grey, Walter de; Marsh, Richard.
Chancery, 67, 94-106; rolls of, 96-106, 207-208; senior clerks of, 63, 65, 78-

79, 80, 83, *see also*, Grey, John de; Camera, Simon de; Branchester, John de; Welles, Hugh de; Welles, Jocelin de; Marsh, Richard; Neville, Ralph de.

Charter of liberties, of Henry I, 217, 220, 286, 300, 303, 312, 327.

Charter of liberties, the great, of 1215, *see* Magna carta.

Charter of liberties, the great, reissue of 1216, 319.

Charter of liberties, the "unknown," 279, 303, 311-315, 317, 323.

Chateau-Gaillard, 23, 32, 39.

Chatillon, Guy de, 107.

Chemillé, William de, 141.

Cheney, C. R.: "King John and the papal interdict," 175; "The alleged deposition of King John," 191.

Chesney, Margery de, wife of Hugh de Cressi and Robert fitz Roger, 219, 251.

Chester, bishop of, Geoffrey Muscamp, 65, 164, 172, 184.

Chester, bishop of, William de Cornhill, 200, 306, 308, 338-339.

Chester, county of, 20, 304.

Chester, earl of, Hugh II, son of Ranulf I, 13.

Chester, earl of, Ranulf I, 13, 20.

Chester, earl of, Ranulf II, son of Hugh II, 13-14, 20-22, 25-29, 31-32, 43, 54-55, 149, 197, 213, 230, 246, 250, 252, 268, 290, 304-305, 337, 355-357, 360, 365, 369-370, 375.

Chesterfield, manor of, 77.

Chichester, bishop of, Richard Poor, 200, 339.

Chichester, bishop of, Simon de Camera, 147, 164, 184.

Chichester, dean and chapter of, 184.

Chichester, see of, 183.

Chilham, castle of, 35, 74, 180, 233, 282.

Chinnor, manor of, 32.

Chinon, castle of, 8-9, 45, 85, 86.

Chokes, barony of, 32.

Christ Church, Canterbury: cathedral priory of, 173-174; monks of, 123, 134, 164-166, 168, 171-173, 178, 189; sub-prior of, Reginald, 165-171.

Christchurch, castle of, 22, 31.

Chronica de Mailros, 47.

Chronica de Melsa, 183.

Cigogné, Engelard de, 206, 235, 265, 304, 324, 329, 336-337, 377.

Cigogné, Guy de, 324.

Cistercian order, 64, 129, 133, 155-156, 175.

Clare, earl of, Richard III, 13, 20-21, 46, 55, 92, 122, 162, 214, 242, 250, 257, 268, 280, 289, 293, 296, 331, 334, 339, 344, 364, 372.

Clare, Adeliza de, daughter of Gilbert I de Clare, wife of Aubrey II de Vere, 291.

Clare, Gilbert III de, son of Earl Richard III, 21, 283, 291-292, 295.

Clare, Richard fitz Gilbert I de, 281.

Clavering, manor of, 251.

Clergy, of England: extortions from, 176, 183, 195-196, 215; mistreatment of, 175-176, 190, 237; property of during interdict, 176, 183, 196.

Clifford, barony of, 239.

Clifford, Roger de, 221, 278, 368.

Clifford, Walter de, 121, 244-245, 278, 357.

Clitheroe, castle of, 23.

Clun, castle of, 357.

Cockermouth, castle of, 40, 252, 370.

Coggeshall, Ralph de, 1.

Coinage of 1205, 145-147.

Colchester, castle of, 59, 332, 337, 352, 371.

Coldingham, Geoffrey de, 187.

Conisborough, castle of, 21.

Constable, of England, 58-59. *See also*, Hereford, earl of, Henry de Bohun.

Constables, hereditary, 29, 36, 40, 59, 251, 264, 302, 331-332, 334.

Constitutions of Clarendon, 151-152.

Copeland, barony of, 252.

Corfe, castle of, 85, 236, 359, 374.

Cornard, John de, 92, 121-122.

Cornhill, Gervase de, 218.

Cornhill, Henry de, son of Gervase de, 68, 218.

Cornhill, Joan de, daughter of Henry de, wife of Hugh de Neville, 68, 231.

Cornhill, Reginald I de, son of Gervase de, 56, 81, 88, 120, 137, 145, 147, 171-173, 222-223.

Cornhill, Reginald II de, son of Reginald I de, 222, 329, 361-362.

Cornhill, William de, 81, 86, 103, 106, 135, 174, 178, 194, 200, 229-230, 270, 283, 300. See also, Chester, bishop of.
Cornwall, earl of, Reginald, illegitimate son of King Henry I, 231, 358.
Cornwall, earldom of, 358-359.
Counties, farm of, 115-124.
Courcy, barony of, 68.
Courcy, Alice de, wife of Henry de Cornhill and Warin fitz Gerold, 68.
Courcy, John de, 46-47, 248.
Court, the king's: common pleas, 61, 81; *coram rege*, 81; on eyre, 81.
Courtenay, Robert de, 290, 359.
Coventry, bishop of, *see* Chester, bishop of.
Coventry, prior and convent of, 184.
Coventry, Walter de, seneschal of Earl Ranulf of Chester, 355.
Coventry, Walter of, 46.
Craon, Guy de, 294.
Craon, Petronilla de, daughter of Guy de, wife of Henry de la Mare and Oliver de Vaux, 294.
Cressi, Hugh de, 251.
Cressi, Roger de, son of Hugh de, 222, 251, 287-288, 292, 307, 353.
Curia regis rolls, 1.
Curterne, Hugh de, nephew of William de Tracy, 38-39, 74.

Danegeld, 125.
Davis, H. W. C., *Regesta regum Anglo-Normannorum*, 331.
Dean, forest of, 238, 241.
Dene, Amfrid de, 48, 168.
Derby, borough of, 20, 26.
Derby, earl of, William de Ferrers, 13, 15, 20, 23-26, 46, 73, 192, 194, 213-214, 242-243, 247, 250, 290-291, 305, 356-357.
Derham, Master Geoffrey de, 166-167.
Devereals, Osmund de, seneschal of Earl William Marshal, 114.
Devizes, castle of, 231, 359.
Devon, earl of, William de Redvers, son of Baldwin I de Redvers, 22, 30-31, 43, 78, 85, 213, 281, 290, 297, 359.
Dialogus de scaccario, 66.
Dieppe, 15-16.

Dinan, Alan de, 53.
Dinan, Hawise de, daughter of Joyce de, mother of Fulk fitz Warin, 49, 53.
Dinan, Joyce de, 49, 53.
Ditton, manor of, 234.
Doncaster, town of, 371.
Donington, castle of, 23, 256, 357.
Dover, barony of, 75-76.
Dover, castle of, 84, 359, 376.
Dover, Fulbert of, 35, 74.
Dover, Rohese I of, daughter of Geoffrey de Lucy, mother of Fulbert of Dover, 75-76.
Dover, Rohese II of, daughter of Fulbert of, wife of Richard fitz Roy, 233, 282.
Downton, castle of, 160.
Dreux, Peter of, son of Count Robert II, *see* Brittany, duke of.
Dreux, Robert of, son of Count Robert II, 215, 285, 375.
Driffield, manor of, 330.
Dublin, archbishop of, Henry of London, 193-194, 337-339, 366.
Dublin, archbishop of, John Cumin, 156, 158-159.
Duffield, castle of, 26.
Dugdale, William: *Monasticon*, 41.
Dunkeswell, abbey of, 78.
Dunstaple, priory of 134.
Dunster, barony of, 85, 359.
Dunwich, town of, 136.
Durand, 186-187, 189, 256.
Durham, archdeacon of, Aimery, 268-269.
Durham, bishop of, Philip of Poitiers, 134-135, 144, 184, 251-252.
Durham, castle of, 354.
Durham, prior and convent of, 184.
Durham, see of, 126, 183.
Duston, William de, 329.

Eardington, Giles de, son of Thomas de, 224.
Eardington, Thomas de, 122, 168-169, 189, 197, 221, 224, 244, 281. 304, 357, 368.
Earliest Lincolnshire assize rolls, 90.
Earliest Northamptonshire assize rolls, 68.
Early charters of St. Paul's, 165.

Index

"Electio Hugonis," 196.
Ely, bishop of, Eustace, 164, 172-179, 181-182, 186, 190, 300.
Ely, bishop of, Nigel, 66.
Ely, bishop of, William de Longchamp, 105.
Ely, see of, 174.
Ely, William of, 66-67, 70, 81-82, 185.
Emperor, Holy Roman, Frederick of Hohenstaufen, 188, 194, 285.
Emperor, Holy Roman, Henry IV, 151.
Emperor, Holy Roman, Otto of Brunswick, 153-155, 158, 187-188, 190, 193, 228, 285.
Empress, Holy Roman, Matilda, *see* England, lady of.
England, king of, Canute, 2.
England, king of, Harold, 2.
England, king of, Henry I, 2, 42, 66, 73, 111, 113, 143, 203-204, 217-219, 223, 233, 276, 300, 330, 332, 334.
England, king of, Henry II, 1-4, 8, 11-13, 17, 20, 23-24, 26, 29-30, 32, 36, 42, 44, 49, 52, 58, 67-68, 71, 74, 89, 94-95, 98, 110-112, 125-129, 141, 145, 151-152, 162, 204, 209, 217, 227, 233, 251, 258, 263, 276, 318, 324, 330, 332-336.
England, king of, Henry III, 224, 232.
England, king of, Henry the young king, son of Henry II, 1, 32, 40.
England, king of, Richard I, 1-14, 17-19, 23-24, 30, 32, 36, 38, 40, 44, 49, 52, 60, 68, 71, 74-75, 78-79, 82, 84, 89, 94, 105, 111, 115, 124-129, 137, 140-141, 148, 152-154, 156, 159, 204, 209, 220, 227, 233, 237, 249, 251, 256, 263, 311, 318, 324, 330, 332-333, 335-336, 358, 373.
England, king of, Stephen, 2, 11, 24, 28, 42, 69, 152, 204, 276, 334.
England, king of, William I, 41, 111, 203, 331.
England, king of, William II, 42, 203, 334.
England, kingdom of, law of succession in, 2-3.
England, lady of, Matilda, daughter of King Henry I, 2, 4, 204, 331, 334.
England, prince of, Eustace, son of King Stephen, 2.
England, prince of, Henry, eldest son of King John, 236, 255, 267. *See also*, England, king of, Henry III.
England, prince of, Richard, second son of King John, 267.
England, prince of, William, son of King Henry I, 2.
England, princess of, Joan, daughter of King John, 236.
England, queen of, Berengeria of Navarre, 1, 9, 159, 197.
England, queen of, Eleanor of Aquitaine, 2, 4, 7-9, 130, 159.
England, queen of, Isabella of Angoulême, 227, 232, 235-236, 267, 369.
Englosam, Master Peter de, 165-167.
Erley, John de, 11, 293, 307.
Essarts, Richard de, 254.
Essarts, Robert de, 254.
Essarts, Roger de, 253-254.
Essendon, manor of, 67.
Essex, countess of, Aveline de Albini, second wife of Geoffrey fitz Peter, 35-36, 282, 293.
Essex, earl of, Geoffrey II de Mandeville, 24, 331, 334.
Essex, earl of, Geoffrey III de Mandeville, son of Geoffrey II, 263, 296.
Essex, earl of, Geoffrey IV de Mandeville, son of Geoffrey fitz Peter, 214, 280, 282-285, 287, 289, 292, 294, 306-307, 333-334, 339, 344, 367-368, 372.
Essex, earl of, Geoffrey fitz Peter, 22, 28, 35-36, 38-39, 50-51, 55, 60-63, 67, 70-71, 73-74, 76, 82, 91, 101-102, 109, 122, 130, 162, 176-180, 189, 192, 194, 205, 218, 228, 230, 234, 237, 242, 258, 261-264, 278-279, 282-283, 292-293, 331, 334.
Essex, earl of, William II de Mandeville, son of Geoffrey II, 10, 263, 284, 296.
Essex, Alice de, daughter of Robert de, mother of Roger de Lacy, 251, 292.
Essex, Henry de, son of Robert de, 251.
Essex, Robert de, 251.
Eu, count of, Ralph de Lusignan, 48, 148, 282.
Eu, countess of, Alice, 282.
Eudes, *dapifer*, 332.
Evreux, bishop of, 159.
Ewyas, barony of, 221.

Ewyas Lacy, castle of, 239.
Exchanges, 110, 144-148.
Exchequer, 59, 61, 66-67, 109-110, 205; of Normandy, 159; rolls of, 96, 101.
Exeter, bishop of, Henry Marshal, brother of Earl William Marshal, 58, 164, 184.
Exeter, bishop of, Simon of Apulia, 199.
Exeter, dean and chapter of, 184.
Exeter, see of, 174, 183.
Eye, honor of, 20.
Eyton, R. W.: *Antiquities of Shropshire*, 49; *Itinerary*, 42.

Falaise, castle of, 85.
Farnham, castle of, 160, 374.
Farrer, William: *An outline itinerary of King Henry the first*, 332; *Early Yorkshire charters*, 294; *Feudal Cambridgeshire*, 333; *Honours and knights' fees*, 20.
Fauconberg, Eustace de, 82.
Feavearyear, A. E., *The pound sterling*, 145.
Ferreby, John de, 345.
Ferrers, William de, *see* Derby, earl of.
Fifteenth on merchants, 136-139.
Fines, 29-30, 31, 34, 36, 38, 44, 49, 64, 74-75, 96-97, 111, 119-121, 135, 157, 218, 245, 248, 255-256, 263, 283, 335; to escape military service, 127-128, 212.
Fines sive pedes finium, 46.
First register of Norwich cathedral priory, 155.
Fitz Ade, Roger, 121.
Fitz Alan, Ruald, 29, 70, 133, 331.
Fitz Alan, William II, 50.
Fitz Alan, William III, 220, 357.
Fitz Count, Henry, illegitimate son of Earl Reginald of Cornwall, 231, 290, 348, 358-359.
Fitz Geoffrey, John, son of Geoffrey fitz Peter, 282.
Fitz Gerold, Henry, brother of Warin, 293.
Fitz Gerold, Warin, 22, 36, 59, 68, 194, 218, 375.
Fitz Henry, Meiler, 123, 159, 183, 239-241.

Fitz Herbert, Matthew, 194.
Fitz Herbert, Peter, 194, 300.
Fitz Hugh, John, 81, 123, 144-145, 229, 269, 375.
Fitz John, William, brother of Henry de Tilly, 150.
Fitz Martin, William, 133.
Fitz Nigel, Richard, son of Nigel, bishop of Ely, 66-67.
Fitz Paien, Robert, 287, 289, 307, 309.
Fitz Peter, Geoffrey, 10-12, 14-15. *See also*, Essex, earl of.
Fitz Ralph, William, 10, 227.
Fitz Renfrew, Gilbert, 208, 252, 255, 274, 296, 300, 355, 362, 370.
Fitz Richard, Roger, father of Robert fitz Roger, 251.
Fitz Robert, John, son of Robert fitz Roger, 255, 280, 287-289, 292, 329, 337, 339, 355.
Fitz Robert, Walter, 22.
Fitz Roger, Robert, son of Roger fitz Richard, 119, 251-252, 255, 268-269, 291-292.
Fitz Roy, Geoffrey, illegitimate son of King John, 232.
Fitz Roy, Henry, illegitimate son of King John, 232.
Fitz Roy, John, illegitimate son of King John, 232.
Fitz Roy, Oliver, illegitimate son of King John, 232-233.
Fitz Roy, Osbert, illegitimate son of King John, 233.
Fitz Roy, Richard, illegitimate son of King John, 233, 282, 303.
Fitz Theobald, Fulk, 120.
Fitz Walter, Alice, *see* Peche, Alice.
Fitz Walter, Matilda, daughter of Robert fitz Walter, wife of Geoffrey IV de Mandeville, 234, 261.
Fitz Walter, Robert, son of Walter fitz Robert, 22-23, 31-35, 54, 59, 76, 109, 188-190, 211, 213, 222, 234, 242, 250, 253, 258-261, 264, 267-274, 278, 280-282, 284, 287, 289, 291-292, 294, 296, 302, 307, 314-315, 331-332, 338-339, 344, 348, 353, 361-364, 367.
Fitz Walter, William, 269, 345.
Fitz Warin, Fulk, 48-54, 84, 157, 280, 289, 294, 358.
Flanders, count of, Baldwin, 6.

Index

Flanders, count of, Ferrand of Portugal, 188, 228, 285.
Fleming, Richard, 84.
Flower, Cyril T., *Introduction to the curia regis rolls*, 81.
Folkingham, 356.
Fontrevault, abbey of, 9.
Ford, abbot of, 176.
Forester, chief, 67-69. *See also*, Neville, Hugh de.
Foresters, 60, 68-69, 333.
Forests, administration of, 68-69, 207-208.
Fortibus, William II de, 41, 235. *See also*, Aumale, count of.
Fossard, William, 8.
Fotheringay, castle of, 22, 70, 268, 331, 365.
Fougères, Clemence de, sister of Geoffrey de, wife of Earl Ranulf of Chester, 26-27.
Fougères, Geoffrey de, 26-27.
Fougères, William de, 26.
Fouke fitz Warin, 49.
Framlingham, castle of, 371.
Frampton, castle of, 294, 371.
France, king of, Philip Augustus, 4-6, 9, 11, 17, 19, 26-27, 29, 32-33, 37, 39, 45, 55, 62, 102, 112, 129, 131, 138-139, 149, 153, 155-159, 163, 170, 188-193, 201, 206, 212-214, 227-228, 234, 250, 253-254, 259, 261, 266, 282, 285, 312, 315, 366-367, 373.
France, prince of, Louis, 215, 232, 289, 297, 351, 353, 359, 367-368, 371-375.
France, princess of, Alis, daughter of King Louis VII, 233.
France, queen of, Ingelborg of Denmark, 153.
Freiston, castle of, 352.
Fulk fitz Warine, 50.
Furnell, Henry, 50.
Furnell, William de, 137.
Furness, abbey of, 133.
Furnival, Gerard de, senior, 7.
Furnival, Gerard de, the younger, 222.

Galway, Alan of, 266.
Gesta Sancti Albani, 259.
Gesta Stephani, 42.
Ghent, Alice de, sister of Robert de, wife of Roger de Mowbray, 257.
Ghent, Gilbert de, son of Robert de, 257, 285, 288, 292, 294, 296, 356, 376.
Ghent, Maurice de, nephew of Gilbert de, 280, 289, 292, 295, 309.
Ghent, Robert de, 257.
Giffard, honor of, 37.
Giraldus Cambrensis, 161; *Opera*, 14.
Glamorgan, lordship of, 44, 239, 241, 283.
Glanvill, Ranulf de, 3, 11, 60, 63, 82, 162; *De legibus*, 3.
Glapion, Warin de, 149.
Gloucester, castle of, 36, 236, 238.
Gloucester, countess of, Isabella, wife of King John and Geoffrey IV de Mandeville, 13, 221, 232, 283-284.
Gloucester, earl of, Amauri VI de Montfort, 34, 283.
Gloucester, earl of, Geoffrey IV de Mandeville, *see* Essex, earl of.
Gloucester, earl of, Robert, 111.
Gloucester, earl of, William, 13, 34, 333.
Gloucester, earldom of, 13, 19-21, 71, 75, 283, 289, 294, 333.
Gloucester, town of, 215.
Gloucester, Bertha of, daughter of Miles of, wife of William II de Briouse, 41.
Gloucester, Miles of, *see* Hereford, earl of.
Gournay, Hugh de, 242.
Gower, lordship of, 13, 44, 239.
Grantham, manor of, 35, 149.
Gresley, Robert de, 285.
Grey, John de, 67, 79, 84. *See also*, Norwich, bishop of.
Grey, Walter de, 64-65, 81, 179, 184-185, 200, 229. *See also*, Worcester, bishop of; York, archbishop of.
Grosmont, castle of, 45, 83, 239.
Gualo, 201, 373.
Guildford, castle of, 374.

Halton, castle of, 23.
Hanley, castle of, 265, 368.
Hanslope, castle of, 364.
Hanslope, Michael of, 332.
Harbottle, castle of, 252.
Harcourt, William de, 87, 307, 355-356.

388 Index

Hardy, T. D., *Itinerary of King John*, 166.
Hartland, barony of, 53.
Hastings, barony of, 48, 282.
Hawise, mistress of King John, 233.
Helmsley, castle of, 370.
Hereford, archdeacon of, *see* Fitz Walter, William.
Hereford, bishop of, Giles de Briouse, 44, 155, 172, 175, 178, 239, 244, 245, 250, 269, 274, 287, 289, 300, 306-307, 309, 345, 352, 358.
Hereford, castle of, 36.
Hereford, earl of, Henry de Bohun, 22, 24, 36, 40, 58-59, 210, 213-214, 239, 242, 250, 253, 258, 262, 264, 275, 280, 287, 289, 292, 296, 307, 330, 339, 367.
Hereford, earl of, Miles of Gloucester, 24, 41, 239.
Hereford, earl of, Roger, son of Miles of Gloucester, 36.
Hereford, see of, 239, 244.
Heriet, Richard de, 234.
Hertford, castle of, 31, 59, 269, 331-332, 352.
Hertford, earl of, *see* Clare, earl of.
Hidage, 113, 125.
Higham Ferrers, manor of, 15, 25, 73.
Histoire de Guillaume le Maréchal, 3.
Histoire des ducs de Normandie, 64.
Ho, manor of, 71.
Holderness, lordship of, 40, 355.
Holy Trinity, London, convent of, 373.
Holy Trinity, London, prior of, 180.
Horsley, castle of, 26, 77, 356.
Hospital, knights of the, 173, 176, 195.
Hostages, 16, 236, 241, 244, 268, 336.
Houbridge, Gervase de, 269.
Houbridge, Philip de, 269.
Houbridge, William de, 269.
Hovedon, Roger of, 2.
Huntingdon, archdeacon of, *see* Cornhill, William de.
Huntingdon, earl of, David, brother of King William of Scotland, 13-14, 22, 36, 70, 214, 253, 267, 331, 365.
Huntingfield, William de, 280, 287, 289, 294, 307.
Hurnard, Naomi Day, " Magna carta, clause 34," 323.

Inquest of 1212, 208-211.
Ireland, expedition to, 246-248, 259, 264.
Ireland, lordship of, 238, 253-254.

Jacob, of London, 141-142.
Jews: debts to, 29, 31-32, 35-36, 44, 221, 258; exploitation of, 139-144, 237; privileges of, 143.
Joigny, Peter de, 236.
Justices, 80-82, 126, 132.
Justices, of the Jews, 142. *See also*, Warren, William de; Neville, Thomas de; Norwich, Geoffrey de.
Justiciar, of England, 60-62. *See also*, Basset, Ralph; Leicester, earl of, Robert I; Lucy, Richard de; Glanvill, Ranulf de; Walter, Hubert; Fitz Peter, Geoffrey; Roches, Peter des; Burgh, Hubert de.
Justiciar, of Ireland, *see* Fitz Henry, Meiler; Norwich, bishop of, John de Grey.

Kendal, barony of, 252.
Kenilworth, castle of, 357.
Kington, barony of, 44, 239.
Kirby Malzeard, castle of, 23.
Kirby's inquest, 294.
Kivelly, Eustace de, 51, 53.
Kivelly, Nicholas de, 53.
Knaresborough, barony of, 257, 336.
Knaresborough, castle of, 265, 334, 356.
Knowles, David, 166-167, 169; *Religious houses*, 77; " The Canterbury Election of 1205-6," 164.
Kyme, Ralph de, 67.
Kyme, Simon de, 135, 273, 294, 296.

La Celle, Geoffrey de, 7.
Lacelles, Geoffrey de, 75-76.
Lacy, Hugh de, 46-47. *See also*, Ulster, earl of.
Lacy, John de, constable of Chester, son of Roger de, 220, 225, 253-256, 258, 268, 280, 287-288, 292, 306, 309, 344, 357, 369-370.
Lacy, Margaret de, *see* Briouse, Margaret de.
Lacy, Robert de, 23.
Lacy, Roger de, constable of Chester,

Index

13-14, 16, 22-23, 27, 32, 39, 119-120, 124, 126, 220, 247, 251-255, 291, 293.
Lacy, Roger II de, son of Roger de Lacy, 369.
Lacy, Walter de, 24, 45-47, 123, 239-240, 242, 244-247, 250, 258, 277, 377.
La Haye, Nichola de, 59, 355.
Laigle, barony of, 35.
Laigle, Gilbert de, 148-149.
Laigle, Master Gilbert de, 184-185.
La Marche, count of, Hugh de Lusignan, 48.
La Mare, Henry de, 88.
Lambourn, manor of, 49.
Lancaster, castle of, 215.
Lancaster, honor of, 255.
Lancaster, William de, son of Gilbert fitz Renfrew, 296, 362.
Landon, Lionel, *Itinerary*, 6.
Langar, manor of, 368.
Langton, Simon, 173-174, 176, 178-179, 181-182, 197, 200.
Langton, Stephen, 123, 151, 169-170. *See also*, Canterbury, archbishop of.
Lanvalay, William II de, 59, 332.
Lanvalay, William III de, 280, 292, 332, 337, 339.
La Poole, Roger de, 78.
Laval, lord of, Guy, 39.
Layettes du trésor des chartes, 9.
Leicester, earl of, Robert I de Beaumont, 58.
Leicester, earl of, Robert II de Beaumont, 21.
Leicester, earl of, Robert III de Beaumont, 21, 26, 28-29, 32, 34-35, 55, 58, 74, 148, 155, 227.
Leicester, earl of, Simon IV de Montfort, 34-35, 58, 267, 338, 366.
Leicester, earl of, Simon V de Montfort, 58.
Leicester, honor of, 34-35, 290, 331.
Leicester, town of, 34.
Leighton-Buzzard, prebend of, 67.
Leinster, lordship of, 239, 241.
Le Mans, 9, 159.
Lenz, Simon de, 51.
Lewes, castle of, 21.
Lichfield, bishop of, *see* Chester, bishop of.
Lichfield, Coventry, and Chester, see of, 183.
Limerick, city of, 44, 240-241.
Limerick, lordship of, 42-43, 221, 239-240, 243, 249.
Limesi, barony of, 14, 71.
Limesi, Amabile de, sister of John de, wife of Hugh Bardolf, John de Briouse, and Robert de Ropsley, 13, 45, 71, 219.
Limesi, John de, 13, 71.
Limoges, bishop of, 158.
Lincoln, bishop of, Hugh of Avalon, 9, 152, 155-156.
Lincoln, bishop of, Hugh de Welles, 300, 338-339, 352, 377.
Lincoln, bishop of, William de Blois, 155, 184.
Lincoln, castle of, 20, 59, 355, 368, 375.
Lincoln, citizens of, 223.
Lincoln, dean and chapter of, 184.
Lincoln, see of, 67, 174, 183.
Lisieux, 5.
Lisle, Brian de, 87, 215, 229, 304, 306, 334, 356.
Llantilio, castle of, 45, 85, 239.
Llywelyn, 43, 48, 232, 246, 264, 266-267, 357-358.
Loches, castle of, 8, 206.
London, bishop of, William de Sainte-Mère-Eglise, 164, 172-179, 181-182, 186, 190, 300, 306, 338-339.
London, citizens of, 138, 308, 323, 344.
London, city of, 308-309, 320, 338, 343-344, 365, 371, 374.
London, mayor of, 143, 364.
London, Tower of, 262, 283, 308, 334, 339, 343.
London, Henry of, 103, 178, 184, 185, 230. *See also*, Dublin, archbishop of
London, Robert of, 235-236.
Longueville, lordship of, 37, 214.
Lot, Ferdinand and Fawtier, Robert, *Premier budget de la monarchie française*, 112.
Loveland, Robert de, 362.
Lucy, Geoffrey de, son of Richard de, 75.
Lucy, Herbert de, son of Geoffrey de, 75.
Lucy, Philip de, 86, 222.
Lucy, Richard de, 35, 73, 75, 332.
Lucy, Richard de, of Egremont, 252, 257, 268.

Ludgershall, castle of, 69.
Ludlow, castle of, 239, 265.
Lundy, island of, 48, 52-53.
Lunt, William E., *Papal revenues*, 160.
Lusignan, Guy de, 108.
Lusignan, Hugh de, *see* La Marche, count of.
Lusignan, Ralph de, *see* Eu, count of.
Luttrel, Geoffrey, 366.

Magna carta, 203-204, 206-207, 211, 213, 230, 237, 275, 286, 297, 303, 309, 311, 313-314, 316-327, 340-341, 345-348, 366.
Magna vita sancti Hugonis, 1.
Maine, county of, 9, 112, 115, 131.
Malebise, Hugh, 222.
Malet, William, 280, 287, 289, 296, 307, 309.
Man, king of, 227.
Mandeville, Beatrice de, daughter of William I de, wife of William I de Say, 263.
Mandeville, Geoffrey II de, *see* Essex, earl of.
Mandeville, Geoffrey III de, *see* Essex, earl of.
Mandeville, Geoffrey IV de, son of Geoffrey fitz Peter, 213, 221, 234, 258, 260-261, 263, 278. *See also*, Essex, earl of.
Mandeville, Geoffrey de, of Merswood, 150.
Mandeville, Matilda de, daughter of Geoffrey fitz Peter, wife of Earl Henry de Bohun, 258, 292.
Mandeville, Robert de, of Merswood, 150.
Mandeville, William I de, 334.
Mandeville, William II de, *see* Essex, earl of.
Mandeville, William III de, son of Geoffrey fitz Peter, 214, 258, 280, 287, 292, 307, 331.
Manors, royal, farms of, 123-124.
Mantel, Matthew, 119.
Marc, Philip, 206, 265, 304, 324, 329, 336, 355-356.
Marlborough, castle of, 69, 231, 359, 375.
Marmion, Robert, 148.
Marriage, right of, 217-219.

Marsh, Richard, 65, 80-81, 86, 103, 106, 109, 183, 197-198, 201, 205, 230, 269, 281, 284, 302, 360, 366.
Marsh, William, 48, 52-54, 84, 157.
Marshal, master, of England, 58, 69, 210. *See also*, Marshal, William.
Marshal, of the exchequer, 58. *See also*, Marshal, Jocelin.
Marshal, of Ireland, 241. *See also*, Marshal, John.
Marshal, Jocelin, 58.
Marshal, John, nephew of Earl William, 241, 304, 329, 359, 366, 377.
Marshal, John fitz Gilbert, 69.
Marshal, William, 3, 10-12, 14-15. *See also*, Pembroke, earl of.
Marshal, William, the younger, 41, 255, 289, 292, 295-297, 339, 375.
Martel, Alan, 197.
Martini, Geoffrey de, 302, 324, 329.
Mauclerk, Walter, 299, 309.
Mauduit, Robert, son of William II, 59, 69, 332-333.
Mauduit, William I, 332.
Mauduit, William II, 332.
Mauduit, William III, son of Robert, 332, 364.
Maulay, Peter de, 86-87, 229, 231, 282, 303, 308, 359, 368.
Mauleon, Savaric de, 299-300, 306-307, 336, 359, 363, 365, 371-372.
McKechnie, William S., 312, 317; *Magna Carta*, 280.
Meath, lordship of, 24, 45, 239, 247.
Memoranda roll 1 John, 1.
Memoranda roll 10 John, 69.
Mercadier, 7, 9.
Mercenary troops, 47, 206, 246, 265-266, 301, 308-309, 336, 360-362, 365, 372, 374.
Merswood, barony of, 150.
Meulan, count of, Robert, 30-31, 99.
Middleham, castle of, 369.
Migne, J. P., *Patrologia*, 46.
Mines, of tin in Devon and Cornwall, 110, 137, 349.
Mints, 110, 144-148.
Mirabeau, castle of, 19, 27.
Mitchell, Sydney Knox, 125, 130, 285; *Studies in taxation*, 126.
Mitford, castle of, 370.
Monasticon Exoniensis, 42.

Index

Monmouth, Baderon de, 239.
Monmouth, John de, 239, 250, 278, 291.
Montaigu, William de, 121, 287, 289, 307-309.
Montbegon, Roger de, 285, 296, 331, 339, 369, 371.
Montchesney, Warin de, 35, 221.
Montchesney, William de, 35.
Montfichet, Avelina de, daughter of Richard I de, wife of William de Fortibus, count of Aumale, 235.
Montfichet, Gilbert de, 333.
Montfichet, Richard I de, son of Gilbert de, 39, 333.
Montfichet, Richard II de, son of Richard I de, 235, 280, 289, 292, 333.
Montfort, Amauri VI de, *see* Gloucester, earl of.
Montfort, Simon III de, 34.
Montfort, Simon IV de, 34. See also, Leicester, earl of.
Montfort, Simon V de, *see* Leicester, earl of.
Moreville, Hugh de, 354.
Morpeth, castle of, 370.
Mortimer, Hugh de, son of Roger de, 46, 239, 250, 278.
Mortimer, Roger de, 239.
Mottisfont, priory of, 78.
Moulton, castle of, 371.
Moulton, Thomas de, 120, 225, 273, 280, 294, 362.
Mountsorrel, castle of, 21, 34-35, 331, 357, 368.
Mowbray, Roger de, son of Nigel de Albini, 29-30, 256-257.
Mowbray, William de, 13-14, 22-23, 29-31, 59, 213, 222, 242, 256, 258, 280, 288, 291-292, 293-294, 296, 321, 333, 339, 344, 353.
Mucegros, Richard de, 243.
Musard, Ralph, 329, 357.
Muscamp, barony of, 67.

Neckton, William de, 183, 270-271.
Nevers, count of, Hervé de Donzy, 228, 376.
Neville, Alan de, 67, 69.
Neville, Geoffrey de, 86-87, 103, 304, 306, 364, 370.
Neville, Henry de, 370.
Neville, Hugh de, 67-70, 73, 86-87, 92, 103, 133, 156, 176, 208, 224, 230-231, 242, 255, 268, 274, 333, 359, 375.
Neville, Joan de, daughter of Henry de Cornhill, wife of Hugh de Neville, *see* Cornhill, Joan de.
Neville, Jocelin de, 103.
Neville, Ralph de, 80.
Neville, Roger de, 329.
Neville, Thomas de, 142, 144.
Newark, castle of, 355, 368, 377.
Newburgh, William of, 6.
Newcastle-on-Tyne, castle of, 265, 354.
Newcastle-on-Tyne, town of, 136, 369.
Newcastle under Lyme, castle of, 356.
Nonant, Henry de, 45-46.
Nonant, Roger de, 42.
Norfolk, earl of, Roger Bigod, 21, 213-214, 251, 280-281, 287, 289, 292, 294, 296, 339, 371-372.
Norham, castle of, 246, 265, 354, 364.
Normandy, duchy of, 1-2, 4, 6, 9-10, 14, 26, 32, 112, 115, 131, 159.
Normandy, duchy of, law of succession in, 1-2.
Normans, English lands of, 148-150, 210.
Normanville, Ralph de, 343.
Northampton, 13, 15.
Northampton, castle of, 302, 306-308, 329, 360-361.
Northampton, citizens of, 268.
Northumberland, archdeacon of, *see* Marsh, Richard.
Northumberland, earl of, Henry, son of David I, king of Scotland, 252.
Norwich, archdeacon of, *see* Burgh, Geoffrey de.
Norwich, bishop of, John de Grey, 51-52, 64, 81, 155, 165-171, 175, 183, 194, 197, 201, 205, 207, 229-230, 237, 242, 245-247, 266.
Norwich, bishop of, John of Oxford, 155.
Norwich, castle of, 287, 360.
Norwich, Geoffrey de, 109, 142, 236, 270-272.
Nottingham, borough of, 20.
Nottingham, castle of, 20, 355, 368.
Nutley, abbey of, 37.

Odiham, castle of, 374-375.
Offaly, castle of, 240-241.

Offices of state, hereditary, 57-60, 68.
Oiry, Fulk de, 133, 135.
Oissel, Hugh, 145, 154.
Ongar, honor of, 35, 75-76, 282.
Orford, castle of, 360.
Orkney islands, 227.
Oxford, castle of, 361.
Oxford, earl of, Aubrey III de Vere, 251.
Oxford, earl of, Aubrey IV de Vere, 24, 36, 55, 178, 208, 213, 220, 230, 251, 281, 295.
Oxford, earl of, Robert de Vere, brother of Aubrey IV, 220, 287, 289, 292, 295, 307, 333-334, 339, 371-372.

Painel, Fulk, of Bampton, son of William I, 73-74.
Painel, Fulk II of Hambye, 26-27, 54, 148, 150.
Painel, Hugh II of West Rasen, 150.
Painel, William I of Bampton, 74.
Painter, Sidney: *Feudal barony*, 113; " Magna Carta," 315; *The scourge of the clergy*, 315; " The sources of Fouke fitz Warin," 50; *William Marshal*, 37.
Pandulf, 186-193, 198, 201, 234, 256, 272, 277, 337, 339, 343-345, 347, 366.
Papal, delegates, 151.
Papal, legates, 152, 158, 200, 201, 202. *See also*, Gualo; Pandulf.
Paris, University of, 169.
Paris, Matthew: *Chronica maiora*, 61; *Historia Anglorum*, 271.
Pattishall, Martin de, 82-83.
Pattishall, Simon de, 82, 141, 268, 287, 307.
Peak, castle of the, 356.
Peche, Alice, sister of Robert fitz Walter, wife of Gilbert Peche, 268.
Peche, Gilbert, 268.
Pembroke, countess of, Isabel de Clare, 37.
Pembroke, county of, 14, 22, 44, 238-239.
Pembroke, earl of, Richard fitz Gilbert de Clare, 14.
Pembroke, earl of, William Marshal, 22, 25-26, 33, 36, 44, 55, 58-59, 69-71, 73, 99, 114, 116, 119, 123, 148-149, 189, 192, 194, 197, 210, 213, 218, 228, 238-245, 247-250, 254-255, 258, 266, 277, 281, 293, 295, 297, 300-301, 303-306, 326, 337, 358, 360, 365, 375.
Perche, count of, Thomas, 148.
Perche, honor of, 232.
Percy, Richard de, 288, 296, 344.
Percy, Robert de, 135, 274.
Percy, William de, 291.
Peterborough, Benedict of, 32.
Peter's pence, 160-161.
Petit-Dutaillis, Ch., *Louis VIII*, 367.
Pevensea, castle of, 35, 149.
Peverel of Nottingham, honor of, 10, 13, 15, 20, 72-73.
Peverel, William, of Bourn, 49.
Peverel, William, of Nottingham, 13.
Pickering, castle of, 355, 370.
Pinkeny, Robert de, 220.
Pipe roll 31 Henry I, 42.
Pipe rolls 2, 3, and 4 Henry II, 42.
Plantagenet, Joan, illegitimate daughter of King John, 232, 267.
Pleshy, castle of, 371.
Plympton, barony of, 30.
Plympton, castle of, 22, 31.
Pointon, Alexander de, 269, 274, 362.
Poitiers, bishop of, 158.
Poitou, expedition to, 1214, 212, 214, 278, 280, 285, 315, 349.
Pòitou, scutage of, 211-212, 214, 280-281, 285.
Polsloe, priory of, 77.
Pomeroy, Henry III de, 74.
Pomeroy, Henry IV de, 220, 290, 307.
Pontefract, barony of, 23.
Pontefract, castle of, 14, 16, 23, 256, 369.
Pontefract, Peter of, 236.
Poor, Richard, 160, 200, 300. *See also*, Chichester, bishop of.
Pope, Gregory VII, 151.
Pope, Innocent III, 54-55, 151, 153-154, 157-161, 164-174, 176-179, 181-189, 191-193, 195, 197-198, 200-201, 237, 270, 272, 274, 277, 285, 299, 301, 305-306, 309, 311, 325, 341-342, 344, 346-348, 365.
Porchester, castle of, 374.
Port, Adam de, 46, 81, 242-243.
Poterna, James de, 82.
Power, Eileen, *Medieval English nunneries*, 77.

Index

Powicke, F. M., 7, 249, 341, 345; *King Henry III and the Lord Edward*, 53; *Loss of Normandy*, 7; "Miramus plurimum," 341; *Stephen Langton*, 170.
Powis, lord of, Gwenwynwyn,, 28-29, 45.
Powis, lord of, Maurice, 49-50.
"Praestito roll of 12 John," 264.
Preaux, Peter de, 30.
Prelates, election of, 155, 158, 184, 199.
Preston, Walter de, 268.
Prudhoe, castle of, 252, 267.

Quency, Robert I de, 32.
Quency, Robert II de, 32.
Quency, Saher I de, 32.
Quency, Saher II de, 31-34. *See also,* Winchester, earl of.

Radnor, barony of, 41-44, 239.
Ramsay, Sir James H., 131; *Revenues of the kings of England*, 111.
Reading, abbot of, 165, 167, 343-345.
Recueil des actes de Philippe Auguste, 149.
Red book of the exchequer, 13.
Redesdale, 252-253.
Redvers, Baldwin I de, son of Richard I de, 42.
Redvers, Baldwin de, son of Earl William, 31, 85, 218.
Redvers, Joan, daughter of Earl William, 30, 78, 85.
Redvers, Richard I de, 111.
Redvers, William de, *see* Devon, earl of.
Reigate, castle of, 21, 374.
Relief, 219-221.
Richard, Alfred, *Histoire des comtes de Poitou*, 8.
Richardson, H. G., 95, 100, 102, 270, 334, 336-337, 343, 345; "Letters of the legate Guala," 109; "The morrow of the great charter," 288; "The morrow of the great charter—an addendum," 342; "William of Ely," 58.
Richmond, archdeacon of, *see* Marsh, Richard.
Richmond, archdeacon of, Honorius, 166-167, 236.
Richmond, castle of, 28-29, 70, 133, 331, 367, 369.
Richmond, honor of, 13, 20-21, 27, 150, 367.
Ridel, Stephen, 154.
Rivers, Richard de, 282.
Rochefort, Chalon de, 108.
Roches, Peter des, 71, 86-87, 107, 160. *See also,* Winchester, bishop of.
Roches, William des, 62, 229.
Rochester, bishop of, Benedict of Sausetum, 306.
Rochester, bishop of, Gilbert de Glanvill, 164, 168, 172, 179, 182.
Rochester, castle of, 162, 350, 361-364, 374.
Rockingham, castle of 59, 69, 265, 332-333, 352, 364.
Rolls of the justices in eyre for Yorkshire in 3 Henry III, 371.
Ropsley, Robert de, 135.
Ros, Robert de, 252-253, 273-274, 280, 288, 292, 296, 300, 334, 337, 350, 353, 355, 369-371.
Roscelin, master, 78.
Rot. chart., 27.
Rot. claus., 25.
Rot. liberate, 28.
Rot. oblatis, 16.
Rot. pat., 27.
Rotuli de dominibus, 296.
Rotuli Normanniae, 84.
"Rotulus misae 14 John," 63.
Rouen, 15, 32.
Rouen, archbishop of, Walter de Coutance, 6, 10-11, 15, 54, 157.
Rouen, tower of, 11.
Roumar, William I de, 20.
Roumar, William III de, 13.
Round, J. H.: *Ancient charters*, 35; *Calendar*, 15; *Feudal England*, 42; *Geoffrey de Mandeville*, 251.
Rouvrai, John de, 149.
Royal letters, 356.
Royal party, 1215-1216, 303-304.
Rufford, abbey of, 215.
Runnymede, 309, 312, 315.
Rymer, Thomas, *Foedera*, 20.

St. Albans, abbey of, 259.
St. Albans, abbot of, 165, 167, 260-261.

St. Andrews, bishop of, Roger de Beaumont, 155.
St. Augustine of Canterbury, abbot of, 168.
St. Bertin, abbey of, 171.
St. Briavel, castle of, 238, 265.
St. Clare, Hamo de, 332.
St. David's, see of, 161.
St. Martin's, London, chapter of, 373.
St. Martin's, London, dean of, see Buckland, Geoffrey de.
Sainte-Mère-Eglise, William de, 141. See also, London, bishop of.
St. Paul's, London, canons of, 109, 269, 373.
St. Paul's, London, dean of, 164-165, 167.
St. Pierre de Semilly, castle of, 27.
St. Valéry, Henry de, 149.
St. Valéry, Thomas de, 149.
St. Vast of Arras, abbot of, 182.
St. Wulstan, cathedral church of, 377.
Saladin tithe, 130-131.
Salisbury, bishop of, Herbert Poor, 164, 172, 175, 179, 182.
Salisbury, castle of, 40, 264.
Salisbury, countess of, Ela, 40, 210, 262-263.
Salisbury, dean of, see Poor, Richard.
Salisbury, earl of, William, illegitimate son of King Henry II, 24, 40, 51-52, 59, 106, 119, 174, 192, 194, 208, 210, 213, 215, 230-231, 242, 262-264, 270-272, 285, 290, 306, 308-309, 330, 359, 361, 365, 371, 374-375.
Salisbury, Edward of, 40, 210, 263.
Salisbury, Maud of, daughter of Edward of, wife of Humphrey I de Bohun, 40, 210, 263.
Saltwood, manor of, 162.
Sanford, Thomas de, 231, 304, 359.
Sauvey, castle of, 265.
Say, Beatrice de, daughter of William II de, wife of Geoffrey fitz Peter, 10.
Say, Geoffrey I de, son of William I de, 62, 262-264, 284, 289, 295.
Say, Geoffrey II de, son of Geoffrey I de, 292, 295, 364.
Say, William I de, 263.
Say, William II de, son of William I de, 263, 296.

Scarborough, castle of, 86, 265, 355, 370.
Scotland, king of, Alexander II, 199, 355, 364, 369, 376.
Scotland, king of, Malcomb IV, 12, 253.
Scotland, king of, William, 12-15, 17, 22, 156, 188, 199, 215, 227, 246, 250-253, 255-256, 264, 267, 292.
Scots, expeditions against, 246, 250, 255-256, 264.
Scutage, 16, 110, 113, 125-128, 211-212.
Seal: the exchequer, 109; the great, 106-107, 110; the small, 107, 110.
Selby, abbey of, 215.
Select pleas of the crown, 352.
Seneschal, of Anjou, see Turnham, Robert de; Roches, William des.
Seneschal, baronial, 113-115.
Seneschal, of England, 58. See also, Leicester, earl of.
Seneschal, of household, 58, 87-88. See also, Cantilupe, William de; Stoke, Peter de; Neville, Geoffrey de; Harcourt, William de; Lisle, Brian de; Bréauté, Fawkes de.
Seneschal, of Normandy, see Fitz Ralph, William; Glapion, Warin de.
Seventh of 1203, 130-131.
Sherborne, castle of, 85.
Sheriff, office of, 89-92, 117-122.
Sheriffs, custodian, 116-122, 124.
Sheriffs, hereditary, 40, 59. See also, Salisbury, earl of, William.
Sicily, king of, Frederick of Hohenstaufen, see Emperor, Holy Roman.
Sicily, king of, Tancred, 5.
Shoreham, 15-16.
Skelton, castle of, 370.
Skenfrith, castle of, 45, 85, 239.
Skipsea, castle of, 40, 355.
Skipton-in-Craven, castle of, 40.
Sleaford, castle of, 355, 368.
Smith, Sidney, 146.
Snaith, manor of, 39.
Sneinton, manor of, 77.
Stafford, archdeacon of, see London, Henry of.
Stamford, baronial muster in, 213, 280, 286-288, 301, 342.
Stamford, castle of, 35, 356.
Stamford, town of, 35, 149.

Index

Stanley, abbey of, 51.
Stenton, Doris, 16.
Stenton, F. M., *English feudalism*, 20.
Stoke, Peter de, 7, 87, 147.
Stoke, Walter de, 258.
Stratford, abbot of, 180.
Striguil, lordship of, 14, 238-239, 243.
Stubbs, William, *Select charters*, 130.
Sturminster, manor of, 99.
Stutville, Nicholas de, son of Robert III de, 221, 257-258, 280, 288, 292, 294, 334-335, 341.
Stutville, Robert III de, 23, 29-30, 256.
Stutville, Robert IV de, son of William de, 335-336.
Stutville, William de, son of Robert III de, 29-30, 92, 113, 157, 163, 217, 221-222, 251, 256, 335-336.
Surrey, earl of, Hamelin Plantagenet, 21, 26, 35.
Surrey, earl of, William II de Warren, 111.
Surrey, earl of, William IV de Warren, 21, 35, 149, 192, 214, 233, 254, 268-269, 290, 297, 300-301, 305-306, 328, 337, 356, 359-360, 364, 374.
Susan, damoiselle, 234.
Sussex, earl of, *see* Arundel, earl of.
Swabia, duke of, Philip of Hohenstaufen, 153.
Swansea, castle of, 44.
Swineshead, abbey of, 133.
Sydenham, manor of, 32.

Talbot, William, 270-272, 371.
Tallage, 16, 110, 113, 125-126, 215, 217.
Talmont, Benedict de, 141-142.
Tamworth, castle of, 368.
Tancarville, chamberlain of, 148.
Tattershall, Robert de, 220.
Taunton, archdeacon of, *see* Wrotham, William de.
Taunton, castle of, 160.
Taxation, *see* aid, carucage, danegeld, fifteenth on merchants, hidage, Saladin tithe, scutage, seventh of 1203, tallage, *tenseriis*, thirteenth of 1207.
Taxon, Ralph, 36, 148.
Temple, knights of, 52-53, 173, 176, 195.
Tenham, manor of, 164.
Tenseriis, 350, 371.

Teutonicus, Terric, 236, 282.
Third penny, 15, 34, 36, 283, 333.
Thirsk, castle of, 23.
Thirteenth of 1207, 130-136, 179, 224.
Thouars, viscount of, Aimery VII, 26.
Thouars, Guy de, brother of Aimery VII, *see* Brittany, duke of.
Tickhill, honor of, 20, 282.
Tidworth, manor of, 210.
Tilly, Henry de, 150.
Tindale, 253.
Tiring, Master Richard de, 189.
Torre, abbey of, 77.
Torrington, barony of, 44.
Totnes, barony of, 42, 45-46, 309.
Totnes, castle of, 46.
Totnes, Alured of, son of Judhaelof, 41-42.
Totnes, Judhael of, 41-42, 45.
Toulouse, count of, Raymond, 188, 228, 279.
Touraine, county of, 8.
Tours, archbishop of, 160.
Tracy, Henry I de, 42.
Tracy, Henry II de, son of Oliver de, 99.
Tracy, Henry de, son of William de, 38-39.
Tracy, Oliver de, son of Henry I de, 38, 43.
Tracy, William de, 38.
Treasurer, of England, 66-67. *See also*, Ely, bishop of, Nigel; Fitz Nigel, Richard; Ely, William of.
Très ancien coutumier de Normandie, 2.
Trowbridge, barony of, 40, 210, 262-263, 330.
Trowbridge, castle of, 40, 330.
Tunbridge, castle of, 162.
Turnham, Isabella de, daughter of Robert de, wife of Peter de Maulay, 282, 302.
Turnham, Robert de, 8-9, 73, 282, 302.
Turnham, Stephen de, 267.
Tusculum, cardinal-bishop of, Nicholas, 195-197, 199, 201-202, 279, 281, 314.

Ulecotes, Philip de, 252, 268-269, 272, 304, 306, 333, 352, 354, 356, 376.

Ulster, earl of, Hugh de Lacy, 47, 239, 241, 246-248.
Ulster, lordship of, 46-47, 239, 247.
Umfraville, Richard de, 252-253, 267-268.

Valognes, Gunora de, daughter of Robert de, wife of Robert fitz Walter, 22, 33, 259.
Valognes, Hamo de, 68.
Valognes, Peter I, de, 331.
Valognes, Philip de, 133.
Valognes, Robert de, son of Roger de, 259.
Valognes, Roger de, son of Peter I, 331.
Vaudey, abbey of, 133.
Vaudreuil, 11.
Vaudreuil, castle of, 32, 259, 261.
Vaux, barony of, 163.
Vaux, Oliver de, 289, 294.
Vaux, Robert de, 222, 252, 257, 337, 350, 355, 370.
Vere, Alice de, daughter of Aubrey II de, wife of Robert de Essex and Roger fitz Richard, 251.
Vere, Alice de, daughter of Aubrey III de and wife of Geoffrey II de Say, 292.
Vere, Aubrey II de, 291.
Vere, Aubrey III de, *see* Oxford, earl of.
Vere, Aubrey IV *de*, see Oxford, earl of.
Vere, Robert de, *see* Oxford, earl of.
Vesci, Eustace de, 14, 189-190, 211, 213, 233, 250, 252-253, 257-258, 261, 267-268, 270, 272, 274, 280-281, 285, 288, 292, 294, 296, 309, 314-315, 333, 339, 344-345, 355, 376.
Vieuxpont, Robert de, 81, 103, 106-108, 119-120, 251-252, 304, 306, 350, 354, 357, 365, 369, 370.
Vieuxpont, William de, 354.
Vire, castle of, 27.
Vivonne, Hugh de, 218.

Wac, Baldwin, 78.
Wagner, Anthony R., *Historical heraldry of Britain*, 36.
Wahull, barony of, 163.
Walensis, Robert, 254.

Wales, marches of, 12, 25, 42, 206, 238, 240, 306, 357-358.
Wallingford, castle of, 85, 359.
Wallingford, honor of, 10.
Walter, Hubert, *see* Canterbury, archbishop of.
Walter, Matilda, wife of Theobald Walter and Fulk fitz Warin, 52.
Walter, Theobald, brother of Hubert Walter, 52.
Walton, barony of, 251.
Wardship, right of, 216-217.
Wark, barony of, 67, 252.
Wark, castle of, 252, 370.
Warkworth, castle of, 251, 370.
Warren, Beatrice de, daughter of William de Warren of Wormegay, wife of Hubert de Burgh, 219.
Warren, Hamelin de, *see* Surrey, earl of, Hamelin Plantagenet.
Warren, William II de, *see* Surrey, earl of.
Warren, William IV de, *see* Surrey, earl of.
Warren, William de, of Wormegay, 142.
Warwick, castle of, 357.
Warwick, countess of, Alice de Harcourt, wife of Earl Waleran and widow of John de Limesi, 13.
Warwick, earl of, Henry II de Beaumont, son of Earl Waleran, 7, 213, 290, 297, 357.
Warwick, earl of, Waleran de Beaumont, 13, 22.
Warwick, earl of, William de Beaumont, 13.
Warwick, earldom of, 7.
Welles, archdeacon of, *see* Camera, Simon de; Welles, Hugh de.
Welles, Hugh de, 79-81, 105, 177-179, 182, 184-186, 205, 232. *See also*, Lincoln, bishop of.
Welles, Jocelin de, 79, 81, 105. *See also*, Bath, bishop of.
Welsh, expeditions against, 246-247, 264, 266.
Wendover, Roger of, 2.
Whitchurch, castle of, 357.
Whittington, castle of, 28, 49-50, 52.
Whitwick, castle of, 352.
Wickenholt, John de, 122.

Wickenton, Henry de, 141.
Wight, isle of, 31, 85.
Wigmore, barony of, 46, 239.
Winchester, bishop of, Godfrey de Lucy, 33, 36, 73, 75-76, 159.
Winchester, bishop of, Peter des Roches, 62, 80, 82, 161, 166-167, 175, 177-178, 180, 183, 197, 205, 228, 230-231, 234, 278-281, 284-285, 300, 305-306, 328, 337, 339, 342-346, 352, 359, 361, 364, 377.
Winchester, castle of, 307, 374.
Winchester, city of, 374.
Winchester, earl of, Saher de Quency, 34-35, 106, 194, 197, 213, 218, 242, 257-258, 264, 280, 287, 289-290, 292, 294, 295-296, 300, 334, 339, 344, 353, 367.
Windsor, castle of, 56, 359, 376-377.
Windsor, Walter de, 85.
Wirksworth, manor of, 26.

Wisbech, castle of, 360.
Wolvsey, castle of, 159, 374.
Worcester, archdeacon of, *see* Branchester, John de.
Worcester, bishop of, Mauger, 164, 172-175, 177-179, 181-182, 186, 190.
Worcester, bishop of, Walter de Grey, 65, 200, 306, 338-339.
Worcester, city of, 375.
Worcester, Philip of, 189.
Wrotham, William de, 81, 137, 139, 147.

York, archbishop of, Geoffrey Plantagenet, 67, 129, 134-135, 156-158, 179, 182, 200.
York, archbishop of, Walter de Grey, 201, 366.
York, castle of, 59, 333, 352, 370.
York, citizens of, 223, 370.
York, dean and chapter of, 200.

JOHNS HOPKINS UNIVERSITY PRESS REPRINTS

An Arno Press Collection

Agard, Walter Raymond. **The Greek Tradition in Sculpture.** 1930

Allen, Don Cameron. **Doubt's Boundless Sea: Skepticism and Faith in the Renaissance.** 1964

Bailey, Thomas A. **The Policy of the United States Toward the Neutrals, 1917-1918.** 1942

Barton, John. **Observations on the Circumstances Which Influence the Condition of the Labouring Classes of Society.** 1934

Beall, Otho T. and Richard H. Shryock. **Cotton Mather: First Significant Figure in American Medicine.** 1954

Beardsley, Grace Hadley. **The Negro in Greek and Roman Civilization.** 1929

Bloomfield, Maurice and Richard Garbe, eds. **The Kashmirian Atharva-Veda.** 1901

Bloomfield, Maurice. **The Life and Stories of the Jaina Savior Parcvanatha.** 1919

Boas, George. **Wingless Pegasus: A Handbook for Critics.** 1950

Carr, Edward Hallett. **German-Soviet Relations Between the Two World Wars, 1919-1939.** 1951

German-Soviet Relations Between the Two World Wars, 1919-1939. 1951

Castiglioni, Arturo. **The Renaissance of Medicine in Italy.** 1934

Chinard, Gilbert, ed. **The Correspondence of Jefferson and Du Pont De Nemours.** 1931

Chinard, Gilbert, ed. **Un Français En Virginie: Voyages d'un François Exilé pour la Réligion avec une Déscription de la Virgine & Marilan dans L'Amérique.** 1932

Chinard, Gilbert, ed. **Houdon in America.** 1930

Chinard, Gilbert, ed. **The Letters of Lafayette and Jefferson.** 1929

Chinard, Gilbert, ed. **Souvenirs D'Édouard De Mondésir.** 1942

Chinard, Gilbert, ed. **The Treaties of 1778 and Allied Documents.** 1928

Chinard, Gilbert, ed. **La Vie Americaine De Guillaume Merle D'Aubigné.** 1935

Chinard, Gilbert, ed. **Voyage dans L'Intérieur des Etats-Unis et au Canada par Le Comte de Colbert Maulevrier.** 1935

Chinard, Gilbert, ed. **Le Voyage de Lapérouse sur les Côtes de L'Alaska et de la Californie.** 1937

Daugherty, William E. **A Psychological Warfare Casebook.** 1958

Drazin, Nathan. **History of Jewish Education from 515 B.C.E. to 220 C.E.** 1940

Dyer, Murray. **The Weapon on the Wall: Rethinking Psychological Warfare.** 1959

French, John C. **A History of the University Founded by Johns Hopkins.** 1946

Galt, John. **The Gathering of the West.** 1939

Gildersleeve, Basil. **The Creed of the Old South, 1865-1915.** 1915

Goodnow, Frank J. **China: An Analysis.** 1926

Hardy, Thomas. **An Indiscretion in the Life of an Heiress.** 1935
Jones, W.H.S. **Philosophy and Medicine in Ancient Greece.** 1946
Korson, George. **Black Rock: Mining Folklore of the Pennsylvania Dutch.** 1960
Korson, George, ed. **Pennsylvania Songs and Legends.** 1949
Lane, Frederic Chapin. **Venetian Ships and Shipbuilders of the Renaissance.** 1934
Langer, Susanne K. **Philosophical Sketches.** 1962
Langer, Susanne K., ed. **Reflections on Art.** 1958
Lumiansky, R.M., ed. **Malory's Originality: A Critical Study of Le Morte Darthur.** 1964
MacKinney, Loren C. **Early Medieval Medicine with Special Reference to France and Chartres.** 1937
Martin-Clarke, D. Elizabeth. **Culture in Early Anglo Saxon England.** 1947
Miller, Genevieve, ed. **Bibliography of the History of Medicine of the United States and Canada, 1939-1960.** 1964
Newsholme, Arthur. **Public Health and Insurance: American Addresses.** 1920
Oliphant, Herman and Theodore S. Hope, Jr. **A Study of Day Calendars.** 1932
Painter, Sidney. **The Reign of King John.** 1949
Qubain, Fahim I. **Education and Science in the Arab World.** 1966
Remer, C.F. **A Study of Chinese Boycotts.** 1933
Ricardo, David. **Letters of John Ramsay McCulloch to David Ricardo** *and* **Three Letters on the Price of Gold,** Two vols. in one. 1931/1903
Ricardo, David. **Minor Papers on the Currency Question, 1809-1823.** 1932
Semmes, Raphael. **Captains and Mariners of Early Maryland.** 1937
Shanks, Lewis Piaget. **Flaubert's Youth, 1821-1845.** 1927
Sigerist, Henry E. **Four Treatises of Theophrastus Von Hohenheim Called Paracelsus.** 1941
Simmons, James Stevens, et al. **Malaria in Panama.** 1939
Simonds, Frank H. **American Foreign Policy in the Post-War Years.** 1935
Spector, Benjamin, ed. **Noah Webster: Letters on Yellow Fever Addressed to Dr. William Currie.** 1947
Suhr, Elmer G. **Sculptured Portraits of Greek Statesmen.** 1931
Suhr, Elmer G. **Two Currents in the Thought Stream of Europe.** 1942
Tabak, Israel. **Judaic Lore in Heine.** 1948
Turnbull, Grace H., ed. **Tongues of Fire: A Bible of Sacred Scriptures of the Pagan World.** 1941
Willoughby, Westel W. **Japan's Case Examined.** 1940
Young, C. Walter. **The International Legal Status of the Kwantung Leased Territory.** 1931
Young, C. Walter. **Japanese Jurisdiction in the South Manchuria Railway Areas.** 1931
Young, C. Walter. **Japan's Special Position in Manchuria.** 1931
Zeeland, Paul van. **A View of Europe, 1932.** 1933
Zimmer, Henry R. **Hindu Medicine.** 1948